Prebiotics and Probiotics in Disease Regulation and Management

Scrivener Publishing
100 Cummings Center, Suite 541J
Beverly, MA 01915-6106

Publishers at Scrivener
Martin Scrivener (martin@scrivenerpublishing.com)
Phillip Carmical (pcarmical@scrivenerpublishing.com)

Prebiotics and Probiotics in Disease Regulation and Management

Edited by

Rajesh K. Kesharwani

Tingirikari Jagan Mohan Rao

and

Raj K. Keservani

Scrivener Publishing

WILEY

This edition first published 2022 by John Wiley & Sons, Inc., 111 River Street, Hoboken, NJ 07030, USA and Scrivener Publishing LLC, 100 Cummings Center, Suite 541J, Beverly, MA 01915, USA

For more information about Scrivener publications please visit www.scrivenerpublishing.com.

Wiley Global Headquarters
111 River Street, Hoboken, NJ 07030, USA

For details of our global editorial offices, customer services, and more information about Wiley products visit us at www.wiley.com.

Library of Congress Cataloging-in-Publication Data

ISBN 978-1-394-16627-5

Cover image: Pixabay.Com
Cover design by Russell Richardson

Set in size of 11pt and Minion Pro by Manila Typesetting Company, Makati, Philippines

Printed in the USA

10 9 8 7 6 5 4 3 2 1

Contents

Preface

The demand for biobased products is increasing enormously, among which are prebiotic oligosaccharides and probiotics, which occupy a major share of the food industry. Even though the majority of agro waste is currently being used for the production of 2G biofuels, agro waste such as citrus peel, sugar beet pulp, copra meal, and wheat husk can be considered for the production of prebiotic oligosaccharides. Prebiotics are dietary fibers which are selectively fermented by the microbes present in the gut and promote the growth of beneficial bacteria in the intestine and regulate the growth of harmful bacteria. Thus, help in maintaining gut homeostasis.

This book highlights the importance of nutraceuticals (prebiotics, and probiotics) in maintaining gut homeostasis, prevention and treatment of gut related disorders, as anti-cancer agent, immune-modulatory agent and in treatment of metabolic disorders. This book brings out the current challenges involved in formulation and development of nutraceuticals, together with the application of nanotechnology and bioinformatics-based approaches to study the effect of nutraceuticals on oral health, and gut microflora in a very precise way.

This book will be very informative not only to those in the scientific community working in various fields associated with disease prevention and treatment in the medical, biopharmaceutical and health sectors; but also as a resource to update budding researchers on the current use of prebiotics and probiotics for the regulation, prevention and management of diseases.

We express our heartfelt appreciation to all the authors on behalf of the entire editorial board and the publisher. It was with your kind co-operation, enthusiasm, and spirit of the authors we could have make this book published. We thank all the authors for considering our request and contributed significantly by sharing their knowledge and expertise in the developing the content of this book. It would be not appropriate if I fail to mention the tireless efforts of Martin Scrivener, and Linda Mohr (Editorial Assistant) of Scrivener Publication for making this book within a short time span. We dream of tremendous citations for your book chapters in near future. We hope that the co-operation of authors will continue in future too.

Editors
Rajesh K. Kesharwani
Tingirikari Jagan Mohan Rao
Raj K. Keservani
July 2022

1

Role of Probiotics in Treatment of Gut-Related Diseases

Kunal Kumar and Rajani Sharma*

Amity Institute of Biotechnology, Amity University Jharkhand, Ranchi, India

Abstract
The living world is well invaded by microbes. Some impart beneficial roles, while others are harmful. The human body also has a number of symbiotic microbes that are beneficial in metabolic activities. Such microbes are categorized under probiotics. Probiotics have a natural mechanism to check the growth of pathogens and favors the growth of essential microbes. Such microbes are involved in major metabolic responses and utilize the residues as nutrition. They are also involved in the absorption of essential minerals from the intestine, repairing epithelial cells, boosting the immune system of our gut environment, and takes part in the treatment of major gastrointestinal diseases. Fermented foods are a natural source of probiotics. With such significance nowadays, it is also available commercially. The chapter has reflected the beneficial effect of probiotics in gut-related diseases.

Keywords: Probiotics, gastrointestinal diseases, inhibit pathogen, immune booster

1.1 Introduction

Microbes are omnipotent. They have adapted even to the adverse conditions. They can survive in hot springs as well as in the Arctic Ocean [1]. Microbes have significance in various life effecting metabolic activities. They have both beneficial and harmful effect on other living as well as the non-living worlds. They are well involved in the demineralization of soil

**Corresponding author*: rsharma@rnc.amity.edu; rajani.bharatiya@gmail.com

Rajesh K. Kesharwani, Tingirikari Jagan Mohan Rao and Raj K. Keservani (eds.) Prebiotics and Probiotics in Disease Regulation and Management, (1–26) © 2022 Scrivener Publishing LLC

to the recycling of nutrition. Microbes also have a significant role in the human body [2]. Few relations are even life taking and other play a central role in healthy living. These microbiomes may include archaea, bacterial, viruses, and even eukaryotes. The microbiomes are also involved in physiological regulations [3]. A significant role of microbes was seen in the gut of humans. It can survive even under adverse condition like in the gallbladder, which consists of antimicrobial activity of gastric juice [4]. They also cast a symbiotic relationship with the gut microenvironment. In the 19th century, a special categorization of microbes was done which has a beneficial role in human health. Such microbes were termed as "probiotics" [5]. Ferdinand Vergin was the first to coin the term "probiotic" in 1954, which is derived from the Greek word meaning "for life." He mentioned probiotics as useful organisms and depicted their nature in his book "Anti-und Probiotika" [6]. In 1995, Gibson and Roberfroid consider probiotics as non-digested food components, which support the growth of microbes that maintain the health of the gastrointestinal tract [7]. Its usefulness was also supported by Fuller in 1989, Guarner and Schaafsma in 1998 [8, 9]. Later in the year 1965 Lilly and Stillwell defined probiotics as a growth promoter of other microorganisms. Few of the microbes promote the growth of probiotics by fermenting the non-digested food and serving the product as nutrition for them. Such organisms are known as 'Prebiotic' [10]. The chapter aims to put together the mechanism of probiotics in serving gut diseases.

1.1.1 Major Gut-Related Diseases and Probiotics Interaction

The beneficial and responsive nature of probiotics contributes to the natural and prescribed treatment of gut-related diseases and syndrome. These microbes have developed strategies to dominate the harmful microbes and colonize our digestive system. Therefore, fermentation of consumed food in the gut to simpler by-products is aided by these microflorae and known to promote our health by mechanisms that remained unexplored to date. Incorrect diet, alcohol, age are the factors triggering the decline of the normal count of these beneficial microbes in the gut. Therefore, a regular diet should include these probiotics as reports suggest the remarkable reductions of the side effect of the pathogens in presence of gut microflora, they also aid in supplying the body with useful by-products, complementing the deficit in our genetic makeup by aiding the gut system to borrow the products of their genes [11]. Some of the useful efforts of probiotics are listed in Table 1.1.

Many probiotic strains cause nonspecific immune response with the release of proinflammatory cytokines, tumor necrosis factor (TNF), and

Table 1.1 Application of probiotics in the treatment of diseases.

Probiotic species	**Diseases**
Bacillus subtilis, Enterococcus faecium	Reflux esophagitis (RE)
Lactobacillus reuteri CGMCC 17942 (LR), *L. plantarum* CGMCC 14407 (LP)	Cholesterol Gallstone
Bifidobacterium breve, Lactobacillus casei, Bifidobacterium longum, and Saccharomyces boulardii	Crohn's Disease
B. longum	Colon cancer
L. gasseri CECT5714 and *L. coryniformis* CECT5711 *S. boulardii*	Diarrhea
B. bifidum W23, *B. animalis* subsp. lactis W52, and *Lactococcus lactis* W58	Eczema in children
L. helveticus R0052 and *B. longum* R0175	Depression
B. fragilis	Autism spectrum disorder (ASD)
Lactobacillus salivarius G1-1	The integrity of cell structure
L. reuteri G8-5	Cell stability
L. reuteri G22-2	Pathogen defenses
Lactobacillus johnsonii No. 1088	Reduce gastric acid production
Bifidobacterium bifidum YIT 10347	Promotes the production of mucin and improves gastric barrier to acidic stomach content
B. bifidum YIT 10347	Control the growth of *H. pylori* by regulating NF–kB signaling
Lactobacillus gasseri LG21	Improves digestion by regulating the secretion of pepsinogen (PGI)
B. animalis and *bifidobacterial*	Lactose digestion

interleukin 6 [12]. *Lactobacillus acidophilus* and *Lactobacillus rhamnosus* strain GG have been instrumental in the phagocytosis of a pathogen entering the gut. Likewise, *Bifidobacterium bifidum*, *Bifidobacterium breve*, and *L. rhamnosus* GG have been found to influence nonspecific and specific humoral immune responses against potentially harmful antigens in the host body. Reduction of diarrheal episodes was observed in infants when administered with *L. acidophilus*– and *Lactobacillus casei*–fermented milk, *Lactobacillus helveticus*– and *Streptococcus thermophilus*–fermented food formula, and formula supplemented with *B. bifidum* and *S. thermophilus* [13].

Thus, with the plethora of benefits it provides, these microbes play a pivotal role in reducing the risks of many guts-related syndrome.

Humans get affected by various gut-related diseases but gastroesophageal reflux disease (GERD), gallstones, Celiac disease, Crohn's disease, and ulcerative colitis are the five major gastrointestinal diseases. GERD is a major disease and is supposed to affect half of all adults once in their lifetime [14]. This is more common in western countries, less common in Asian countries, and completely absent in Africa. This is being characterized by heart burning. The diseases are associated with lower esophageal sphincter and prone in the person with high body mass index (BMI), less physical activity, and consumption of acidic food. The symptoms of GERD become serious when it leads to chronic inflammation of the esophagus and gastrointestinal (GI) bleeding due to esophagitis [15]. Overgrowth of intestinal bacteria was also being seen to be associated with GERD [16]. Prevention is preferred for such diseases by following a healthy lifestyle, cutting down proteins and fats from the routine diet, and care should be taken to avoid allergens. Pharmaceutical science prefers to use medicine that can suppress the acidic secretion by inhibiting the proton pump. Dietary supplements are also preferred like digestive enzymes, magnesium, and probiotics. GERD has been associated with the upper digestive tract. There are very few supportive data that support the function of probiotics in this region. Probiotics target the immune response toward the pathogenic microbes by secretion of lactic acid. Secretion of lactic acid modulates the pH of the system inhibiting the growth of pathogenic microbes, which are supposed to grow in response to GERD. Further, probiotics also relieve the symptoms of GERD [17]. They speed up the emptying of the gastric tract by interaction with stomach receptors and acceleration protein digestion by increasing the release of pepsinogen.

Helicobacter pylori colonization is a major concern in GERD. Probiotics do not check out the growth of *H. pylori* but suppress its activity [18].

Gallstone is supposed to be the second most prominent gut disease, which is the result of the imbalance between the bile acid and the cholesterol composition in the gallbladder. The composition of bile acid and cholesterol in the gallbladder is regulated by the liver [19]. The imbalance in cholesterol is because of the metabolic disorder. Moreover, microbial activity was also seen to be associated with gallstone formation. Urease and β-glucuronidase activity of microbes were involved in the formation of cholesterol and pigmented gallstones, respectively [20]. The activity of bacteria is not limited to their enzymatic activity, rather they also disrupt the enterohepatic circulation by epimerization of bile acid. Cholecystectomy is the only preferred treatment for gallstones. During this treatment, process gallbladder is removed. The loss of the gallbladder causes indigestion of fats and develops the gastric condition. An attempt has also been taken to include probiotics in regulating cholesterol to bile acid concentration in the gallbladder. Probiotics may target the FXR receptor to regulate the bile and cholesterol concentration, which may relieve gallstones. Some probiotics like lactulose and *Bifidobacterium breve* can decrease β-glucuronidase activity [1]. *Lactobacilli* also can inhibit urease activity [1]. In combination, probiotics can be used to control the factors causing the formation of gallstone and may prevent cholecystectomy.

Celiac is another major gut disease that is categorized as autoimmune disease. It is common in both adults and children. In this, there is indigestion of alcohol-soluble protein gluten, which is present in various cereals, including wheat, barley, kamut, and spelt. This disease is predominant in a person who has the allele for HLA-DQ2 or HLA-DQ8 or the hybrid of these two alleles [21]. To date, the only solution to a celiac is to exclude gluten diet. Further, the allele HLA genetically favors the growth of *Bacteroides* spp. and decreases the colonies of *Bifidobacterium* spp [22]. This evidence that probiotics can be involved in the improvement of gut digestion and can play an efficient role to overcome celiac disease. A study states that a cocktail of eight strains can be effective in decreasing the toxic effect of wheat. But when used alone they do not show any effectiveness. The cocktail includes three species of *Bifidobacterium*, four species of *Lactobacillus*, and *Streptococcus thermophilus* probiotics [23]. Contradicting the previous study *in vivo* inoculation of *B. longum CECT7347* alone can induce the level of IL-10 and reduce TNF-α, which impairs with an inflammatory response in presence of gliadin. Inoculation of *B. longum* prevents the movement of gliadin to the lamina propria by alteration in jejunal structure [24].

Another major gastrointestinal disease is Crohn's disease and ulcerative colitis, which belongs to inflammatory bowel disease (IBD). People with age groups 30 to 39 are more prone to Crohn's disease [25]. Like other gastrointestinal diseases, IBD also has imbalanced microbiomes. There is an influence in the metabolism of microbes and the mucosal immune system. There is also the variation in short-chain fatty acid, bile acid, and certain amino acid metabolites. All these symptoms also favor the researcher to administer probiotics for IBD. In IBD, there is damage to an epithelial barrier or M-cell (microfold cell), which activates the innate immunity. During this process, proinflammatory cytokines are released by dendritic cells and macrophages, leading to chronic inflammation. The inflammation can be fatal. Probiotics, like *B. adolescentis IM38,* were seen to regulate the NF-κB pathway and reduce the inflammation [26]. During the metabolic pathway of probiotics, short-chain fatty acid is produced, which replaces the depleted fatty acid due to IBD. Pathogenic microbial growth, which includes *Proteus, E. coli, Mycobacterium avium,* and *Helicobacter pylori* were seen to be controlled on the administration of probiotics.

Irritable bowel syndrome (IBS) is another most common reason for referral to gastroenterology clinics. Abdominal pain, diarrhea, constipation are the common symptoms along with mucus discharge in stools and changes in their appearance. The main cause of the disease is not entirely apparent as various factors play key roles in its etiology [27].

The pathogenesis of IBS has been believed to get instigated by aberrations in small and large bowel motility, visceral hyperalgesia; a case of hypersensitivity in the viscera, brain-gut interactions, reactivity in response to postinfection, changes in fecal microflora, bacterial overgrowth, sensitivity to certain foods, improper absorption of carbohydrates, and intestinal inflammation all have been associated in the pathogenesis of IBS [28]. It is estimated that IBS affects around 11% of the population globally, and it is the most common disorder among 15% of Americans [29]. A small number of the affected population visits physicians accounting for 30% of the total patients. The total annual direct medical cost of IBS in the USA alone has been projected at $1.7 to $10 billion [30]. Probiotics-mediated therapy could reduce the complications associated with IBS as evident from the work of Kim, Tsuchiya, Saggioro. Strains of *Lactobacillus* species, *Bifido bacterium* species, and *Propioni bacterium* species, along with different probiotic combinations, such as VSL#3 (combination of probiotics that contains live bacteria, including *Bifidobacterium* (*B. longum, B. infantis,* and *B. breve*); *Lactobacillus* (*L. acidophilus, L. casei, L. delbrueckii ssp. bulgaricus,* and *L. plantarum*); and *Streptococcus salivarius ssp. Thermophilus)* and SCM-III (*L. acidophilus, Lactobacillus helveticus,* and *Bifidobacterium sp.*), led to a decline in episodes of flatulence and an improvement in colonic transit time, improvement in bloating, abdominal pain, and bowel habits [31–33].

Table 1.2 Probiotics assist in the absorption of minerals from the intestine [44].

Probiotics	Minerals absorbed
Bifidobacterium lactis HN019 + oligosaccharide (Synbiotics), *Lactobacillus plantarum* 299v	Iron
Lactobacillus reuteri strains ATCC PTA 6475 and ATCC 55730	Vitamin B12 and folate synthesis
L. reuteri strain ATCC 55730	Thiamine
Bacillus subtilis, L. lactis pNZGBAH	Riboflavin

supplement, the probiotics should be harsh enough to tolerate the processing, storage, and stress conditions while passing across the buccal cavity to enter the gut environment. Microbiomes show the symbiotic relation to producing vitamin B, which is absorbed by host cells. Along with the production of nutrition, probiotics also maintain the permeability of the intestine by the production of butyrate. Further, it maintains the strength of TJ proteins, a protein involved in maintaining the integrity of the epithelial layer. Table 1.2 presents few of the probiotics involved in the absorption of essential nutrients from the intestine irrespective of the age group and gender [44]. The TJ proteins consist of cytoskeleton, including claudins, zonulin, and regulatory proteins.

A study in an animal model has been seen to increase the expression of proteins involved in the maintenance of cell integrity, stability, and defense mechanism.

1.3 Symbiotic Relation of Probiotics in the Gut

The probiotics show a symbiotic relationship with the gut. The gut provides essential nutrition to the probiotics whereas in turn, it gets essential factors that are involved in immune regulation. It has been seen that probiotics are involved in the stimulation of cytokines, which play a central role in immune regulation. Interleukin 10 and interleukin 12 are one of the major examples, which are activated by Lactobacillus spices. Probiotics produce various vitamins and minerals as the product of their metabolism, which is utilized by the host cells.

1.3.1 Mechanism of Interaction

There are various probiotics which predominate in the human gut. *Firmicutes* and *Bacteroidetes* constitute 90% of such probiotic colonies. Interaction of such probiotics changes the microenvironment, which promotes the colonization of healthy gut microbes [45]. They have the mechanism to improve the immune system by regulating toll-like receptor signaling pathways for inflammation.

The presence of probiotics inhibits the binding of other pathogenic microbes. The probiotics binding is regulated by the number of factors like steric forces, lipoteichoic acids that provide specificity to interact with receptor, whereas pathogenic microbes do not have such interaction. Further, presence of probiotics causes steric hindrance at binding receptor. Probiotics also lead to the expression of MUC2/3, which secretes mucin [45]. The presence of mucin inhibits the adhesion of enteropathogenic microbes. The antimicrobial proteins secreted by probiotics also check the growth of pathogenic organisms. The protein include lysozyme, α and β defensins and cathelicidins. Lysozyme is involved in the hydrolysis of glycosidic linkage of peptidoglycans layers leading to the lysis of pathogenic cell [46]. α and β defensins and cathelicidins establishes electrostatic interaction which disrupt the membrane and α-helical surface protein respectively. The capability of the metabolites of probiotics to interact with surface protein also provides repair mechanism for epithelial layer. They regulate P38 and kinase pathway and zonula occludens to reconstruct

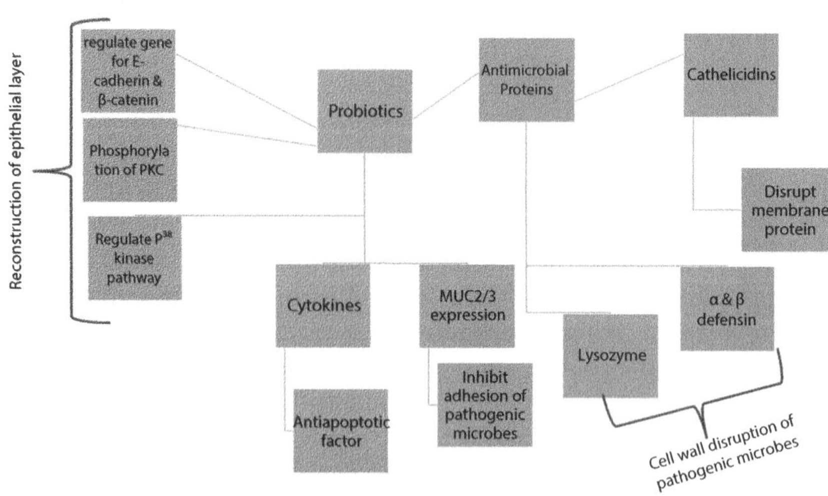

Figure 1.1 Action of probiotics in controlling gut diseases.

tight junctions. They also target the adherence junction by regulating cytoskeleton including E-cadherin, β-catenin, and PIP (phosphotidylinositol biphosphate) pathway (Figure 1.1) [47].

1.3.2 Escaping Mechanism of Probiotics From Immune Cells

The microenvironment of the gut varies concerning pH, oxygen availability, chemical environment, and microbiota. These microenvironments influence the abundance of healthy gut microbiota. Microbiomes must survive to vary pH. Secretion of various chemicals also influences the pH across the intestine. As duodenum has acidic pH because of the secretion of acidic chyme from the stomach. While ascending toward the terminal ileum the pH is basic due to the secretion of bicarbonate from the liver and pancreas. Along with the physical factors, our immune system must have developed the capability not to respond against commensal microbiota. Probiotics can survive the variable physical changes in the gut [48].

1.4 Probiotics Role in Boosting Host Immunity

Probiotics play an influential role in the regulation and modulation of the immune system against pathogens, thereby boosting immune health. Probiotics genes and their expressed proteins do involve in the prevention of diseases and treatment of allergic reactions and viral infections. Work on immunomodulatory capacities of *Lactobacillus plantarum* strains revealed that six genes express proteins of the *N*-acetyl-glucosamine/galactosamine phosphotransferase system, the LamBDCA quorum-sensing system, components of bacteriocin biosynthesis, and transport pathway [49]. These proteins stimulate cytokine production of IL-10 and IL-12 by dendritic cells. *Lactobacillus rhamnosus GG*-derived soluble protein, p40, has been known to treat intestinal injury and acute colitis in a mouse model. This soluble protein p40 was found to reduce to the expression of (TNF), IL-6, keratinocyte chemoattractant, and interferon (IFN)-γ. TNF, IL-6, IFN-γ is known to exaggerate cases of inflammation and can have an indirect detrimental effect on the host, with the development of intravascular thrombosis, hypotension, pulmonary edema, and hemorrhage [50].

Mutants of L. acidophilus NCFM were seen to downregulate IL-12 and TNF but enhanced IL-10 production in dendritic cells. Mouse model treated with mutants of *L. acidophilus* NCFM significantly decreased dextran sulfate sodium-induced colitis. Upregulation of IL-10 by these mutant bacteria was associated with decreased mucosal inflammation.

Another report suggested *L. acidophilus* NCFM-stimulated genes in murine bone marrow-derived dendritic cells, which are related to viral defense and are known to trigger the expression of IFN-β, IL-12, and IL-10 [50]. Recent work of [51] identified *L. acidophilus* to modulate the transcriptional regulation of IL 23, a mediator in mucosal inflammatory bowel disease. *L. rhamnosus is involved in* wound healing, IFN response, and ion homeostasis. *L. casei* enhanced the development of natural killer cells with the stimulation of IL 21 and IL-17D, thus shifting Th1/Th2 balance to a Th2 type and/or Th17 type. Human volunteers fed with fermented milk products harboring *L. acidophilus* and bifidobacteria strains had significantly elevated total IgA, and specifically *Salmonella enterica* subsp-specific IgA.

Cell surface proteins of L. casei have also been identified in the prevention of inflammation through inhibition of protein (IP-10) secretion aided by TNF. Specific *Lactobacillus helveticus* strains protect against enterohemorrhagic *Escherichia coli* strains with the activation of transcription 1 signaling in intestinal epithelial cells.

1.5 Commercial Probiotic Products Possessing Beneficial Properties

The plethora of health benefits being offered by probiotics has been widely accepted. This has opened new avenues for probiotic health food products. Further, this has led to the establishment of industries targeting different applications of probiotics in a range of food products from health drinks to desserts.

1.5.1 Probiotics in Dairy Products

Dairy products are the oldest means for the delivery of probiotics in the human system. Microbes of probiotics get a suitable environment for growth and viability in dairy products. The first commercial probiotics-based dairy food product is dairy drinks or beverages. Functional dairy beverages have been classified into two categories: fortified dairy beverages and whey-based beverages [52]. The commercially available milk-based probiotic fortified dairy beverages including acidophilus milk, bifidus milk, acidophilus-yeast milk, acidophilin have witnessed market success in countries of Europe, Asia-Pacific, and North America. Other potential sources of probiotic-based dairy beverages include cheese whey and buttermilk whey and these products offer a suitable medium for the growth and viability of probiotic microorganisms. Fortification of dairy beverages with *L. rhamnosus* GG has drawn attention owing to the acid and bile resistance of the strain. Therefore, among all the probiotic bacteria used in the manufacture of dairy beverages, *L. rhamnosus* GG is mostly accepted for industrial application. Frozen fermented dairy desserts, ice cream, sour cream, chocolate mousse, and quark have all been listed in dairy beverages fortified with improved strains of lactobacillus. *L. paracasei* subsp. *paracasei* LBC 82 in chocolate mousse was found to remain viable imparting health benefits to the food [53, 54].

Ice creams are also significant carriers of probiotics making them a functional health food. Moreover, the general viability of probiotics in ice creams has been found significantly better compared to a few other dairy products. Strains *Lactobacillus casei, L. plantarum, L. acidophilus* used in ice creams remained viable with better shelf life and acceptable CFU count. The addition of *L. acidophilus* La5 in ice cream mix before fermentation led to a significantly higher level of total solids (42%), titratable acidity (2.2%), and proteins (16.5%), compared to the ice creams without any supplementation of probiotics [55].

There are several probiotic-based commercially produced yogurts like Activia yogurt, Greek yogurt plain, Brown cow yogurt, Wallaby organic yogurt that is widely used in France, the U.K., U.S.A., and Australia respectively involving strains of *Bifidobacterium* sps., *Lactobacillus acidophilus, L. casei*, and *L. rhamnosus*. Yogurts produced by many probiotic strains are comparable with traditionally produced yogurts, and in many cases, are much better with appealing physicochemical, sensory, and microbial properties [54].

Cheese is known as a better medium of probiotic supplement compared to many other dairy products, which is probably due to its requirement of low storage temperature, low water activity, relatively higher pH, and textural characteristics (e.g., high fat content, which protects probiotics during gastrointestinal transit). Probiotics in cheese are not typically incorporated for imparting better technological and physiological qualities of cheese, but in general, to give nutritive value to the product and enhance consumer attention [54]. Spanish pasteurized sheep milk cheese with *Bifidobacterium* sps. significantly enhanced overall proteolysis and enhanced the concentration of some free amino acids. Likewise, cheddar cheese had increased antioxidant activity in presence of *Lactobacillus casei* and *Lactobacillus plantarum*. Similarly, Minas Frescal cheese exhibited a better fatty acid profile, higher ACE inhibitory, and antioxidant activities, lower pH, and higher proteolysis and organic acid levels on inoculation with *L. casei* 01 strains [56, 57].

1.5.2 Fermentation of Fruit Juices With Fortified Probiotic Lactobacilli

The work of Nguyen *et al.*, revealed that two *Lactobacillus* isolates, viz. *L. plantarum* and *L. acidophilus* could be able to survive in fruit juices and utilize the nutritional content for their cell synthesis, as shown by a decrease in fruit sugar and pH and an increase in acidity. Therefore, it could be concluded that such probiotic-fortified fruit juices could be considered as a medium for the supplement of probiotics and could be used as a functional healthy beverage among individuals allergic to milk-based products. Thus, these findings open avenues to encourage better health and nutrition for the population. Fermentation of pineapple juice with probiotic strains of *Lactobacillus* and *Bifidobacterium* also displayed good growth without supplementation of any nutrient compounds and demonstrated increased total phenolic content and antioxidant capacity during fermentation [58].

1.5.3 Probiotics as Pharmaceutics

Several probiotic strains have also been introduced in the market in pharmaceutical forms. Lactic acid bacteria (*Lactobacillus*) and *Bifidobacterium* constitute the main group of probiotics commercialized in pharmaceutics and biologics. VSL 3 with freeze-dried lactic acid bacteria and bifidobacteria is one among the many commercial pharmaceutics of probiotics with 112.5 billion CFU (https://www.vsl3.com/assets/v1/patient/files/VSL3Leaflet-PI.pdf). This drug is effective against acute cases of Ulcerative colitis [59]. Enterogermina® is another probiotic capsule of 2 billion Spores of poly-antibiotic–resistant *Bacillus clausii*, a friendly bacterium usually present in the gut [60] recommended for the treatment of diarrhea and its symptoms in adults and children. Vibact-DS Capsule recommended for treatment of irritable bowel syndrome (IBS) and inflammatory bowel disorders (IBD) and reduces clinical symptoms of gastroenteritis (infectious diarrhea) as well as traveller's diarrhea. It comprises *Lactobacillus sporogenes, Clostridium butyricum, Streptococcus faecalis*, and *Bacillus mesentericus* as major active ingredients. (https://www.1mg.com/otc/vibact-ds-capsule-otc173930). Some of the commercially available probiotics products are depicted in Table 1.3.

Table 1.3 Lists of commercially available probiotics.

Commercial name of probiotics	Microbial colony content (Billion CFU)	No. of strains present	Extra content	Bacterial strain
Wellbeing Nutrition Daily Probiotic + Prebiotic	6 Billion CFU,	3 6 Strains	Chicory root extract, Apple Pomace fiber	*Lactobacillus Acidophilus, Lactobacillus Casei, Lactobacillus rhamnosus, Bifidobacterium lactis, Bifidobacterium bifidum, Streptococcus thermophilus*
Setu Tummy Probiotic	15 Billion CFUs	9 strains		*Lactobacillus & Bifidobacterium*
Healthy Hey Nutrition Probiotics	50 Billion		Cranberry fruit extract (*Vaccinium oxycoccos*), fructooligosaccharides (FOS), vitamin C (ascorbic acid), Zinc (as zinc sulphate)	*Lactobacillus acidophilus, Lactobacillus rhamnosus, Lactobacillus plantarum, Lactobacillus paracasei, Bifidobacterium longum, Bifidobacterium bifidum, Bifidobacterium breve* and *Saccharomyces boulardii*

(*Continued*)

Table 1.3 Lists of commercially available probiotics. (*Continued*)

Commercial name of probiotics	Microbial colony content (Billion CFU)	No. of strains present	Extra content	Bacterial strain
BBETTER Probiotics	24 Billion CFU	10		*Lactobacillus spp., Bifidobacterium spp., Streptococcus thermophilus*
EXERFIT Synbiotics	30			300 mg Unique Prebiotic Blend, 200 mg Spirullina, 150 mg Digestive Enzyme Blend, and a 110 mg Extract Blend
Gut Eze Probiotic	1			*Lactobacillus & Bifidobacterium*

(*Continued*)

Table 1.3 Lists of commercially available probiotics. (*Continued*)

Commercial name of probiotics	Microbial colony content (Billion CFU)	No. of strains present	Extra content	Bacterial strain
Carbamide Forte Probiotics	50	20	Ginseng Extract (Panax Ginseng Korean) 21.25 mg, Ginkgo Biloba Extract 5000 mcg, Grape Seed Extract 5000 mcg, Lycopene (6 %) 500 mcg, Lutein 1000 mcg, Selenium (from Sodium Selenate) 40 mcg, biotin (D-biotin) 30 mcg, vitamin E (D-alpha-tocopherol) 50% 10 mg, vitamin C (ascorbic acid) 40 mg, Alfalfa 10 mg, calcium (from dicalcium phosphate) 100 mg, magnesium (from magnesium Oxide) 105 mg, vitamin D (ergocalciferol) 400 IU, vitamin K2 (MK-7) (menaquinone) 55 mcg, CissusQuadrangularis Extract (Stem) 25 mg,	Lactic Acid Bacillus 100 Million Spores, Fructooligosaccharides 10 mg

(*Continued*)

Table 1.3 Lists of commercially available probiotics. (*Continued*)

Commercial name of probiotics	Microbial colony content (Billion CFU)	No. of strains present	Extra content	Bacterial strain
			Phosphorus (from dicalcium phosphate) 59 mg, vitamin A (retinol) 600 mcg, vitamin B1 (thiamine mononitrate) 1.4 mg, vitamin B2 (riboflavin) 1.6 mg, vitamin B3 (nicotinamide) 18 mg, vitamin B5 (calcium D-pantothenate) 5 mg, vitamin B6 (pyridoxine HCl) 2 mg, vitamin B12 (cobalamin) 1 mcg, folic acid 117.65 mcg, zinc (from zinc sulphate) 12 mg, Iron (from carbonyl iron) 8.5 mg, manganese (from manganese chloride) 4 mg, copper (from copper sulphate) 1.7 mg, iodine (from potassium iodide) 150 mcg, chromium (from chromium picolinate) 50 mcg, molybdenum (from sodium molybdate) 45 mcg, boron (from boron proteinate) 75 mcg.	

(*Continued*)

Table 1.3 Lists of commercially available probiotics. (*Continued*)

Commercial name of probiotics	Microbial colony content (Billion CFU)	No. of strains present	Extra content	Bacterial strain
Simply Nutra Probiotics	25 Billion			*L. plantarum, L. fermentum, L. casei*
Billion Cheers Probiotic Drink	25			*Lactobacillus and bifidobacterium*
Himalayan Organics Probiotics	35		Bulking agent (INS 1401, INS341), Class II preservatives (INS211, INS217 & INS219)	*L. plantarum, B. bifidum, B. lactis, L. acidophilus, S. thermophilus, B. longum, L. rhamnosus, L. fermentum, B. Breve, L. salivarius, L. casei, S. boulardii, L. gasseri L. reuteri, B. infantis, L. paracasei*

(*Continued*)

Table 1.3 Lists of commercially available probiotics. (*Continued*)

Commercial name of probiotics	Microbial colony content (Billion CFU)	No. of strains present	Extra content	Bacterial strain
WOW Life Science Probiotics Capsules	20	14		*L. plantarum, L. fermentum, L. acidophilus, B. lactis, L. reuteri, L. salivarius, L. paracasei, L. gasseri, S. thermophillus, B. bifidum and B. breve*
HealthKart Pre & Probiotics				*L. plantarum, L. fermentum, L. acidophilus, B. boulardii, L. Casei, L. rhamnosus, B. lactis, L. reuteri, L. salivarius, L. paracasei, L. gasseri, S. thermophilus, B. bifidum, B. breve*

(*Continued*)

Table 1.3 Lists of commercially available probiotics. (*Continued*)

Commercial name of probiotics	Microbial colony content (Billion CFU)	No. of strains present	Extra content	Bacterial strain
INLIFE Probiotic Forte	25			*L. plantarum*, *L. fermentum*, *L. acidophilus*, *B. infantis*, *L. shamnosus*, *B. lactis*, *L. reuteri*, *L. salivarius*, *L. paracasei*, *L. gasseri*, *S. thermophilus*, *B. bifidum*, and *B. bereve*
Nutrabay Wellness Pre & Probiotic Digestive	50			*B. bifidum*, *B. lactis*, *B. breve*, *B. longum*, *L. acidophilus*, *L. reuteri*, *L. rhamnosus*, *L. plantarum*, *L. casei*, *L. brevis*
Swisse Ultibiotic Probiotic				*Bifidobacterium lactis* and *Lactobacillus acidophilus*

1.6 Controversial/Side Effects of Probiotics

The application of probiotics is still controversial in certain diseases like encephalopathy, necrotizing enterocolitis, and ventilator-associated pneumonia. Apart from these, it has been seen that in a person with multiple organ failure, the infection becomes more severe on the administration of probiotics. Rather the situation may become more severe that can result in fatality.

1.7 Conclusion

Probiotics contribute immensely to the natural and prescribed treatment of gut-related diseases and syndrome with their beneficial and constructive role. These microbes have developed an inbuilt mechanism to overshadow the harmful microbes and colonize our digestive system. Therefore, the consumed food undergoes fermentation in the gut to simpler by products with the aid of these microflorae and thus known to promote our health through mechanisms that remained unexplored till date. With the adoption of incorrect food habits and improper lifestyle, the normal count of these beneficial microbes in the gut is bound to decline. Therefore, a regular diet should include these probiotics in the form of fermented drinks, yoghurt, probiotics ice creams, and probiotic fruit juice. A body with a normal and safe count of the microbes in the gut would experience remarkable immunity against pathogens.

1.8 Future Prospect

Probiotics are involved in boosting the immune system and controlling major gut diseases. The exact mechanism adopted by probiotics in such beneficial effects is still unexplored. Further, the factor that prevents the immune system to recognize probiotics as pathogens also needs a detailed investigation. All these factors can contribute to modern medicine and health improvement.

References

1. Rampelotto, P., Extremophiles and extreme environments. *Life*, 3, 482–485, 2013.

2. Paul, E.A., The nature and dynamics of soil organic matter: Plant inputs, microbial transformations, and organic matter stabilization. *Soil Biol. Biochem.*, 98, 109–126, 2016.
3. Martin, A.M., Sun, E.W., Rogers, G.B., Keating, D.J., The influence of the gut microbiome on host metabolism through the regulation of gut hormone release. *Front. Physiol.*, 10, 428, 2019.
4. Sharma, R., Sachan, S.G., Sharma, S.R., *In vitro* analysis of gallstone formation in the presence of bacteria. *Indian J. Gastroenterol.*, 39, 4763–480, 2020.
5. Fijan, S., Microorganisms with claimed probiotic properties: An overview of recent literature. *Int. J. Environ. Res. Public Health*, 11, 4745–4767, 2014.
6. Vergin, F., Antibiotics, and probiotics. *Hippokrates*, 25, 116–9, 1954.
7. Gibson, G.R. and Roberfroid, M.B., Dietary modulation of the human colonic microbiota: Introducing the concept of prebiotics. *J. Nutr.*, 125, 1401–12, 1995.
8. Guarner, F., Probiotics. *Int. J. Food Microbiol.*, 39, 237–238, 1998.
9. Fuller, R., Probiotics in man and animals. *J. Appl. Bacteriol.*, 66, 365–78, 1989.
10. Lilly, D.M. and Stillwell, R.H., Probiotics: Growth-promoting factors produced by microorganisms. *Science*, 147, 747–748, 1965.
11. Amara, A.A. and Shibl, A., Role of Probiotics in health improvement, infection control and disease treatment and management. *Saudi Pharm. J.*, 23, 107–114, 2015.
12. Miettinen, M., Vuopio-Varkila, J., Varkila, K., Production of human tumor necrosis factor alpha, interleukin-6, and interleukin-10 is induced by lactic acid bacteria. *Infect. Immun.*, 64, 5403–5405, 1996.
13. Saavedra, J.M. *et al.*, Feeding of Bifidobacterium bifidum and Streptococcus thermophilus to infants in hospital for prevention of diarrhoea and shedding of rotavirus. *Lancet*, 344, 1046–1049, 1994.
14. Clarrett, D.M. and Hachem, C., Gastroesophageal reflux disease (GERD). *Mo. Med.*, 115, 214–218, 2018.
15. Broderick, R. *et al.*, Clinical presentation of gastroesophageal reflux disease: A prospective study on symptom diversity and modification of questionnaire application. *Dig. Dis.*, 38, 188–195, 2020.
16. Okereke, I. *et al.*, Associations of the microbiome and esophageal disease. *J. Thorac. Dis.*, 11, S1588–S1593, 2019.
17. Mu, Q., Tavella, V.J., Luo, X.M., Role of Lactobacillus reuteri in Human Health and Diseases. *Front. Microbiol.*, 9, 757, 2018.
18. Pace, F. and Porro, G.B., Gastroesophageal reflux and Helicobacter pylori: A review. *World J. Gastroenterol.*, 6, 311–314, 2000.
19. Sharma, R., Soy, S., Kumar, C., Sachan, S.G., Sharma, S.R., Analysis of gallstone composition and structure in Jharkhand region. *Indian J. Gastroenterol.: Official Journal of the Indian Society of Gastroenterology*, 34, 29–37, 2015.

20. Sharma, R., Sachan, S.G., Sharma, S.R., Urease positive and slime producing bacterial activity: Results in gallstone precipitation and solidification. *Arch. Clin. Infect. Dis.*, 8, e17090, 2013.
21. Cecilio, L.A. and Bonatto, M.W., The prevalence of HLA DQ2 and DQ8 in patients with celiac disease, in family and in general population. *Arq. Bras. Cir.: ABCD = Braz. Arch. Dig. Surg.*, 28, 183–5, 2015.
22. Martín, R. *et al.*, Human milk is a source of lactic acid bacteria for the infant gut. *J. Pediatr.*, 143, 754–758, 2003.
23. Seiler, C.L. *et al.*, Probiotics for celiac disease: A systematic review and meta-analysis of randomized controlled trials. *Am. J. Gastroenterol.*, 115, 1584–1595, 2020.
24. Laparra, J.M., Olivares, M., Gallina, O., Sanz, Y., Bifidobacterium longum CECT 7347 modulates immune responses in a gliadin-induced enteropathy animal model. *PLoS One*, 7, e30744, 2012.
25. Prelipcean, C.C., Mihai, C., Gogalniceanu, P., Mihai, B., What is the impact of age on adult patients with inflammatory bowel disease? *Clujul Med. (1957)*, 86, 3–9, 2013.
26. Lim, S.-M. and Kim, D.-H., Bifidobacterium adolescentis IM38 ameliorates high-fat diet–induced colitis in mice by inhibiting NF-κB activation and lipopolysaccharide production by gut microbiota. *Nutr. Res.*, 41, 86–96, 2017.
27. Everhart, J.E. and Renault, P.F., Irritable bowel syndrome in office-based practice in the United States. *Gastroenterology*, 100, 998–1005, 1991.
28. Aragon, G., Graham, D.B., Borum, M., Doman, D.B., Probiotic therapy for irritable bowel syndrome. *Gastroenterol. Hepatol.*, 6, 39–44, 2010.
29. Camilleri, M. and Choi, M.-G., Review article: Irritable bowel syndrome. *Aliment. Pharmacol. Ther.*, 11, 3–15, 1997.
30. Sandler, R.S. *et al.*, The burden of selected digestive diseases in the United States. *Gastroenterology*, 122, 1500–1511, 2002.
31. Saggioro, A., Probiotics in The Treatment of Irritable Bowel Syndrome. *J. Clin. Gastroenterol.*, 38, S104106, 2004.
32. Tsuchiya, J. *et al.*, Single-blind follow-up study on the effectiveness of a symbiotic preparation in irritable bowel syndrome. *Chin. J. Dig. Dis.*, 5, 169–174, 2004.
33. Kim, H.J. *et al.*, A randomized controlled trial of a probiotic combination VSL# 3 and placebo in irritable bowel syndrome with bloating. *Neurogastroenterol. Motil.*, 17, 687–696, 2005.
34. Davis, B.R., Lee-Kong, S.A., Migaly, J., Feingold, D.L., Steele, S.R., The American society of colon and rectal surgeons clinical practice guidelines for the management of hemorrhoids. *Dis. Colon Rectum*, 61, 284–292, 2018.
35. Sakai, T. *et al.*, Effect of fermented milk containing *Lactobacillus casei* strain Shirota on constipation-related symptoms and haemorrhoids in women during puerperium. *Benef. Microbes*, 6, 253–262, 2015.

36. Lohsiriwat, V., Hemorrhoids: From basic pathophysiology to clinical management. *World J. Gastroenterol.*, 18, 2009–2017, 2012.
37. Malik, T.F. and Panuganti, K.K., *Lactose Intolerance*, StatPearls Publishing, Treasure Island (FL), 2021.
38. Oak, S.J. and Jha, R., The effects of probiotics in lactose intolerance: A systematic review. *Crit. Rev. Food Sci. Nutr.*, 59, 1675–1683, 2019.
39. Plaza-Diaz, J., Ruiz-Ojeda, F.J., Gil-Campos, M., Gil, A., Mechanisms of action of probiotics. *Adv. Nutr. (Bethesda, Md.)*, 10, S49–S66, 2019.
40. Sharma, R., Garg, P., Kumar, P., Bhatia, S.K., Kulshrestha, S., Microbial fermentation and its role in quality improvement of fermented foods. *Fermentation*, 6, 106, 2020.
41. Santocchi, E. *et al.*, Effects of probiotic supplementation on gastrointestinal, sensory and core symptoms in autism spectrum disorders: A randomized controlled trial. *Front. Psychiatry*, 11, 944, 2020.
42. Sarkar, P., Lohith Kumar, D.H., Dhumal, C., Panigrahi, S.S., Choudhary, R., Traditional and ayurvedic foods of Indian origin. *J. Ethn. Foods*, 2, 97–109, 2015.
43. Markowiak, P. and Śliżewska, K., Effects of probiotics, prebiotics, and synbiotics on human health. *Nutrients*, 9, 1021, 2017.
44. Sheridan, P.O. *et al.*, Can prebiotics and probiotics improve therapeutic outcomes for undernourished individuals? *Gut Microbes*, 5, 74–82, 2014.
45. Magne, F. *et al.*, The firmicutes/bacteroidetes ratio: A relevant marker of gut dysbiosis in obese patients? *Nutrients*, 12, 1474, 2020.
46. Vermassen, A. *et al.*, Cell wall hydrolases in bacteria: Insight on the diversity of cell wall amidases, glycosidases and peptidases toward peptidoglycan. *Front. Microbiol.*, 10, 331, 2019.
47. Liu, Q. *et al.*, Surface components and metabolites of probiotics for regulation of intestinal epithelial barrier. *Microb. Cell Fact.*, 19, 23, 2020.
48. Tannock, G.W., A special fondness for Lactobacilli. *Appl. Environ. Microbiol.*, 70, 3189–3194, 2004.
49. van Hemert, S. *et al.*, Identification of Lactobacillus plantarum genes modulating the cytokine response of human peripheral blood mononuclear cells. *BMC Microbiol.*, 10, 293, 2010.
50. Yan, F. and Polk, D.B., Probiotics and immune health. *Curr. Opin. Gastroenterol.*, 27, 496–501, 2011.
51. van Baarlen, P. *et al.*, Human mucosal *in vivo* transcriptome responses to three lactobacilli indicate how probiotics may modulate human cellular pathways. *Proc. Natl. Acad. Sci.*, 108, 4562, 2011.
52. Song, D., Ibrahim, S.A., Hayek, S.A., Recent application of probiotics in food and agricultural science, in: *Probiotics*, R. Everlon (Ed.), pp. 123–141, INTECH publisher, Croatian, 2012.
53. Turkmen, N., Akal, C., Özer, B., Probiotic dairy-based beverages: A review. *J. Funct. Foods*, 53, 62–75, 2019.

54. Gao, J. *et al.*, Probiotics in the dairy industry—Advances and opportunities. *Compr. Rev. Food Sci. Food Saf.*, 20, 3937–3982, 2021.
55. Senanayake, S.A., Fernando, S., Bamunuarachchi, A., Arsekularatne, M., Application of Lactobacillus acidophilus (LA 5) strain in fruit-based ice cream. *Food Sci. Nutr.*, 1, 428–431, 2013.
56. Sperry, M.F. *et al.*, Probiotic Minas Frescal cheese added with L. casei 01: Physicochemical and bioactivity characterization and effects on hematological/biochemical parameters of hypertensive overweighted women – A randomized double-blind pilot trial. *J. Funct. Foods*, 45, 435–443, 2018.
57. Langa, S. *et al.*, Human Bifidobacterium strains as adjunct cultures in Spanish sheep milk cheese. *J. Dairy Sci.*, 103, 7695–7706, 2020.
58. Nguyen, B.T. *et al.*, Probiotic beverage from pineapple juice fermented with lactobacillus and bifidobacterium strains. *Front. Nutr.*, 6, 54, 2019.
59. Linares, D.M. *et al.*, Lactic acid bacteria and bifidobacteria with potential to design natural biofunctional health-promoting dairy foods. *Front. Microbiol.*, 8, 846, 2017.
60. de Castro, J.-A.A., Guno, M. J. V.-R., Perez, M.O., Bacillus clausii as adjunctive treatment for acute community-acquired diarrhea among Filipino children: A large-scale, multicenter, open-label study (CODDLE). *Trop. Dis. Travel Med. Vaccines*, 5, online, 23, 14, 2019.

2

Immune Response of Fructo and Galacto-Oligosaccharides

Muthu Vijayasarathy[1], Yesudass Antony Prabhu[2], Selvan Pavithra[3], Selvaraj Jothi Prabha[4] and Tingirikari Jagan Mohan Rao[5]*

[1]*Department of Microbiology, Thiagarajar College of Arts and Science, Madurai, Tamil Nadu, India*
[2]*Department of Biochemistry, Rathnavel Subramaniam College of Arts and Science, Coimbatore, India*
[3]*Department of Microbiology, Sri Ramakrishna College of Arts and Science for Women Coimbatore, Coimbatore, Tamil Nadu, India*
[4]*Department of Microbiology, PSG College of Arts and Science, Coimbatore, India*
[5]*Department of Biotechnology, NIT Andhra Pradesh, Tadepalligudem, India*

Abstract
Gastrointestinal (GI) tract infections are mainly influenced by the improper immune function associated with several factors, which comprise dietary constituents, commensal bacteria, and many other vital components. Over the decades, consumption of prebiotic oligosaccharides displayed great potential in the treatment of numerous illnesses in humans and animals and serve as the best alternative to antibiotics. Therefore, the comprehensive understanding of the cellular and molecular mechanisms responsible for the direct and indirect effect of dietary oligosaccharides on intestinal immunity will help improve immune ailments and also GI tract infections. This chapter will provide the current knowledge of the immunomodulatory role of oligosaccharides by influencing the microbes present in the intestine to mount an immune response. The role of fructooligosaccharides and galactooligosaccharides in the activation of receptors present on immune cells, and gut-associated lymphoid tissue is to be discussed. Detailed evidence for the immune-modulatory role of fructooligosaccharides and galactooligosaccharides concerning the gastrointestinal disorder, antiallergic, and anticancer properties has been elaborated. The anti-inflammatory properties influencing immune

**Corresponding author*: tjmr@nitandhra.ac.in

Rajesh K. Kesharwani, Tingirikari Jagan Mohan Rao and Raj K. Keservani (eds.) Prebiotics and Probiotics in Disease Regulation and Management, (27–60) © 2022 Scrivener Publishing LLC

stimulation, mineral absorption, lipid metabolism, cholesterol reduction, and other immune effects are also discussed in this chapter.

Keywords: FOS, GOS, Immunomodulation, microbiota, SCFA, NF-κB, TLR

Abbreviations

AD	Atopic Dermatitis
AMPK	AMP-Activated Protein Kinase
APC	Antigen Presenting Cells
BCR	B-Cell Receptor
CASR-PLC	Calcium Sensing Receptor-Phospholipase C
CAMKKB	$Ca2^{+}$/Calmodulin-Dependent Protein Kinase Kinase-B
CD	Crohn's Disease
CD3	Cluster of Differentiation
CRC	Colorectal Cancer
DC	Dendritic Cells
DSS	Dextran Sulfate Sodium
FOS	Fructo – Oligosaccharide
GABA	Gaba-Amino Butyric Acid
GOS	Galacto - Oligosaccharide
GI	Gastrointestinal Tract
GE	Gastric Emptying
GPCR	G-Protein-Coupled Receptors
HDAC	Histone Deacetylases
IG	Immunoglobulin
IL	Interleukins
IEC	Intestinal Epithelial Cells
IFN	Interferons
IBD	Inflammatory Bowel Disease
LDL	Low Density Lipoprotein
LPS	Lipopolysaccharides
MAPK	Mitogen-Activated Protein Kinases
MCP	Monocyte Chemo Attractant Protein
MHC	Major Histocompatibility Complex
NLRP	Nod-Like Receptor Proteins
NDO	Non-Digestible Oligosaccharide
NEC	Necrotizing Enterocolitis
NF-κB	Nuclear Factor Kappa-Light-Chain-Enhancer of Activated B Cells

NK	Natural Killer Cell
PAMP	Pathogen Associated Molecular Pattern
PBMC	Peripheral Blood Mononuclear Cell
PI	Prebiotic Index
SCFA	Short Chain Fatty Acids
TCR	T- Cell Receptor
TLR	Toll-Like Receptors
TNBS	2, 4, 6-Trinitro Benzene Sulfonic acid
TNF- α	Tumor Necrosis Factor- α
UC	Ulcerative Colitis
VLDL	Very Low Density Lipoprotein
ZO	Zonula Occludens

2.1 Introduction

Numerous bioactive compounds that are identified in natural products possess vast health benefits [1]. However, bad dietary habits with consumption of excessive saturated fats, sugar, and very low intake of dietary fibers lead to the occurrence of chronic degenerative disease. The diseases associated with poor dietary habits are Obesity, Cardiovascular diseases, Cancer, and Diabetes [2]. Therefore, public healthcare policies have gained major interest in improving people's health by changing dietary habits, physical activity, and reduction in tobacco use [3]. Consumption of natural bioactive compounds as functional foods is an emerging trend in public health [4]. Many reports have highlighted the role and application-wide variety of dietary carbohydrates in resolving gastrointestinal and metabolic disorders [5]. Oligosaccharides are one such example of natural carbohydrates, which can be considered functional foods and improve the quality of foods manufactured by the food industry [1]. Oligosaccharides are a sort of "prebiotic" which are defined as nondigestible food ingredients that are fermented and foster the growth of beneficial bacteria in the gut [4]. Generally, these prebiotics acts as a substrate for probiotic bacteria, such as *Lactobacilli* and *Bifidobacteria* sp. and produce short-chain fatty acids (SCFA), Gaba-amino butyric acid (GABA), and other beneficiary products [6]. The above metabolites will diffuse through the blood circulation via enterocytes and bring enormous changes in the host immune system of distant site organs. For instance, SCFA could impact immune cells, such as macrophage and dendritic cells (innate) in the bone marrow and T cells (adaptive) in the airway [7]. Some common prebiotic oligosaccharides are categorized into fructans (fructooligosaccharides and inulin), galactooligosaccharides, and glucose-derived oligosaccharides (resistant starch and polydextrose). Among those FOS (fructo-oligosaccharide) and GOS (Galacto-Oligosaccharide) are of particular interest with safe history and commercialized on an industrial scale [8]. The market value of oligosaccharides globally increasing and is expected to reach 7.37 billion USD by 2023 [9]. In 2015, the global market value of FOS reached 1.2 billion dollars at a 10.4% annual growth rate and expect to reach 3.9 billion dollars in the year 2027 [10]. As a prebiotic characteristic, FOS and GOS are resistant to gastric juice and not hydrolyzed by digestive enzymes [11]. During food formulations, individuals are subjected to a single or combination of oligosaccharides. However, studies with GOS are limited but the reports with a mixture of FOS and GOS or FOS alone were investigated to a large extent [12–14]. The rationale of using oligosaccharides in host well-being is primarily due to their stimulatory effects on probiotic bacteria in the gut. These microbes could normalize intestinal metabolism and integrity thereby regulating intestinal function [15, 16]. Several *in vitro* evidence suggested that oligosaccharides inhibit pathogenic invasion by mimicking glycol-conjugate structure on cell surface receptors and prevent pathogen adhesion [17]. As a result, the oligosaccharides could establish normal gut microflora and subsequently maintain intestinal homeostasis, influencing the development of the host immune system [11]. In the gut environment, the oligosaccharides show a direct impact on the local immune system thereby exhibiting therapeutic potential against inflammatory disorders [18]. Hence, prebiotic oligosaccharides exert direct or indirect effects on the host immune system.

This chapter will focus on the production of FOS as well as GOS, and their physicochemical characteristics because of their nutritional and functional importance of oligosaccharides. The physiological effects of FOS and GOS on intestinal barrier functioning in a microbiota-dependent and independent manner are summarized. This chapter also narrates the modulation of immune response concerning regular intake of FOS and GOS in humans and animals.

2.2 Sources of FOS and GOS

Fructans are naturally available in different forms, such as inulin type-fructans found in plants constituting β-(2, 1)-D-fructo-furanosyl units and the corresponding FOS obtained by fungal synthesis [19].

However, bacterial-mediated synthesis of FOS is achieved from plants with levan-type fructans comprising β-(6, 2)-D-fructo-furanosyl units [20]. Galactose is an oligomer made of lactose, which is a significant component of mammalian milk that gives rise to β-GOS [21]. These β-GOS are composed of a variable number of galactose units with the terminal glucose and galactose units linked together by β (1 → 4) and β (1 → 6) glycosidic bonds. Another plant-based GOS is named α-GOS mainly found in pulses with terminal sucrose units [8].

2.3 Synthesis of FOS and GOS

Various techniques are used to produce FOS including chemical glycosylation, de novo synthesis using glycosidase, and glycosyltransferase activities [8]. These processes are slow and complicated, as they require expensive chemicals, and yield is found to be quite low, making commercial manufacturing less plausible [22]. Transfructosylation of sucrose can be used in the industrial synthesis of FOS, which involves the action of microbial enzymes, such as β-D-fructosyltransferase (FTASE) and β-fructofuranosidase (FFASE). Using the transfructosylation process, FTASE cleaves sucrose at β-1, 2 linkages involving the transfer of fructosyl group results in FOS formation [23]. However, for FFASE mediated transfructosylation activity, more than 500 g/L of sucrose is required. FTASE can be produced by a variety of microorganisms, but fungal species, such as *Aspergillus, Aureobasidium, Fusarium*, and *Penicillium* respectively. In the case of bacteria species, such as *Lactobacillus, Arthrobacter, Bacillus macerans*, and *Zymomonas mobilis.* While yeast species, such as *Rhodotorula, Candida, Cryptococcus, Kluyveromyces*, and *Saccharomyces cerevisiae* are also reported to produce FTASE enzyme [22]. For the generation of FOS, either the complete microorganism or extracted enzymes either in a suspended or immobilized state are being employed. Various methods of FOS production have been reported so far. The difference in composition of FOS is mainly influenced by catalytic and physicochemical properties of enzymes involved, production conditions, and type of microbial strains. According to the studies, the highest possible yield for FOS is only between 55% and 60% in hydrolytic activity, since during hydrolytic activity the byproducts, such as glucose and fructose, are released [8]. To avoid trans-glycosylation inhibition, glucose is being converted to gluconic acid (using glucose oxidase) or into fructose (using glucose isomerase). While gluconic acid can be separated by using ion-exchange resins and strains with transfructosylating activity improves the FOS yield to up to 98% [24].

Like FOS, GOS can be derived through chemical means, but due to uneconomical process preference goes to enzymatic synthesis. Galactosyltransferase and galactosidase are noted to be vital enzymes involved in GOS production from lactose and lactulose [21]. Nevertheless, galactosyltransferase is more stereoselective, produces higher quantities of GOS as compared to galactosidase. However, the complexity of the process with galactosyltransferase is due to the requirement of nucleotide sugar, a costlier and unstable donor. Henceforth, β-galactosidase is assigned as an appropriate enzyme in converting lactose to GOS in a kinetically controlled mechanism. Generally, several microbial species are capable of producing β-galactosidase enzymes, such as *Aspergillus oryzae*, *Sterigmatomyceselviae*, *Bifidobacteria sp*., and *Lactobacilli sp* [22]. Versatile enzymatic production of GOS is investigated by applying either whole cell or using enzymes or its recombinant forms. However, factors, such as source, pH, and temperature, mainly influence β-galactosidase activity during the synthesis of oligosaccharides through the varied glycosidic bond formation and degree of polymerization [8].

2.4 Bifidogenesis of FOS and GOS

Administration of nondigestible oligosaccharides, such as FOS, GOS, and inulin stimulates the desired bacterial population, such as *Bifidobacteria* and *Lactobacilli*, in the gut [25]. The scientific research on gut identified that *Bifidobacteria* is the prominent bacteria capable of expressing a higher quantity of β-galactosidase and β-fructofuranosidase enzymes [26]. Genome sequencing and annotations of different Bifidobacterium species recognize several β-galactosidase encoding genes. Of those, many forms of these enzymes are proven with lactases activity, while strains, such as *B. adolescentis* DSM20083, possess a tendency to hydrolyze GOS. Similarly, enzyme β-fructofuranosidase was isolated from *B. infantis* JCM no. 7007, *B. adolescentis* G1, and *B. infantis* ATCC 15697 [27]. Depending on the enzyme family in *Bifidobacteria* species, they liberate either fructose or galactose moieties from appropriate oligosaccharides. Therefore, the tendency of *Bifidobacteria sp* to degrade oligosaccharides structure is based on its access to these degrading isoenzymes. Subsequently, the sugar transport system participates in the incorporation of fructose or galactose moieties that exist in the extracellular environments. Wei *et al.* [28] demonstrated the fructose-specific ABC transport system induced in *Bifidobacterium longum* NCC2705. Furthermore, the health-promoting effect of bifidogenic oligosaccharides is evident with: (i) its contribution to host nutrition, (ii) short-chain fatty acid productions, which are major fuel for colonocytes and responsible for pH decrease, (iii) decreasing bacterial putrefaction and toxin production from pathogenic bacteria, (iv) gastrointestinal motility and function improvements, (v) involved in synthesizing complex vitamins (B and K), (vi) local immune system stimulation. The fermentative end-products of bifidogenic oligosaccharides, such as butyric acid, play a significant role against colon cancer and ulcerative colitis (UC) [16, 28–31]. Moreover, the other SCFA, such as propionic acid, influences lipid metabolism. SCFA mediated pH reduction develops mineral absorption in the colon, thereby rises local blood flow. In addition, SCFA plays a significant role in nuclear factor kappa-light-chain-enhancer of activated b cells (NF-κB) suppression and thus promotes anti-inflammatory response.

2.5 Mechanisms of Oligosaccharides Mediated Immune Effects

The GI constitutes the largest immunologic site in higher organisms, which controls pathogenic invasion and damage associated inflammation. It involves maintaining gut homeostasis through digestion of nondegradable carbohydrates, regulating serum cholesterol and nutrient absorption, productions of fatty acids and other beneficial products [26]. Thus, the overall functioning of the immune system in the human body is mainly driven through an intestinal environment. Specifically, prebiotics (nondegradable oligosaccharides) are reported to play a key role in modulating gut homeostasis by microbiota independent or dependent effects [17]. In microbiota independent mode, oligosaccharides interact directly with the surface receptors of intestinal epithelial cells or immune cells (Figures 2.1 and 2.2). Consequently, these phenomena regulate intestinal barrier integrity and immune functions. Alternatively, oligosaccharide enables the promotion/inhibition of commensals/pathogenic microbes, and oligo-derived short-chain fatty acids production (Figures 2.1 and 2.2) in a microbiota-dependent approach [18].

2.5.1 Intestinal Immune Cells

The tendency of a host system in preventing infections and limiting tumor formations is more prevalent in higher vertebrates [17]. Such a destructive system encompasses mechanisms, such as innate and adaptive responses. Innate immunity provides the early phase of host defenses against invading microorganisms without prior antigen exposure. In this arm of the immune

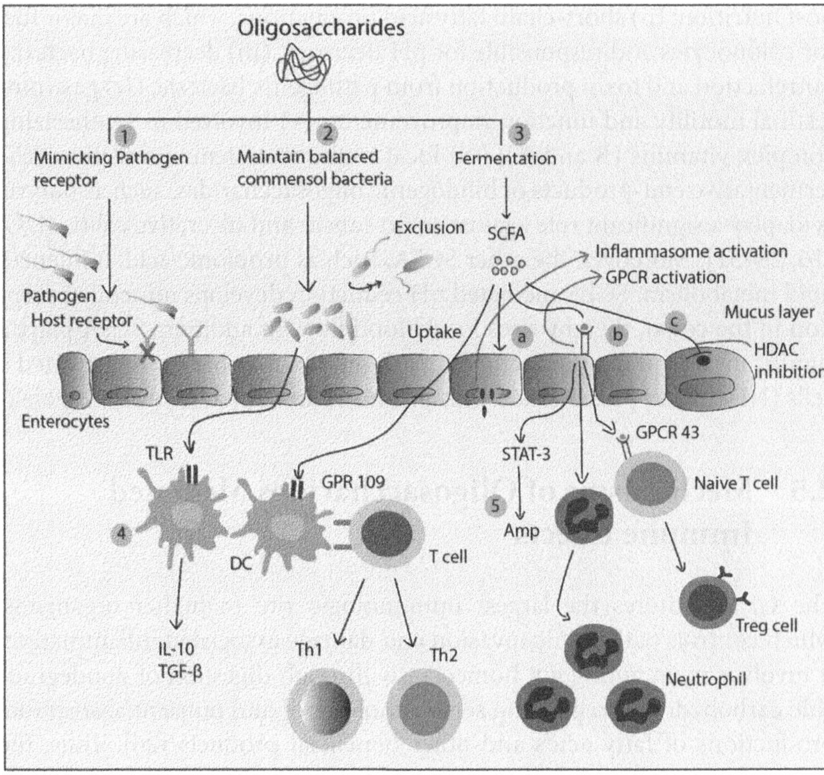

Figure 2.1 Indirect effect of oligosaccharides on the immune system. This figure demonstrates the regulatory effect of prebiotic oligosaccharides in the intestinal immune system by alleviating gut microbial homeostasis. Such a mechanism is driven through the reduction in microbial-mediated cytotoxicity, preventing pathogenic growth and adhesion. (1). Oligosaccharides possess characteristics of decoy receptors thus eliciting anti-adherence and elimination of pathogenic microbes, (2). Oligosaccharides maintain the growth and activity of intestinal commensals, which could enhance the balance between pro-and anti-inflammatory responses, (3). SCFA produced from microbial fermentation of oligosaccharides are capable of interacting with MAPK, mTOR, and STAT3 and brings improvement in the intestinal immune response by a. Formation of inflammasome complex b. Elevation of naive T cells polarization to regulatory phenotype and c. HDAC activity inhibition, (4). Oligosaccharides amplify intestinal commensals thereby triggering DC cells secretion for regulatory cytokines, such as IL-10 and TGF-β. (5). Microbial metabolites SCFA regulate the expression of an antimicrobial peptide in intestinal epithelial cells based on the activation of mTOR and STAT3.

system, innate immune cells recognize pathogen-associated molecular pattern (PAMPs) patterns in microbial surfaces [32]. These receptor-mediated microbial interactions are more prevalent in innate immune cells, such as macrophages, neutrophils, and dendritic cells. The further step involves

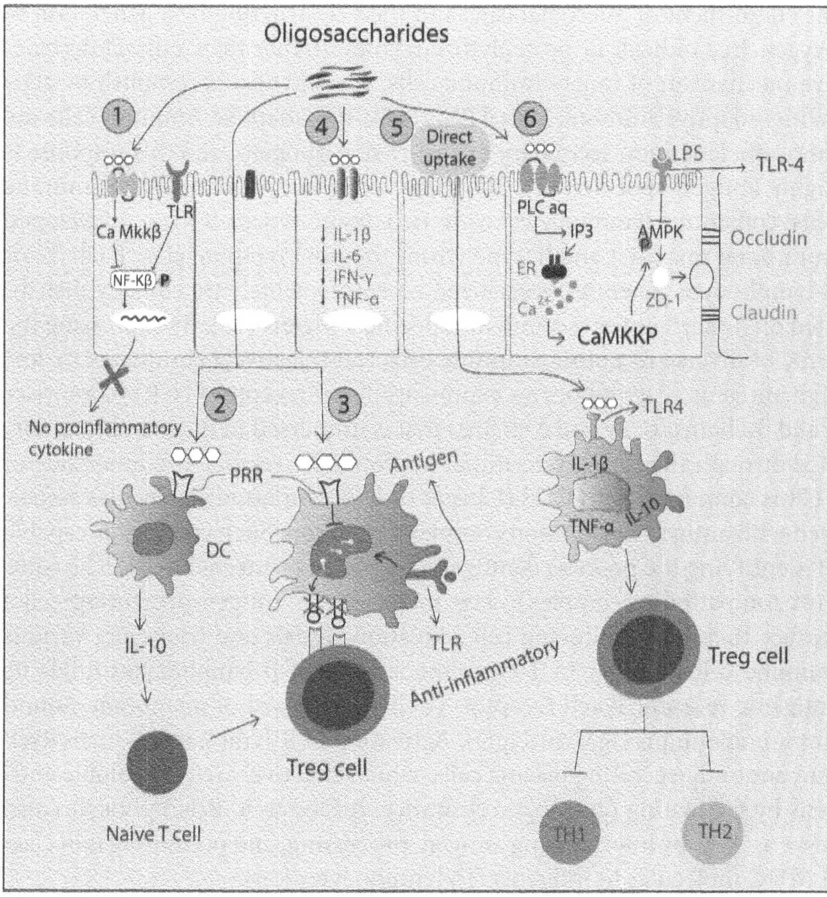

Figure 2.2 Direct effect of oligosaccharides on the immune system. Oligosaccharides could directly modulate the intestinal epithelial cells and immune cells independent of microbiota. It involves regulation of epithelial cell maturation, epithelial cell barrier function improvement, inducing specific PPRs in the intestinal immune system or other regulatory molecules. (1). Oligosaccharides will have direct interaction with the immune cells through PRR eventually activating NF-κB and enhancing cytokine production (IL-10, IL-1β, and TNF-α). (2). Antigen-induced changes in the DC phenotype can be modulated by oligosaccharides during the maturation stage. (3). Oligosaccharide-mediated CaSR- CaMKKβ activation selectively inhibits NF-κB in epithelial cells and so prevents pro-inflammatory response. (4). In intestinal epithelial cells, oligosaccharides diminish the expression of pro-inflammatory cytokines (IL-10, IL-1β, and TNF-α) release thereby attenuating APC mediated inflammatory response. (5). Oligosaccharides intercede anti-inflammatory response by interaction with dendritic cells via pattern recognition receptors (PRRs) and promoting regulatory T cells with subsequent Th1 and Th2 cells suppression. (6). Prebiotic oligosaccharides can effectively reciprocate LPS induced AMPK inhibition and so promotes tight junction re-assembly via activation of CaSR-PLC-IP_3 receptor channel-mediated calcium release.

the engulfment of microbial cells and their destruction by a generation of oxygen-free radicals or proteolytic enzymes. Rather than a direct destructive mechanism of innate immune cells, it could also accomplish by activating adaptive immune cells [17]. Thus, the adaptive immune cells are more efficient upon secondary exposure of pathogens, and this response is highly antigen-specific [32]. The major components of adaptive immune cells constitute lymphocytes with two main types: B type (developed from bone marrow) and T type (from thymus) lymphocytes. Each T- or B-lymphocyte generates specialized receptors, which are clonally distributed on its surface for recognizing specific antigens [18]. By expressing the array of diverse receptors, immune cells can selectively eliminate any foreign antigens. T lymphocytes express its T-cell receptor (TCR) (comprises α and β-chains (or) γ and δ chains) that is immersed in the membrane surface through the carboxy-terminal hydrophobic region. The inner side of TCR is connected with CD3 (Cluster of Differentiation) molecules associated with antigen recognition complex formation. Such complex is capable of identifying the processed antigenic peptides connected to MHC (major histocompatibility complex) class molecule on antigen-presenting cells) surface thereby transducing cell activation signals and triggering various immune cells. Similar to T-type, the surface of B-lymphocytes holds its antigenic receptor B cell receptor (BCR) composed of membrane-bound immunoglobulins (IgM and IgD). Activation of B-lymphocytes turns itself into antibody-secreting plasma cells, which effectively release soluble antigens by facilitating phagocytic clearance. Added to it, B-lymphocytes also serve as APC by internalizing antigen, processing, and presenting it in class II MHC molecules to influence Th lymphocytes [33].

2.5.2 Intestinal Epithelial Barrier

The intestinal epithelial barrier covers mucosal epithelium, underlying lamina propria, and the well-organized gut-associated lymphoid tissue, such as Peyer's patches and mesenteric lymph nodes [17]. Mucosal epithelial is composed of epithelial and intraepithelial cells (Paneth cells). Epithelial cells exhibit proinflammatory function by secreting Interleukin-8 (IL), Tumor necrosis factor-α (TNF-α), IL-6 also acts as a selective barrier for pathogens and bacterial toxins. Paneth cells prevent microbial entry by generating antimicrobial peptides, such as β-defensins [18]. The immune cells, such as dendritic cells (DCs), macrophages, mast cells, activated T cells, and plasma cells, are well populated among subepithelial lamina propria. Moreover, intestinal epithelial cells are capable of secreting glucagon-like peptides, which control inflammation and other metabolic disorders [34].

Therefore, the primary cause of the inflammatory and autoimmune disorder is closely associated with a disruption in the intestinal barrier function. And the consequence of intestinal barrier function was evidenced with penetration of pathogenic markers (like Lipopolysaccharides (LPS) through the mucosal membrane of the GI tract [35]. Standing line of evidence suggests that the health-promoting action of prebiotics is proficient in repairing tight junction protein and promoting barrier integrity [11, 31, 36, 37]. Generally, prebiotics act either by direct interaction with the epithelial cells or through their metabolite interactions.

2.5.3 Microbiota-Dependent Effects of Oligosaccharides

2.5.3.1 Indirect Effect of Oligosaccharides on Intestinal Epithelial Cells

Oligosaccharides assist in maintaining intestinal homeostasis by enriching the beneficial bacteria and declining the pathogenic forms [22]. Figure 2.1 demonstrates the microbiota-dependent role of oligosaccharides modulating immune effects on epithelial cells. Oligosaccharides, such as FOS and GOS, have been recommended as the best fibers stimulating the growth of *Lactobacillus species*, and *Bifidobacterium species* respectively [8]. Table 2.1 illustrates some of the evidence of the therapeutic effect of oligosaccharides on epithelial cells based on selective stimulation of intestinal microbes. These microbial strains efficiently produce SCFA with oligosaccharides that help improve intestinal epithelial barrier function [7]. A study in obese mice reveals that oligo-fructose enriched *Lactobacillus sp* and *Bifidobacteria* sp improve intestinal barrier function through the production of glucagon-like peptide-2 [34]. Oligosaccharides induce preferential growth of beneficial microbes and mediate competitive adhesion in intestinal epithelial cells (IECs) against pathogenic bacteria. Ruiz *et al.* [38] demonstrated that GOS induced *Bifidobacterium infantis* IM-1 capable of displacing pathogenic bacteria, such as *Cronobacter sakazakii* and *Salmonella enterica* from the enterocyte layer. Many intestinal pathogens, such as *Salmonella*, *E. coli*, and *Cronobacter sakazakii* expresses specific adhesins for binding to carbohydrate moiety in IECs. Oligosaccharides, such as GOS, FOS acts as soluble decoy receptors in mimicking pathogenic adhesin binding sites and so preventing the pathogen binding to IECs [19]. GOS inhibits adherence of enteropathogenic *E. coli*, and *Cronobacter sakazakii* to gut epithelium by competitive binding. Similarly, the adherence of *Vibrio cholera* toxin binding to intestinal epithelial cell surface receptor is also inhibited by GOS [18]. Oligosaccharides-derived microbial

Table 2.1 Overview of microbiota-dependent effect of oligosaccharides on immune system.

S. no	Types of prebiotics	Clinical/pre-clinical studies	Effect on microbiome	Mechanism of action	Diseases and treatment	Reference
1	GOS	S mad3-deficient mice	Increases fecal *Bifidobacterium*	Stimulate colonic IL- 15 production	Reduces Colitis, modulatory function and of NK cells	[41]
2	FOS	Patient with Crohn's disease	Increases fecal *Bifidobacterium*	Increase lamina propia DC IL-10 production and TLR expression	Capable of reducing Crohn's disease	[82]
3	GOS	IBS patients	Stimulate gut Bifidobacteria in IBD patients		IBS symptoms	[83]
4	FOS & Inulin	HLA- B27 transgenic mice	Increase *Bifidobacterium* and decrease *Clostridium* cluster II population	SCFA mediated anti-inflammation effect	Reduces chronic intestinal inflammation	[84]

(Continued)

Table 2.1 Overview of microbiota-dependent effect of oligosaccharides on immune system. (*Continued*)

S. no	Types of prebiotics	Clinical/pre-clinical studies	Effect on microbiome	Mechanism of action	Diseases and treatment	Reference
5	GOS	Healthy elderly individual	Increase *Bifidobacteria* population	Increase in Phagocytosis, NK cell activity, and IL- 10 production	Improve GI health and immune function	[26]
6	GOS	Neonatal rat model and rat colon cells	Reduce adherence of *Citrobacter rodentium*	Anti adherence independent mechanism	Protects against intestinal inflammation	[85]
7	GOS	HEPC human cell line	Reduce adherence of *Cronobacter sakazakii*	Anti adhesive effects		[86]

metabolites also play a key role in maintaining the intestinal epithelial barrier integrity. Short-chain fatty acids (SCFA) is a major metabolite of oligosaccharide fermentation mainly acts as an inducer of mucin synthesis and promotes secretion by intestinal epithelial cells thereby regulating gut homeostasis. GOS consumption enhances intestinal mucosa-associated mucin production through the *in vivo* rodent model [39]. SCFA regulates signaling of intestinal epithelial cell functioning through a G-protein-coupled receptor (GPCR) dependent or independent pathway. In GPCR-dependent pathway, SCFA activates signaling molecule mitogen-activated protein kinase (MAPK) through GPCR41 and GPCR43 for triggering cytokine production. SCFA binding to GPCR on the intestinal epithelial surface also activates the nod-like receptor proteins (NLRP3) inflammasome pathway linked to gut epithelial integrity and homeostasis. In GPCR independent way, SCFA plays a key role in gut homeostasis through inhibition of histone deacetylases (HDAC) in intestinal cells [19].

2.5.3.2 An Indirect Effect of Oligosaccharides on Immune Cells

Many *in vitro* and *in vivo* studies validated the microbial-dependent effect of oligosaccharides in regulating immune cell function. Some of the mechanistic evidence for a casual microbiota-dependent role of oligosaccharides on immune cells is highlighted in Figure 2.1. For instance, GOS-enriched *Bifidobacterium species* can induce natural killer cell (NK) function and IL-15 production by reverting goblet cell depletion. It is concluded by enhanced functions of mucosal dendritic cells with IL-10 release [18]. Thus, the oligosaccharide effects reduce the inflammatory cell infiltration and immune cell depletion by increasing the microbial population (Table 2.1). Rather than oligosaccharide itself, its metabolic product, such as SCFA can also modulate the functionality of immune cells [8]. The activation of immune cells, such as DCs, macrophages, regulatory T cells, NK cells, and neutrophils, is well documented for SCFA functionality. Intestinal DCs are in gut-associated lymphoid tissues expressing pattern recognition receptors, such as TLR-2 and TLR-4 through which SCFA binds and triggers DCs maturation. A recent study by Logtenberg *et al.* [25] investigated that the FOS-derived SCFA binding to GPR109 receptor on dendritic cells attenuates proinflammatory cytokine release further influencing T-cell polarization. In the intestine, macrophages more preferably reside on the site of antigen entry (subepithelial region) specialized in phagocytosing harmful microbes and apoptotic cells. However, FOS-derived SCFA is capable of improving macrophage activation manifesting enhanced superoxide anion production and phagocytosis [40]. Oligosaccharides mediated produced SCFA could interact with Naive T cells and elicit enhanced functionality and memory potential. In *in vivo* mice studies, administration of oligosaccharide mixture (scGOS and lcFOS) tends to accelerate Treg populations. Since the oligo-derived SCFA recognizes Treg through the surface receptors GPCR43, and GPCR109A to induce expansion and trafficking of regulatory T cells. Similarly, in neutrophils cells surface, the expression of GPCR43 is indicative of an oligosaccharide-induced inflammatory response. However, the SCFA interaction with GPCR43 also inhibits the migratory potential of neutrophils to mitigate inflammations [41]. The increasing body of evidence suggests that oligosaccharides and the associated SCFA positively influence the NK cell activity. For instance, in the *in vivo* study of *smad-3*–deficient mice, GOS consumption significantly reduce colitis severity by modulating NK cell functions and trafficking [42].

2.5.4 Microbiota Independent Effects of Oligosaccharides

2.5.4.1 Direct Effect on Intestinal Epithelial Cells

Prebiotic oligosaccharides have direct interaction with intestinal epithelial cells, thereby involved in protecting intestinal barrier function and promoting homeostasis (Figure 2.2). Table 2.2 provides some of the available data from preclinical studies on the direct effects of oligosaccharides on immune cells and intestinal epithelial cells. Accumulating evidence suggests that GOS upsurge the gene expression responsible for goblet cell secretory products and Golgi-sulfotransferase, thus enhancing mucosal barrier function [43]. It also stabilizes the expression of sealing protein claudin-3 and thus regulates tight junction reassembly and cellular distribution [44]. Moreover, GOS supplementation in mice attenuates LPS-induced intestinal barrier damage and inflammation in the jejunum and ileum. It is obvious with the upregulation of tight junction protein (zonula occludens [ZO-1] and claudin-1) and downregulation of pro-inflammatory cytokines (IL-1β, IL-6, interferons (IFN-γ), and TNF-α) leads to increasing villus height and villus to crypt ratio [35]. In another way, oligosaccharides accomplish intestinal barrier function by altering epithelial signaling pathways. Perhaps, FOS activates CaSR- Ca2+/calmodulin-dependent protein kinase kinase-B (CaMKKβ)–AMP-activated protein kinase (AMPK) dependent pathway to regulate intestinal tight junction assembly. AMPK signifies AMP-activated protein kinase that assists in regulating tight junction assembly and barrier function in intestinal epithelial cells. Furthermore, the FOS-induced calcium-sensing receptor (CaSR)-phospholipase C (PLC) pathway thereby

Table 2.2 Overview of microbiota independent effect of oligosaccharides on immune system.

S. no	Type of oligosaccharide	*In vitro* cell model	Effect of oligosaccharide	Mechanism of action	Reference
1	GOS	Colonic adenocarcinoma LS174T	Stimulation of goblet cells	Induction of MUC2, TFF3, RETNCB, and CHST5	[42]
2	GOS	Mucosal epithelial cell (NCM- 60)	Anti-inflammatory response	Attenuate TNF- α, induce MIP- 3α and inhibits NF- Kb activation	[79]
3	FOS, GOS, GMO1, Inulin	Intestinal epithelial cells (CaCo2 cells, IEC18 CELLS)	Immunomodulatory effects	Induction of TLR4 expression and stimulates cytokine release	[46]
4	FOS & Inulin	Primary rat monocytes and lymphocytes	Immunomodulatory effects	Induced TNF- α, IL- 4, IL- 10 and growth related oncogene- α	[48]
5	Primary GOS & FOS	Human monocyte derived dendritic cells	Immunomodulatory effects	Stimulates F0XP^{3+} T cells expression and activates T reg cells	[47]

(*Continued*)

Table 2.2 Overview of microbiota independent effect of oligosaccharides on immune system. (*Continued*)

S. no	Type of oligosaccharide	*In vitro* cell model	Effect of oligosaccharide	Mechanism of action	Reference
6	GOS & Chicory inulin	Human epithelial cells & Dendritic cells ($CaCO_2$)	Anti-inflammatory and regulatory effects	Increase in IL- 10/ IL- 12 ratio in T cell response	[50]
7	FOS	Human intestinal cells ($CaCO_2$)	Anti-inflammatory effects	Induce PG1Yrp$_3$ PPARγ and regulates PG1Yrp3	[80]
8	Primary FOS & Secondary GOS	Intestinal epithelial cells (HT- 29, T84 cells)	Alleviation of allergic activity and inflammatory response	Galactose- 9 dependent Th1 and T reg polarization through IFN- γ and IL- 10 secretion	[81]

inhibits NF-κB activation. These potentials prove reverting ability of FOS against LPS-induced AMPK suppression [45]. Moreover, the combination of oligosaccharides (scGOS/lcFOS) could proficiently restrain both proinflammatory and regulatory responses. Since the oligosaccharide mixture is capable of enhancing IFN-γ, and IL-10 production. Declining TNFα and IL-13 production are evident through the co-culture model using IEC and peripheral blood mononuclear cell (PBMC) [46]. Oligosaccharides are capable of modulating cytokine and chemokine release from intestinal epithelial cells. For instance, GOS and FOS elevate the secretion of growth-related oncogene-α, monocyte chemoattractant protein (MCP-1), macrophage inflammatory protein (MIP-2), IL-8 [47]. Thus, the IEC-derived signals could also influence innate and adaptive immune cells, such as dendritic cells (DCs), macrophages, and mast cells.

2.5.4.2 *Direct Effects on Immune Cells*

Like IECs, the activation of intestinal immune cells has been mediated by the direct interaction of prebiotics on its signaling pathways. Several research findings have revealed the direct effects of oligosaccharides on immune cells as shown in Figure 2.2. Such mechanism in immune cells involves TLR ligation enabling cytokines release like TNF-α, IL-10, and growth-related oncogene-α subsequently ends with classical NF-κB pathway [47]. For instance, scGOS/lcFOS stimulate monocyte-derived DCs via TLR-4 ligation inducing IL-10 release and evoking Tregs stimulation [48]. Also, TLR signaling activates mitogen-activated protein kinase and phosphatidylinositol-3-kinase associated pathways of pro-inflammatory response [29]. In contrast, some oligosaccharides might exert an anti-inflammatory milieu by interacting with other recognition molecules. The anti-inflammatory molecules, such as peroxisome proliferator-activated receptor-γ are elevated by interactions of FOS and α3-sialyl lactose [18]. Such molecules are capable of inhibiting pro-inflammatory cytokines, such as IL-12, IL-10, and TNF-α and so halting the NF-κB pathway [47]. Therefore, the prebiotics interaction may suggest the complexities of its signaling events between the pro and anti-inflammatory response. Various preclinical studies have renowned the immunomodulatory effects of oligosaccharides in immune cells, such as DCs, and macrophages are as follows.

2.5.4.2.1 Intestinal Dendritic Cells

Antigen presentation is the major role played by dendritic cells and it also acts as an interesting target for certain oligosaccharides (Figure 2.2).

For instance, Hayen *et al.* [49] demonstrated that the allergen-induced changes in DC phenotype during the maturation stage are efficiently modulated by oligosaccharide mixture (scFOS/lcFOS). Such phenotypic modulation improves the allergen-induced discrepancy in Th1/Treg through successive T-cell responses. Oligosaccharides, such as GOS, influencing the regulatory status of DCs are evident through elevated ratios of IL-10/IL-12. For instance, a coculture study by Bermudez *et al.* [50] revealed that dietary fibers like GOS could impact cytokine (IL-2, IFN-γ, IL-8, MCP-1, and TNF-α) release from IECs derived DCs.

2.5.4.2.2 Macrophage

Oligosaccharide detection by macrophage takes place through specific carbohydrate receptors, such as galactose specific lectin, Ca^{+}-dependent, or -independent C-type lectin receptor. These interactions activate intracellular signaling pathways, which promote and trigger proinflammatory cytokine release. FOS interactions with human and rat monocytes tend to secrete inflammatory cytokines, such as TNF-α and IL-10 [51]. But, a decline in LPS-induced secretion of IFN-γ and IL-17 in mouse splenocytes is evident through TLR-mediated signaling pathways [29]. Moreover, the effect of FOS on peritoneal exudate cells is evident with enhanced production of nitric oxide, free radicals, and phagocytic activity in the *in vivo* rat model study [51].

2.6 Immunomodulatory Effects of Fructooligosaccharides and Galactooligosaccharides

2.6.1 Gastrointestinal Disease

Generally, consumption of nondigestible oligosaccharide (NDO) improves viscosity, fermentability, and water solubility index of gastric content consequently normalizing intestinal transit, maintaining homeostasis, regularizing intestinal functions, and increasing fecal volume [11]. A single-center, prospective, double-blind randomized controlled trial with 144 healthy, exclusively breast-fed infants evaluated the effect of the mixture of FOS, GOS, and polyunsaturated fatty acids. Compared with the control group, the infants in the experimental group tend to have amended gut comfort by the route of stool consistency, GE time, GI symptoms, and stool microbiota [12]. Oligosaccharides possess great potential to alleviate enteral infections by decreasing an absolute number of harmful bacteria families, such as *Clostridiaceae* and *Enterococcacea* and increasing

Bifidobacteriaceae and *Lactobacillecea*. Li *et al.* [26] demonstrated that bifidobacteria shows relatively higher selectivity and prebiotic index (PI) for GOS, whereas FOS possesses a higher PI value toward lactobacilli in an *in vitro* simulated intestinal digestion. Hopkins and Macfarlane [52] identified the suppressing ability of GOS against *Clostridium difficile* growth and its toxin production. Necrotizing enterocolitis (NEC) is a gastrointestinal emergency that primarily affects premature neonates and causes necrosis of the bowel [53]. It is claimed that prebiotics, such as FOS and GOS, can prevent preterm infants by stimulating the growth of gut microbiota (e.g., *Bifidobacteria*) and reducing pathogenic bacteria [54].

2.6.2 Immune Stimulation

Prebiotic oligosaccharides pose direct interaction with the microbiota further modifies the inflammatory process in the intestinal environment (Figure 2.3). Several reports about the immune-enhancing effect of oligosaccharides come from the experimental trial of FOS, GOS, and inulin [29, 55]. Furthermore, the oligosaccharides supplementation will change the composition and metabolic features of gut bacteria which in turn stimulates immune cell functions possibly through varied cytokine expression. Experiment evidence demonstrated that a FOS-based diet effectively stimulates distinct subpopulations of T lymphocytes and dendritic cells in the GI tract by increasing IL-10 and IFN-c production [29]. In AOM-treated mice, administration of a fructan-based diet (FOS/inulin) had a lower risk of colon cancer as well as a reversal in the inhibition of NK cell activity [55]. Mice fed with a fructan-rich diet showed an increase in NK cell functioning and macrophage activation, thereby diminishing the *Salmonella* and *Listeria* infections, and suppressing tumor development [32]. Intestinal mucus bilayer comprises an outer layer, which plays a vital role in reducing mucosal shear stress and trapping pathogenic bacteria, whereas the inner adherent layer role in barrier function. These intestinal mucus bilayers have largely controlled by oligosaccharides, such as GOS. Mice fed with GOS had a significantly thicker adherent layer and higher mucus (*MUC2*) secretion in the lumen [56]. Moreover, the structure of oligosaccharides can resemble pathogen receptors on intestinal epithelial cells and may act as antiadhesive molecules that completely inhibit bacterial adherence. GOS inhibited the adhesion of microcolony-forming enteropathogenic *Escherichia coli* E2348/69 on HEp-2 and Caco-2 cells. But in a dose-dependent manner, it reduced the invasion and adherence of *Salmonella typhimurium* in three dimensions cultured HT-29-16E cells [21].

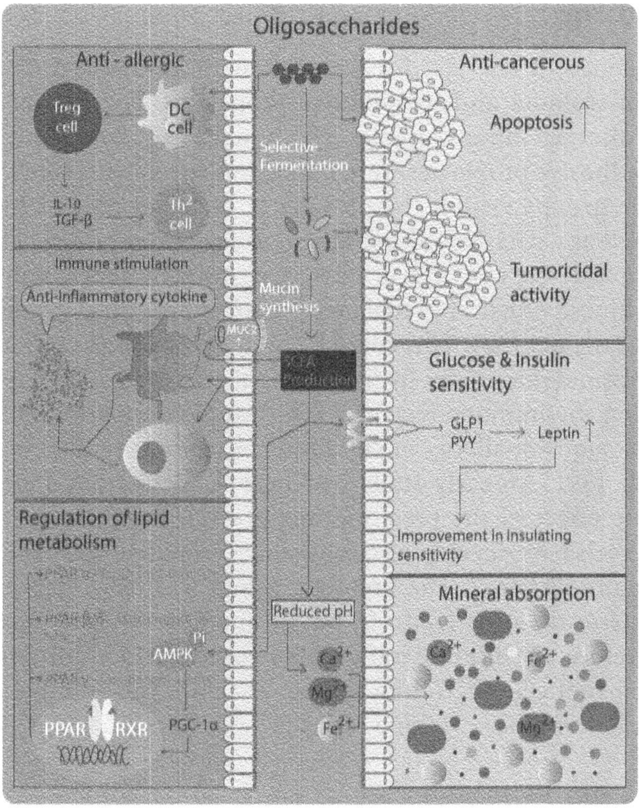

Figure 2.3 Overview of immune-modulatory action of oligosaccharides. The figure illustrates that oligosaccharides pass through the gut and induce selective microbial growth and functionality of specific genera or species. Selective microbial growth produces metabolic end-products, including organic acids, mucin can lower intestinal pH eliciting subsequent effects on microbial pathogens and mineral absorption. Oligosaccharides promote the secretion of mucin and tight junction protein thereby enhancing epithelial barrier function. Oligosaccharide metabolic products like SCFA contribute to the expansion of anti-inflammatory response mainly through the signaling of innate immune cells, such as DC cells and NK cells. SCFAs can also regulate lipid metabolism through the PPAR pathway. SCFAs activate PPAR isoforms by phosphorylating uncoupling protein AMPK and recruiting PPAR-RXR dimerization thereby regulating the expression of PPAR response elements in different regions. For instance, PPAR α activation prevents lipid accumulation by fatty acid oxidation, PPAR β/δ induces mitochondrial biogenesis and metabolism and PPAR γ activates insulin secretion. Oligosaccharides are efficient in triggering cancer cell apoptosis and tumoricidal activity. Metabolic products of oligosaccharides improve peptide hormone (PYY, GLP-1) secretion capable of regulating host cell metabolism. Like appetite reduction is regulated by PYY and GLP-1 escalates insulin secretion and so lowers blood glucose level. pH decrease due to SCFA production improves mineral solubility and mediates subsequent improvement in active and passive mineral transfer routes. Oligosaccharides are capable of initiating a Treg differentiation program to encourage cytokine-mediated polarization of Th2 cells.

2.6.3 Allergy

The incidence of allergic disease deals with an association between colonic microbiota and its adhesive properties. For instance, in the feces of allergic infants, lower cell numbers of *Bifidobacteria* with reduced adhesive properties were found compared with control groups [57]. Such groups exhibit the prevalence of IgE-mediated food allergies, as well as a Th2-biased immune response (Figure 2.3). The babies have a skewed Th2 response at birth due to the mother's high levels of Th2 cytokines, which are rebalanced after appropriate stimulation by bacteria at the gut [58]. This could be because prebiotics influences the gastrointestinal microflora by increasing the number of *Bifidobacteria*, rebalancing the immune response [16]. Atopic dermatitis (AD) is one of the first signs of allergy in childhood, affecting 10–20% of children worldwide [59]. An early study by Roger & McCartney [60] demonstrated the effect of the prebiotic mixture (90% GOS and 10% FOS) in infants' risk of developing atopy and compared with the placebo group (maltodextrins). The prebiotic group was observed with more *Bifidobacteria* than the controls, but no increase in *Lactobacillus* species. Therefore, the administration of oligosaccharides positively influences the beneficial microflora and so rebalance the immune response by anti-inflammatory cytokine release.

2.6.4 Mineral Absorption

The absorption of calcium and magnesium in the body has a significant impact on osteoporosis and other bone-related diseases [61]. Several reports in preclinical studies suggest that dietary fibers, such as FOS, GOS, and inulin improve bone density (Figure 2.3) by bioavailability and mineral absorption [13, 61]. An earlier study by Delzenne *et al.* [62] reported that consumption of oligofructose and inulin (on 10% weight) significantly improved intestinal absorption of calcium and magnesium by 60% as proved in rat model studies. Oligosaccharides are believed to play a significant role in influencing the prevalence of osteoporosis in postmenopausal women. In postmenopausal women, oligofructose administration increases calcium and magnesium absorption and prevents bone loss caused by estrogen deficiency [63]. Whereas in the case of FOS and GOS alone is concerned, its beneficial effect on mineral absorption is well studied in rat models. However, studies are limited in human trials with inconsistent results [64]. In an early study, teenage boys consumed with FOS, inulin, and V-GOS (15 g per day) for 3 weeks, showed no effect on iron and calcium absorption for tested prebiotics [65]. Conversely, postmenopausal women given V-GOS (15 g per day) for 9 days, have shown a significant increase in calcium absorption [66]. Besides, consumption of oligofructose-enriched inulin in individuals with poor bone density displays improved mineral absorption [36].

2.6.5 Inflammatory Bowel Diseases

Inflammatory bowel disease (IBD) is categorized into UC and Crohn's disease (CD), which are caused due to inappropriate immune responses against intestinal commensals [67]. Consequently, under inflammatory disease conditions, a family of beneficial bacteria (*Bifidobacteriaceae, Bacteroidaceae, Lachnospiraceae, Ruminococcaceae,* and *Eubacteriaceae*) decreased and nonbeneficial forms (*Enterobacteriaceae, Pseudomonadaceae, Clostridiaceae,* and *Desulfo vibrionaceae*) are enriched in the colonic mucosa [68]. Moreover, in IBD patients, the immune-mediated tissue injury disrupts gut integrity thereby unbalances pro-inflammatory and anti-inflammatory cytokines. Therefore, CD develops response profile via Th1 pattern of cytokine (TNF-α, interferon-γ, IL-12, and IL-1β) formation, whereas Th2 pattern of cytokines (IL-5 and IL-10) is expressed in UC [69]. Henceforth, the use of oligosaccharides is successful in therapeutic modulation of IBD evident through *in vivo* studies. For instance, GOS administration ameliorates dextran sulfate sodium (DSS) induced murine colitis by regulating intestinal flora and inhibiting NF-κB activation [31]. Similarly, in the 2,4,6-trinitrobenzene sulfonic acid (TNBS) induced rat model of colitis, GOS derived from lactulose results in a better anti-inflammatory profile by improving luminal microbiota balance compare to lactulose [37]. However, in humans with active CD, FOS intake for 2 to 4 weeks decreased the inflammatory markers, such as fecal calprotectin, C-reactive protein, and inflammatory cytokines [14].

2.6.6 Cancer

Immunomodulatory effects of oligosaccharides provide an opportunity to prevent cancer by modulating gut microflora, decreasing cell proliferation, apoptosis stimulation, angiogenesis inhibition (Figure 2.3), prevention of pro-carcinogenic to carcinogenic conversion [16, 70]. Possibly, SCFA produced from oligosaccharides exert histone deacetylation inhibition, thereby stimulating apoptosis and cell cycle arrest in tumor cell environment [71]. Several recent studies used FOS and GOS as a choice of prebiotics for reducing cancer development in animal studies.

For instance, Fernandez *et al.* [72] demonstrated that lactulose-derived GOS are effective against colorectal cancer (CRC) onset by influencing DNA damage, inflammation, and apoptosis. Although early studies with a model system of the human gut [15] used GOS to reveal reduced activities of genotoxic enzymes (β-glucosidase and β-glucuronidase and aryl sulphatase) produced by colonic microorganisms linked to CRC. Another study [73], illustrates GOS feeding in humans exhibits a marked reduction in nitroreductase, indole, and isovaleric acid. However, epidemiological evaluation and subsequent demonstration on the specific anti-cancer effects of either GOS or FOS and the colonic microbiota in humans are still lacking.

2.6.7 Cholesterol and Triglyceride Reduction

A high-fat hypercaloric diet induces dyslipidemia, such as hypertriglyceridemia and insulin resistance, that retains a linear relationship with the risk of atherosclerotic cardiovascular disease [74]. A growing body of evidence in human studies and animal model suggest that oligosaccharide consumption helps lower blood cholesterol levels and improves lipid profile in cardiovascular patients [2, 75]. For example, in Figure 2.3 (section d) we have shown the process of oligosaccharide metabolites in regulating lipid metabolism. Hashmi *et al.*, [75] demonstrated that hypercholesterolemia female Sprague-Dawley rats administered with GOS for 2 months evident with a significant reduction in serum triglycerides, low-density lipoprotein (LDL-C), and very-low-density lipoprotein (VLDL-C) compared with the control group. Prebiotic oligosaccharides enhance cholesterol reduction through two mechanisms, such as increasing fecal cholesterol excretion by decreasing its absorption, and SCFA drove inhibition of hepatic cholesterol and fatty acid synthesis by suppressing lipogenic enzymes [2, 5]. A recent study by Dai *et al.* [76] demonstrated that mice administrated with α-GOS derived from galactose (α-GOSg) significantly reduce total cholesterol and LDL-cholesterol alanine aminotransferase and liver lipids. Furthermore, the α-GOSg treatment decreases the histopathological score for liver steatosis and downregulation of the hepatic fatty acid synthesis gene acetyl CoA carboxylase-α. An early investigation of parallel reports is also evidenced with FOS-induced reduction of triglyceride synthesis in the liver [77]. Similarly, reductions in triacylglycerol and gradual reduction in total cholesterol and LDL levels are also obvious in an animal model of hyperlipidemia [32]. As a consequence, subsequent GOS/FOS consumption is capable of preventing/reducing the risk of cardiovascular disease.

2.7 Conclusion

Oligosaccharides, such as FOS and GOS, are the most investigated prebiotic compounds with demonstrated health benefits in humans. Many clinical and preclinical studies validate the implications of oligosaccharides in regulating the proinflammatory and anti-inflammatory response in controlling inflammatory diseases (IBD, cancer, allergy, and others). Many kinds of literature evidence state that oligosaccharides, such as FOS and GOS, capable of enriching gut microbiota, such as bifidobacteria and lactic acid bacteria, play a significant role in immune system regulation. The intricate relationship between the gut, intestinal immune cells, and epithelial cells involves the release of cytokines, metabolite production, and interference of gut microbiota. Thus, the prebiotic oligosaccharides initiate a network of signaling and cell-cell communications thereby controlling systemic inflammatory response via functional microbiome interventions and epigenetic mechanisms. Indirect effects of oligosaccharides on the immune system through enriching beneficial microbes and depressing pathogenic forms are well documented. However, the direct immunomodulatory effects of oligosaccharides are not well explored. Hence, further research is encouraging to study the immunomodulatory role of oligosaccharides independent of microbiota.

Acknowledgment

The authors would like to thank their respective institutes for providing the facilities to write this book chapter successfully.

References

1. Jovanovic-Malinovska, R., Kuzmanova, S., Winkelhausen, E., Oligosaccharide profile in fruits and vegetables as sources of prebiotics and functional foods. *Int. J. Food Prop.*, 17, 5, 949, 2014.
2. Florowska, A., Krygier, K., Florowski, T., Dluzewska, E., Prebiotics as functional food ingredients preventing diet-related diseases. *Food Funct.*, 7, 5, 2147, 2016.
3. Mozaffarian, D., Dietary and policy priorities for cardiovascular disease, diabetes, and obesity: A comprehensive review. *Circulation*, 133, 2, 187, 2016.

4. Gibson, G.R. and Roberfroid, M.B., Dietary modulation of the human colonic microbiota: Introducing the concept of prebiotics. *J. Nutr.*, 125, 6, 1401, 1995.
5. Ul Haq, Z. and Khan, A.A., Prebiotics: The gut ecology modifiers. *J. Entomol. Zool. Stud.*, 6, 3, 1816, 2018.
6. Tingirikari, J.M.R., Sarathy, M.V. *et al.*, Impact of probiotics in human health and disease treatment, in: *Nutraceutical and Functional Foods in Disease Prevention*, R. Keservani, A. Sharma, R. Kesharwani (Eds.), pp. 35–67, IGI Global, Hershey, PA, 2019.
7. Hee, B.V.D. and Wells, J.M., Microbial regulation of host physiology by short-chain fatty acids. *Trends Microbiol.*, 29, 8, 700, 2021.
8. Martins, G.N., Ureta, M.M., Tymczyszyn, E.E., Castilho, P.C., Gomez-Zavaglia, A., Technological aspects of the production of fructo and galacto-oligosaccharides enzymatic synthesis and hydrolysis. *Front. Nutr.*, 6, 78, 2019.
9. Santibanez, L., Henriquez, C., Corro-Tejeda, R., Bernal, S., Armijo, B., Salazar, O., Xylo-oligosaccharides from lignocellulosic biomass: a comprehensive review. *Carbohydr. Polym.*, 251, 117118, 2021.
10. Zeng, J., Hu, Y., Gao, H., Sun, J., Ma, H., Fructo-oligosaccharides impact on the hydration and retro-gradation of wheat starch and gel. *Int. J. Food Prop.*, 19, 12, 2682, 2016.
11. Muller, M., Canfora, E.E., Blaak, E.E., Gastrointestinal transit time, glucose homeostasis and metabolic health: modulation by dietary fibers. *Nutrients*, 10, 3, 275, 2018.
12. Vivatvakin, B., Mahayosnond, A., Theamboonlers, A., Steenhout, P.G., Conus, N.J., Effect of a whey-predominant starter formula containing LCPUFAs and oligosaccharides (FOS/GOS) on gastrointestinal comfort in infants. *Asia Pac. J. Clin. Nutr.*, 19, 4, 473, 2010.
13. Bryk, G., Coronel, M.Z., Pellegrini, G., Mandalunis, P., Rio, M.S., Portela, M.L.P.M.d., Zeni, S.N., Effect of a combination GOS/FOS® prebiotic mixture and interaction with calcium intake on mineral absorption and bone parameters in growing rats. *Eur. J. Nutr.*, 54, 913, 2015.
14. Benjamin, J.L., Hedin, C., Koutsoumpasm, A., Ng, S.C., McCarthy, N.E., Hart, A.L., Kamm, M.A., Sanderson, J.D., Knight, S.C., Forbes, A., Stagg, A.J., Whelan, K., Lindsay, J.O., Randomized, double blind, placebo-controlled trial of fructo oligosaccharides in active Crohn's disease. *Gut*, 60, 7, 923, 2011.
15. Mcbain, A.J. and Macfarlane, G.T., Modulation of genotoxic enzyme activities by non-digestible oligosaccharide metabolism in *in-vitro* human gut bacterial ecosystems. *J. Med. Microbiol.*, 50, 9, 833, 2001.
16. Macfarlane, G.T., Steed, H., Macfarlane, S., Bacterial metabolism and health-related effects of galacto-oligosaccharides and other prebiotics. *J. Appl. Microbiol.*, 104, 2, 305, 2008.

17. Cai, Y., Folkerts, J., Folkerts, G., Maurer, M., Braber, S., Microbiota-dependent and-independent effects of dietary fibre on human health. *Br. J. Pharmacol.*, 177, 6, 1363, 2020.
18. Pujari, R. and Banerjee, G., Impact of prebiotics on immune response: From the bench to the clinic. *Immunol. Cell Biol.*, 99, 3, 255, 2021.
19. Tashiro, Y., Ueno, H., Takaba, M., Hayashi, S., Production of functional inulin-type fructo-oligosaccharides by an Enzyme from *Penicillium citrinum. Curr. Microbiol.*, 74, 9, 1114, 2017.
20. Xavier, J.R. and Ramana, K.V., Optimization of levan production by cold-active *Bacillus licheniformis* ANT 179 and fructo-oligosaccharide synthesis by its levansucrase. *Appl. Biochem. Biotechnol.*, 181, 3, 986, 2017.
21. Bruno-Barcena, J.M. and Azcarate-Peril, M.A., Galacto-oligosaccharides and colorectal cancer: Feeding our intestinal probiome. *J. Funct. Foods*, 12, 92, 2015.
22. Davani-Davari, D., Negahdaripour, M., Karimzadeh, I., Seifan, M., Mohkam, M., Masoumi, S.J., Berenjian, A., Ghasemi, Y., Prebiotics: Definition, types, sources, mechanisms, and clinical applications. *Foods*, 8, 3, 92, 2019.
23. Choukade, R. and Kango, N., Production, properties, and applications of fructosyltransferase: A current appraisal. *Crit. Rev. Biotechnol.*, 41, 1–16, 2021.
24. Nobre, C., Teixeira, J.A., Rodrigues, L.R., New trends and technological challenges in the industrial production and purification of fructo-oligosaccharides. *Crit. Rev. Food Sci. Nutr.*, 55, 10, 1444, 2015.
25. Logtenberg, M.J., Akkerman, R., An, R., Hermes, G.D.A., Haan, B.J.d., Faas, M.M., Zoetendal, E.G., Schols, H.A., Vos, P.d., Fermentation of chicory fructo-oligosaccharides and native inulin by infant fecal microbiota attenuates pro-inflammatory responses in immature dendritic cells in an infant-age-dependent and fructan-specific way. *Mol. Nutr. Food Res.*, 64, 13, 2000068, 2020.
26. Li, W., Wang, K., Sun, Y., Ye, H., Hu, B., Zeng, X., Influences of structures of galacto-oligosaccharides and fructo-oligosaccharides on the fermentation *in vitro* by human intestinal microbiota. *J. Funct. Foods*, 13, 158, 2015.
27. Avila-Fernandez, A., Cuevas-Juarez, E., Rodriguez-Alegria, M.E., Olvera, C., Lopez-Munguia, A., Functional characterization of a novel β-fructofuranosidase from *Bifidobacterium longum* subsp. *infantis* ATCC 15697 on structurally diverse fructans. *J. Appl. Microbiol.*, 121, 1, 263–276, 2016.
28. Wei, X., Guo, Y., Shao, C., Sun, Z., Zhurina, D., Liu, D., Liu, W., Zou, D., Jiang, Z., Wang, X., Zhao, J., Shang, W., Li, X., Liao, X., Huang, L., Riedel, C.U., Yuan, J., Fructose uptake in Bifidobacterium longum NCC2705 is mediated by an ATP-binding cassette transporter. *J. Biol. Chem.*, 287, 1, 357, 2012.

29. Capitan-Canadas, F., Ocon, B., Aranda, C.J., Anzola, A., Suarez, M.D., Zarzuelo, A., Medina, F.S.D., Martinez-Augustin, O., Fructo-oligosaccharides exert intestinal anti-inflammatory activity in the $CD4^+$ $CD62L^+$ T cell transfer model of colitis in C57BL/6J mice. *Eur. J. Nutr.*, 55, 1445, 2016.
30. Vulevic, J., Juric, A., Walton, G.E., Claus, S.P., Tzortzis, G., Toward, R.E., Gibson, G.R., Influence of galacto-oligosaccharide mixture (B-GOS) on gut microbiota, immune parameters and metabolomics in elderly persons. *Br. J. Nutr.*, 114, 4, 586, 2015.
31. Chu, H., Tao, X., Sun, Z., Hao, W., Wei, X., Galacto-oligosaccharides protects against DSS-induced murine colitis through regulating intestinal flora and inhibiting NF-κB pathway. *Life Sci.*, 242, 117220, 2020.
32. Delgado, G.T.C., Tamashiro, W.M., Pastore, G.M., Immunomodulatory effects of fructans. *Food Res. Int.*, 43, 5, 1231, 2010.
33. Junior, D.M., Araujo, J.A.P., Catelan, T.T.T., Souza, A.W.S.D., Cruvinel, W.D.M., Andrade, L.E.C., Silva, N.P.D., Immune system-part II: Basis of the immunological response mediated by T and B lymphocytes. *Rev. Bras. Reumatol.*, 50, 552, 2010.
34. Cani, P.D., Possemiers, S., Wiele, T.V.D., Guiot, Y., Everard, A., Rottier, O., Geurts, L., Naslain, D., Neyrinck, A., Lambert, D.M., Muccioli, G.G., Delzenne, N.M., Changes in gut microbiota control inflammation in obese mice through a mechanism involving GLP-2-driven improvement of gut permeability. *Gut*, 58, 8, 1091, 2009.
35. Wang, G., Sun, W., Pei, X., Jin, Y., Wang, H., Tao, W., Xiao, Z., Liua, L., Wang, M., Galactooligosaccharide pretreatment alleviates damage of the intestinal barrier and inflammatory responses in LPS-challenged mice. *Food Funct.*, 12, 4, 1569, 2021.
36. Holloway, L., Moynihan, S., Abrams, S.A., Kent, K., Hsu, A.R., Friedlander, A.L., Effects of oligofructose-enriched inulin on intestinal absorption of calcium and magnesium and bone turnover markers in postmenopausal women. *Br. J. Nutr.*, 97, 2, 365, 2007.
37. Algieri, F., Rodriguez-Nogales, A., Garrido-Mesa, N., Vezza, T., Garrido-Mesa, J., Utrilla, M.P., Montilla, A., Cardelle-Cobas, A., Olano, A., Corzo, N., Guerra-Hernandez, E., Zarzuelo, A., Rodriguez-Cabezas, M.E., Galvez, J., Intestinal anti-inflammatory effects of oligosaccharides derived from lactulose in the trinitro benzenesulfonic acid model of rat colitis. *J. Agric. Food Chem.*, 62, 4285, 2014.
38. Ruiz, L., Florez, A.B., Sanchez, B., Moreno-Munoz, J.A., Rodriguez-Palmero, M., Jimenez, J., Gavilan, C.G.d.l.R., Gueimonde, M., Ruas-Madiedo, P., Margolles, A., *Bifidobacterium longum* subsp. *infantis* CECT7210 (*B. infantis* IM-1®) Displays *in vitro* activity against some intestinal pathogens. *Nutrients*, 12, 3259, 2020.
39. Leforestier, G., Blais, A., Blachier, F., Baglieri, A.M., Gay, A.M.D., Perrin, E., Tome, D., Effects of galacto-oligosaccharide ingestion on the

mucosa-associated mucins and sucrase activity in the small intestine of mice. *Eur. J. Nutr.*, 48, 457, 2009.
40. Delgado, G.T.C., Thome, R., Gabriel, D.L., Tamashiro, W.M.S.C., Pastore, G.M., Yacon (Smallanthus sonchifolius)-derived fructooligosaccharides improves the immune parameters in the mouse. *Nutr. Res.*, 32, 884, 2012.
41. Kamp, M.E., Shim, R., Nicholls, A.J., Oliveira, A.C., Manson, L.J., Binge, L., Mackay, C.R., Wong, C.H.Y., G protein-coupled receptor 43 modulates neutrophil recruitment during acute inflammation. *PLoS One*, 11, e0163750, 2016.
42. Gopalakrishnan, A., Clinthorne, J.F., Rondini, E.A., McCaskey, S.J., Gurzell, E.A., Langohr, I.M., Gardner, E.M., Fenton, J.I., Supplementation with galacto-oligosaccharides increases the percentage of NK cells and reduces colitis severity in Smad3-deficient mice. *J. Nutr.*, 142, 7, 1336, 2012.
43. Bhatia, S., Prabhu, P.N., Benefiel, A.C., Miller, M.J., Chow, J., Davis, S.R., Gaskins, H.R., Galacto-oligosaccharides may directly enhance intestinal barrier function through the modulation of goblet cells. *Mol. Nutr. Food Res.*, 59, 3, 566, 2015.
44. Akbari, P., Braber, S., Alizadeh, A., Verheijden, K.A., Schoterman, M.H.C., Kraneveld, A.D., Garssen, J., Fink-Gremmels, J., Galacto-oligosaccharides protect the intestinal barrier by maintaining the tight junction network and modulating the inflammatory responses after a challenge with the mycotoxin deoxynivalenol in human Caco-2 cell monolayers and B6C3F1 mice. *J. Nutr.*, 145, 7, 1604, 2015.
45. Wongkrasant, P., Pongkorpsakol, P., Ariyadamrongkwan, J., Meesomboon, R., Satitsri, S., Pichyangkura, R., Barrett, K.E., Muanprasat, C., A prebiotic fructo-oligosaccharide promotes tight junction assembly in intestinal epithelial cells via an AMPK-dependent pathway. *Biomed. Pharmacother.*, 129, 110415, 2020.
46. Hayen, S.M., Otten, H.G., Overbeek, S.A., Knulst, A.C., Garssen, J., Willemsen, L.E.M., Exposure of intestinal epithelial cells to short- and long-chain fructo-oligosaccharides and CpG oligodeoxynucleotides enhances peanut-specific T helper 1 polarization. *Front. Immunol.*, 9, 923, 2018.
47. Ortega-Gonzalez, M., Ocon, B., Romero-Calvo, I., Anzola, A., Guadix, E., Zarzuelo, A., Suarez, M.D., Medina, F.S.D., Martinez-Augustin, O., Nondigestible oligosaccharides exert nonprebiotic effects on intestinal epithelial cells enhancing the immune response via activation of TLR 4-NF κB. *Mol. Nutr. Food Res.*, 58, 2, 384, 2014.
48. Lehmann, S., Hiller, J., Bergenhenegouwen, J.V., Knippels, L.M.J., Garssen, J., Traidl-Hoffmann, C., In vitro evidence for immune-modulatory properties of non-digestible oligosaccharides: direct effect on human monocyte derived dendritic cells. *PLoS One*, 10, e0132304, 2015.
49. Hayen, S.M., Knulst, A.C., Garssen, J., Otten, H.G., Willemsen, L.E.M., Fructo-oligosaccharides modify human dc maturation and peanut-induced

autologous t-cell response of allergic patients in vitro. *Front. Immunol.*, 11, 600125, 2020.

50. Bermudez-Brito, M., Sahasrabudhe, N.M., Rosch, C., Schols, H.A., Faas, M.M., Vos, P.D., The impact of dietary fibers on dendritic cell responses in vitro is dependent on the differential effects of the fibers on intestinal epithelial cells. *Mol. Nutr. Food Res.*, 59, 4, 698, 2015.
51. Kumar, V.P., Prashanth, K.V., Venkatesh, Y.P., Structural analyses and immunomodulatory properties of fructo-oligosaccharides from onion *(Allium cepa). Carbohydr. Polym.*, 117, 115, 2015.
52. Hopkins, M.J. and Macfarlane, G.T., Nondigestible oligosaccharides enhance bacterial colonization resistance against Clostridium difficile in vitro. *Appl. Environ. Microbiol.*, 69, 1920, 2003.
53. Garg, B.D., Balasubramanian, H., Kabra, N.S., Bansal, A., Effect of oropharyngeal colostrum therapy in the prevention of necrotizing enterocolitis among very low birthweight neonates: A meta-analysis of randomized controlled trials. *J. Hum. Nutr. Diet.*, 31, 5, 612, 2018.
54. Armanian, A.M., Sadeghnia, A., Hoseinzadeh, M., Mirlohi, M., Feizi, A., Salehimehr, N., Saee, N., Nazari, J., The effect of neutral oligosaccharides on reducing the incidence of necrotizing enterocolitis in preterm infants: A randomized clinical trial. *Int. J. Prev. Med.*, 5, 11, 1387, 2014.
55. Roberfroid, M., Gibson, G.R., Hoyles, L., McCartney, A.L., Rastall, R., Rowland, I., Wolvers, D., Watzl, B., Szajewska, H., Stahl, B., Guarner, F., Respondek, F., Whelan, K., Coxam, V., Davicco, M.J., Leotoing, L., Wittrant, Y., Delzenne, N.M., Cani, P.D., Neyrinck, A.M., Meheust, A., Prebiotic effects: metabolic and health benefits. *Br. J. Nutr.*, 104, 2, S1, 2010.
56. Arnold, J.W., Roach, J., Fabela, S., Moorfield, E., Ding, S., Blue, E., Dagher, S., Magness, S., Tamayo, R., Bruno-Barcena, J.M., Azcarate-Peril, M.A., The pleiotropic effects of prebiotic galacto-oligosaccharides on the aging gut. *Microbiome*, 9, 1, 1, 2021.
57. Sangwan, V., Tomar, S.K., Singh, R.R.B., Singh, A.K., Ali, B., Galacto-oligosaccharides: novel components of designer foods. *J. Food Sci.*, 76, 4, R103, 2011.
58. Vandenplas, Y., Zakharova, I., Dmitrieva, Y., Oligosaccharides in infant formula: More evidence to validate the role of prebiotics. *Br. J. Nutr.*, 113, 9, 1339, 2015.
59. Weidinger, S. and Novak, N., Atopic dermatitis. *Lancet*, 387, 10023, 1109, 2016.
60. Roger, L.C. and McCartney, A.L., The application of prebiotics and synbiotics in pediatrics, in: *Probiotics in Pediatric Medicine*, S. Michail and P.M. Sherman (Eds.), pp. 307–322, Nutrition and health series, Humana Press, Totowa, New Jersey, 2009.
61. Whisner, C.M. and Castillo, L.F., Prebiotics, bone and mineral metabolism. *Calcif. Tissue Int.*, 102, 443, 2018.

62. Delzenne, N., Aertssens, J., Verplaetse, H., Roccaro, M., Roberfroid, M., Effect of fermentable fructo-oligosaccharides on mineral, nitrogen and energy digestive balance in the rat. *Life Sci.*, 57, 17, 1579, 1995.
63. Slevin, M.M., Allsopp, P.J., Magee, P.J., Bonham, M.P., Naughton, V.R., Strain, J.J., Duffy, M.E., Wallace, J.M., Sorley, E.M.M., Supplementation with calcium and short-chain fructo-oligosaccharides affects markers of bone turnover but not bone mineral density in postmenopausal women. *J. Nutr.*, 144, 297, 2014.
64. Weaver, C.M., Martin, B.R., Nakatsu, C.H., Armstrong, A.P., Clavijo, A., McCabe, L.D., McCabe, G.P., Duignan, S., Schoterman, M.H.C., Galacto-oligosaccharides improve mineral absorption and bone properties in growing rats through gut fermentation. *J. Agric. Food Chem.*, 59, 12, 6501, 2011.
65. Heuvel, E.G.V.D., Schaafsma, G., Muys, T., Dokkum, W.V., Nondigestible oligosaccharides do not interfere with calcium and nonheme-iron absorption in young, healthy men. *Am. J. Clin. Nutr.*, 67, 445, 1998.
66. Heuvel, E.G.V.D., Schoterman, M.H., Muijs, T., Trans galacto-oligosaccharides stimulate calcium absorption in postmenopausal women. *J. Nutr.*, 130, 2938, 2000.
67. Mendoza, J.L., Lana, R., Taxonera, C., Alba, C., Izquierdo, S., Diaz-Rubio, M., Extraintestinal manifestations in inflammatory bowel disease: Differences between Crohn's disease and ulcerative colitis. *Med. Clin. (Barc)*, 125, 8, 297, 2005.
68. Nagao-Kitamoto, H. and Kamada, N., Host-microbial cross-talk in inflammatory bowel disease. *Immune Netw.*, 17, 1, 1, 2017.
69. Brown, S.J. and Mayer, L., The immune response in inflammatory bowel disease. *Am. J. Gastroenterol.*, 102, 9, 2058, 2007.
70. Mahdavi, M., Laforest-Lapointe, I., Masse, E., Preventing colorectal cancer through prebiotics. *Microorganisms*, 9, 6, 1325, 2021.
71. Chang, P.V., Hao, L., Offermanns, S., Medzhitov, R., The microbial metabolite butyrate regulates intestinal macrophage function via histone deacetylase inhibition. *Proc. Natl. Acad. Sci. U.S.A.*, 111, 6, 2247, 2014.
72. Fernandez, J., Moreno, F.J., Olano, A., Clemente, A., Villar, C.J., Lombo, F., A galacto-oligosaccharides preparation derived from lactulose protects against colorectal cancer development in an animal model. *Front. Microbiol.*, 9, 2004, 2018.
73. Ito, M., Deguchi, Y., Miyamori, A., Matsumoto, K., Kikuchi, H., Matsumoto, K., Kobayashi, Y., Yajima, T., Kan, T., Effects of administration of galacto-oligosaccharide on the human feacal microflora, stool weight and abdominal sensation. *Microb. Ecol. Health Dis.*, 3, 285, 1990.
74. Huynh, K., Martins, R.N., Meikle, P.J., Lipidomic profiles in diabetes and dementia. *J. Alzheimers Dis.*, 59, 2, 433, 2017.

75. Hashmi, A., Naeem, N., Farooq, Z., Masood, S., Iqbal, S., Naseer, R., Effect of prebiotic galacto-oligosaccharides on serum lipid profile of hypercholesteremic. *Probiotics Antimicrob. Proteins*, 8, 1, 19, 2016.
76. Dai, Z., Feng, S., Liu, A.B., Wang, H., Zeng, X., Yang, C.S., Protective effects of α-galacto-oligosaccharides against a high-fat/western-style diet-induced metabolic abnormalities in mice. *Food Funct.*, 146, 2, 358–367, 2016.
77. Delzenne, N.M. and Kok, N.N., Biochemical basis of oligofructose induced hyperlipidemia in animal models. *J. Nutr.*, 129, 7, 1467S, 1999.
78. Newburg, D.S., Ko, J.S., Leone, S., Nanthakumar, N.N., Human milk oligosaccharides and synthetic galactosyl-oligosaccharides contain 3'-, 4-, and 6'-galactosyllactose and attenuate inflammation in human T84, NCM-460, and H4 cells and intestinal tissue *ex vivo*. *J. Nutr.*, 146, 2, 358, 2016.
79. Zenhom, M., Hyder, A., Vrese, M.D., Heller, K.J., Roeder, T., Schrezenmeir, J., Prebiotic oligosaccharides reduce proinflammatory cytokines in intestinal Caco-2 cells via activation of PPARγ and peptidoglycan recognition protein 3. *J. Nutr.*, 141, 5, 971, 2011.
80. Kivit, S.D., Tobin, M.C., Forsyth, C.B., Keshavarzian, A., Landay, A.L., Regulation of intestinal immune responses through TLR activation: Implications for pro-and prebiotics. *Front. Immunol.*, 5, 60, 2014.
81. Lindsay, J.O., Whelan, K., Stagg, A.J., Gobin, P., Al-Hassi, H.O., Rayment, N., Kamm, M.A., Knight, S.C., Forbes, A., Clinical, microbiological, and immunological effects of fructo-oligosaccharide in patients with Crohn's disease. *Gut*, 55, 3, 348, 2006.
82. Silk, D.B.A., Davis, A., Vulevic, J., Tzortzis, G., Gibson, G.R., Clinical trial: The effects of a trans-galactooligosaccharide prebiotic on faecal microbiota and symptoms in irritable bowel syndrome. *Aliment. Pharmacol. Ther.*, 29, 5, 508, 2009.
83. Koleva, P.T., Valcheva, R.S., Sun, X., Ganzle, M.G., Dieleman, L.A., Inulin and fructo-oligosaccharides have divergent effects on colitis and commensal microbiota in HLA-B27 transgenic rats. *Br. J. Nutr.*, 108, 9, 1633, 2012.
84. Kittana, H., Quintero-Villegas, M.I., Bindels, L.B., Gomes-Neto, J.C., Schmaltz, R.J., Munoz, R.R.S., Cody, L.A., Moxley, R.A., Hostetter, J., Hutkins, R.W., Ramer-Tait, A.E., Galacto-oligosaccharide supplementation provides protection against *Citrobacter rodentium*-induced colitis without limiting pathogen burden. *Microbiology*, 164, 2, 154, 2018.
85. Quintero, M., Maldonado, M., Perez-Munoz, M., Jimenez, R., Fangman, T., Rupnow, J., Wittke, A., Hutkins, R., Adherence inhibition of *Cronobacter sakazakii* to intestinal epithelial cells by prebiotic oligosaccharides. *Curr. Microbiol.*, 62, 5, 1448, 2011.
86. Cheng, W., Lu, J., Li, B., Lin, W., Zhang, Z., Wei, X., Sun, C., Chi, M., Bi, W., Yang, B., Jiang, A., Yuan, J., Effect of functional oligosaccharides and ordinary dietary fiber on intestinal microbiota diversity. *Front. Microbiol.*, 20, 1750, 2017.

87. Desjardins, M.L., Roy, D., Toupin, C., Goulet, J., Uncoupling of growth and acids production in *Bifidobacterium* ssp. *J. Dairy Sci.*, 73, 6, 1478, 1990.
88. Warchol, M., Perrin, S., Grill, J.P., Schneider, F., Characterization of a purified β-fructo-furanosidase from *Bifidobacterium infantis* ATCC 15697. *Lett. Appl. Microbiol.*, 35, 6, 462, 2002.

3

Human Mucosal Organ and Application of Probiotics

Tanuja Mohanty[†], Bhanu Pratap Gurjar[†], and Usha Nagarajan*

Department of Biochemistry, School of Interdisciplinary and Applied Sciences, Central University of Haryana, Mahendergarh, India

Abstract

In the last few decades, a lot of interest have revolved around the science of probiotics, which propelled intensive research aiming to comprehend its role in strengthening the barriers and improving the Host health. The human mucosal organ provides the first line of defense and also maintains Intestinal Homeostasis. The interaction between the mucosal barrier and Gut microbiome is crucial for Host health. Previous metagenomic studies have already revealed the significance of the microbiome in maintaining gut equilibrium. Hence, some of these beneficial microbiotas are proposed to be promising candidates for probiotics. They augmented the effectiveness of the mucosal ecosystem against the pathogenic invasion and also upregulated the mucus-related factors. The review summarizes the current perspective on the effect of probiotics on mucin, a glycoprotein, and other components of Goblet cells. The underlying core mechanism of some well-known probiotics, such as *Bifidobacterium, Lactobacillus, Streptococcus* is also elucidated. Their contribution in combating some life-threatening diseases through their action on the mucosal surface is also discussed. The review aims to gather more knowledge about the strategies utilized by the probiotics for designing more improved versions in the future. However, there is a need for more clinical trials to confirm strain-specific outcomes.

***Keywords*:** Probiotics, prebiotics, gut microbiome, mucosal organ, mucin, immune system, *bifidobacterium* and *Lactobacillus*

**Corresponding author*: usha@cuh.ac.in

[†]Authors contributed equally

Rajesh K. Kesharwani, Tingirikari Jagan Mohan Rao and Raj K. Keservani (eds.) Prebiotics and Probiotics in Disease Regulation and Management, (61–94) © 2022 Scrivener Publishing LLC

3.1 Introduction

Usually, the epithelial tissue employs two protective mechanisms against the pathogens, i.e., coating of the dead cells and lamination by mucus layer. Most of the volume of villi is coated with mucus. It is rich in antibacterial peptides by Paneth cells, located at the end of crypts [1]. Mucus layer provide the first layer of defense against gut pathogens as it inhibits bacterial translocation, hence its integrity must be maintained for fighting against some serious inflammatory diseases [2]. Mucus comprises 95% of water, including some salts, lipids, growth factors, cytokines, and proteins like defensin, providing defensive properties. Humans secrete mucus, which accounts for up to 10 L per day [3]. Mucin is a glycoprotein that makeup mucus and acts as a barrier between the intestinal lumen and epithelium. It is composed of two layers—outer and inner, each bearing a different composition of microbial cells. These glycoproteins are found in different parts of the body, such as the kidneys, bladder, respiratory tracts, and urinary tracts, and are expressed from the 20 different MUC genes. The gut microbiome mainly exploits them for attachment and nutritive reasons [4]. Mucins are categorized into two types—transmembrane and gel forming [5]. Among all the mucin genes, *MUC-2, MUC5AC* is majorly secreted by Goblet cells, whereas MUC1, MUC3, MUC4, MUC13, and/or MUC17 are secreted by the absorptive cells and are membrane-bound. Lack of *muc-2* expression or mutation in the glycosyltransferase enzyme generates a defective mucus layer which has several deleterious effects, such as the surge in the permeability for the pathogens to invade, making it more prone to inflammation and colitis. Goblet cells are not only restricted to mucin; rather, they secrete other components, such as intestinal trefoil factor (ITF), Resistin-like molecule β, and Fc-γ binding protein. Each component has its function and contributes to mucus production. ITF increases mucus viscosity and structural integrity of mucus layers, resistin-like molecule beta upregulates MUC2 expression, and Fc-γ binding protein aids in the stabilization and cross-linking of MUC2 mucin [6]. Moreover, intestinal trefoil factor 3 is observed to be coexpressed with the mucin as it also helps in wound repairing [7]. Trefoil Factors (TFFs) secreted in the mucus gels play a crucial role in cell migration and downregulating intestinal apoptosis. TFFs are of several subtypes like TFF1, TFF2, and TFF3. Of these, TFF1 and 2 are mainly produced by stomach mucosa, whereas TFF3 is by intestinal goblets whose elevated amount is correlated with the inflammatory responses [8] production of toxins in the lumen and any shift in the goblet cell function aid in the impairment of the intestinal barrier. Overexpression of muc-2 has been correlated with human cancers [9]. When there is a lack of adequate nutrients, the enteric microbiome feeds on the mucin. Mucin is composed of N-acetylgalactosamine, N-acetylglucosamine, and galactose. The breakdown of mucin provides food for other microbes to thrive [10]. Both the terminal of the mucin protein is not equally glycosylated, rather consists of cysteine residues. This residue causes the formation of interdisulfide and intradisulfide linkages in the glycan part. This provides hydrophilicity and resistance against proteolytic degradation [7]. Among all the mucins, MUC-2 remains attached until cleaved by the protease meprin β followed by detachment. The uncleaved mucin favors the growth of Bacteroidetes, whereas detached mucin propels the growth of firmicutes. Hence, it is quite evident that Mucus can be one of the factors for bringing about a shift in the intestinal microbiota. Mucus is found to be in high concentration at the distal ileum. Many commensal microbes metabolize the monosaccharides present in the outer layer of colonial mucus and extract energy for their proliferation [11]. Thus, Mucus has been the main target for both the pathogenic microbes and probiotics but for different purposes. The probiotics strengthen this layer by altering the permeability and reinforcing the tight junction as minute loss of the barrier can result in a huge imbalance in host's metabolism. They are the beneficial microorganisms that are introduced along with the food for improving the gut environment by bringing certain modulations in the commensal microbiome. Probiotics are also reported to collaborate with the host microbiome and produce by-products, such as organic acids and bacteriocins, which are potent immunomodulators. These acids reduce the pH of the lumen for inhibitory effects. Many probiotics are also reported to produce neurotransmitters such as GABA, Dopamine, Serotonin, thereby regulating the neural activities and management of Stress [12]. The current chapter describes the mode of action followed by some of the well-known probiotics. It also evaluates probiotics' application in mucus-related disorders.

3.2 Mode of Action of Probiotics on Human Mucosa

Lilly and Stillwell first established the term "probiotic" for the substance secreted by one organism to favor the growth of another. There are several representatives of bacterial genes, such as *Lactobacillus*, *Bifidobacterium*, *Bacillus* which are employed for the probiotic preparation. There are several parameters to decide the efficacy of probiotics, such as tolerance level to variable pH level, bile acid concentration, and influence on the immune response [13]. Probiotic mode of action includes a) competitive exclusion method (Competing for same binding sites and nutrients); b) lowering pH or secreting organic acids, thereby making the environment conducive for other pathogenic microbes to grow; c) obstructing quorum sensing hence indirectly controlling the thriving process [8]. Many researchers have conducted placebo studies to understand the true effects of probiotics on health. Out of numerous probiotic-related mechanisms postulated, some of them have been described in the current review and are summarized

Table 3.1 Mode of action of probiotics.

S. no.	Probiotic	Species	Mode of action	Reference
1.	*Bifidobacterium*	*B. dentium*	• Promote MUC-2 expression • Calcium stimulated mucin release • Target tight junction protein	[15]
2.	*Streptococcus*	*S. thermophilus*	• Modify Glycosylation in Mucus • Increase RELMβ, TFF3 and AGR2	[18, 19]
3.	*Lactobacillus*	*L. johnsonni*	• Release Cytokines • Aggregation of *H. pylori*	[3, 21]
		L. rhamnosus	• Revive TEER level • Increase expression of zonula occludens-2 • Increase MUC-2	[2, 8]

(Continued)

Table 3.1 Mode of action of probiotics. (*Continued*)

S. no.	Probiotic	Species	Mode of action	Reference
		L. plantarum	• Increase MUC-2 and MUC-3 • Inhibit adherence of Pathogenic *E. coli*	[8]
		L. farciminis	• Alter stress induced glycosylation	[27]
		L. acidophilus DDS1	• Increase MUC-2 • Decrease RELMβ, TFF3 and AGR2	[19]

in Table 3.1. More emphasis has been given to the action of probiotics on mucous and its related factors.

3.2.1 Bifidobacterium

In 2002, the Food and Drug Administration entitled the bacterial genus *Bifidobacterium* for GRAS (Generally Regarded As Safe) status indicating its safe use [14]. Although many species of *Bifidobacterium* which are isolated so far consists of mucin degrading enzymes, however *Bifidobacterium dentium* consists of few mucins degrading enzyme glycosyltransferase, which makes it unfit to use mucin carbon as its source of nutrition. They lack the gene which removes the terminal sialic acid from the O-linked glycosylated mucin. Rather, *B. dentium* has been proposed to treat patients suffering from ulcerative colitis as it enhances mucus production and produces beneficial products such as acetate and GABA. Acetate promotes MUC-2 expression, whereas GABA increases calcium-dependent migration of stored mucin granules from the goblet cells. Calcium stimulates autophagy which is essential for the release of mucin. The release of acetate generates a low pH environment for the organization of MUC2. Studies also suggest the increase of secretory peptides from the goblet cells in the presence of this microbe. However, no impact was seen on the Mucus associated cytokines such as IL-22, IL-33 and IL-13, indicating the role of *B. dentium* restricted to mucus layer only rather than immunostimulatory function. Experimental data also confirm the fact that the *B. dentium* colonized mice showed an increase in the MUC-2 mRNA level as well as terminal sialic acid than control suggesting the pivotal role of bacteria in enriching the mucus layer.

Further comparative studies revealed that germ-free mice or heat-killed *B. dentium* mice showed no effect on the MUC expression [15]. It has also been reported to target the tight junction-associated protein to exert its action as a probiotic. It also secretes a thick mucus layer which is continuously replaced in order to prevent the adherence of pathogens [16]. Another strain of *Bifidobacterium,* i.e., *B. bifidum* or BF-1 has also been reported to be effective in preventing catastrophic effect of *Heliobacter pylori* on mucus and its related factors. The mRNA level of both mucin, as well as sugar concentration was found to be elevated in the stomach of rats after 2 hours of oral administration of BF-1. The presence of polysaccharide in its cell wall further provided gastric protective effects. Moreover, if compared to other strains, BF-1 was observed to have more tightly adhered to the mucus layer. BF-1 thus provided an immediate-early response to the gastric injury in rats which indicated about its probiotic action [17]. Moreover, other two of the bifidobacterial species, i.e., *B. longum* and *B. breve* are also found to be quite effective in pediatric diarrhea [14].

3.2.2 Streptococcus

European Food Safety Authority (EFSA) claimed the probiotics *Streptococcus thermophilus* and *L. bulgaricus* to be the essential component found in the Yoghurt. *Streptococcus thermophilus* in the yogurt secrete certain enzymes such as bile salt hydrolase and β-galactosidase, which aids in the digestion of lactose in the host [12]. It produces lactic acid from the lactose in the milk, and this organic acid lowers the pH, which helps in the coagulation of the milk protein casein. Lactate produced favors the selective growth of lactate-consuming microbes in the gut. *Streptococcus* also produces SCFA such as Propionate and butyrate. Few literatures have also described the mucophilic potential of *Streptococcus* and have tried to evaluate its Mucus producing abilities.

Experimental studies on animal models have confirmed role of *Streptococcus* in modifying glycosylation in the Mucus. Mice treated with it showed exaggerated sulfate structures in the glycan part, which protect against inflammation in the colon region. Some experimental data suggest that *S. thermophilus* show very poor adherence to mucus layer and degrade the sugar residue of mucus to a very low extent when compared with other probiotic, like Lactobacillus. However, it does stimulate mucus-related pathways via lactate production [18]. One of its strains, i.e., *S. thermophilus UASt-09* has been reported to elevate the level of the secretory antimicrobial peptides of the goblet cells such as RELMβ, TFF3, and AGR2 [19]. These lactic acid-producing bacteria ferment milk and produce many bioactive peptides. One of them is beta-casomorphin-7 (β-CN), which affects goblet cells and regulates the mucin gene expression. *In Vitro* experiments have shown that these peptides induce MUC-2 and MUC-4 production. It was also observed in rats that oral administration of these peptides of around 0.1–100 μmol/L concentration elevated goblet cell production; however, no effect was seen on colonic mucus level. β-CN(94-123) is composed of 30 amino acids, and the presence of proline in the sequence protects it from degradation by the digestive enzyme. Moreover, the presence of L-glutamate maintains the thickness of mucus in the lumen as it stimulates the activation of afferent nerves, thereby triggering the activity of mucus cells. However, this effect of glutamate is concentration-dependent and is diminished when the peptide is present at a very low concentration. Thus, further research on such bioactive peptides would propel its synthesis and usage for improving the nutritional status [20].

3.2.3 Lactobacillus

The first step of the lactic acid bacteria to showcase its probiotic activity is its binding to the mucous layer. Few proteins like GroEL (found in *Lactobacillus johnsonni*) are involved in adherence and this attachment aids in pathogen (e.g., *H. pylori*) clearance. These proteins on the cell surface not only trigger cytokine production in macrophages and epithelial cells but also contribute to *H. Pylori* aggregation, thus reflecting upon its probiotic action. However, the binding to the host mucus was found to be pH-dependent as strong binding was seen in acidic pH, whereas no binding was seen in the neutral environment [21]. Various clinical studies have depicted the role of probiotics such as *Lactobacillus rhamnosus* in reviving the trans-epithelial electrical resistance (TEER) level and also uplifted the expression level of the tight junction protein zonula occludens-2 (ZO-2) [8]. It has been reported to regulate this layer by elevating the MUC2 gene expression. The molecular mechanism behind the action of *Lactobacillus* was analyzed by isolating and evaluating the soluble protein p40 from it. This protein was found to activate the Epidermal growth factor receptor, thereby initiating the downstream cascade, which prevented epithelial damage due to cytokine production and downregulating the disastrous effects of hydrogen-peroxide on the epithelial barrier. When P40 was delivered to the mouse's gut using hydrogen beads, it significantly reduced colon epithelial cell injury and inflammation. P40 acted as an activator for the Transcription Factors (TFs) of goblet cells, which indirectly contributed to the increased production of mucin; however, the effect was concentration dependent. Thus, the evidence proved the requirement of EGFR kinase activity for p40-mediated MUC-2 production [2]. EGFR on binding with its ligand undergoes dimerization and recruit's adapter proteins, such as phospholipase C, which further initiate the cascade of reaction and activate cellular processes, such as goblet cell proliferation and growth. The entire pathway was revealed when rat conjunctiva goblet cells were cultured and stimulated. EGF stimulates the secretion of calcium ions which enhances mucin production from the goblet cells [22]. Another soluble protein, p75 along with p40 has been reported to impair the hydrogen peroxide-induced damaging effects of tight junction and its associated proteins, which disrupts the integrity of the epithelial barrier. MAP kinase and PKC pathways are usually employed by the probiotics to lessen the reactive oxygen species production and redistribution of tight junction protein under the influence of hydrogen peroxide. However, p40 and p75 do not degrade the H2O2 rather only focus on eliminating the deleterious effects of the compound [23]. Another species of *Lactobacillus*, i.e., *Lactobacillus plantarum* regulate the synthesis of mucin by escalating *MUC-2* gene expression and secretion of MUC-3 extracellularly. Such modulation at the genetic level is very advantageous as it inhibits the adherence of enteric pathogens, such as *E. coli* [8]. *Lactobacillus plantarum KCC-10* has been reported to produce an antifungal compound 3-phenyllactic acid (PLA). This compound is most active against filamentous fungi and dermatophytes. This species is found to be functional in low pH (around 2) environment in the stomach, thereby enhancing its probiotic property [24]. PLA is involved in the progression of carcinogenesis and was even identified as marker in the patients suffering from Oral Squamous Cell Carcinoma. Conducted saliva metabolomics to characterize markers of patients afflicted with Oral squamous cell carcinoma. These compounds seem to use IKK/NF-κB signaling pathway for cell migration, which confers them to the invasion and metastasis ability, as demonstrated in the experiment with HeLa cells. They inhibit the expression of a few oncoproteins aiding in cell migration. In contrast, it escalates the expression of matrix metalloproteinases, which invade ECM for invasion [25, 26]. However, a detailed understanding of the substrate is required to understand the shift from optimum to hyperproduction of PLA. Various other strains of *Lactobacillus* are also involved in mucus alteration. Many clinical studies have illustrated the stress-induced effects which deranged the intestinal barrier integrity and even suggested the probiotic measure to lessen the induced effects. Psychological Stress exerted an influence on the O-linked glycosylation of mucin as more expanded O-glycan structures containing neutral polylactosamine chains were noticed in stressful rats. Flattened mucus and decrease in roughness were also observed in these rats, contrasting to control, which possessed structurally organized and cohesive mucus. Among the probiotics, *Lactobacillus farciminis* have been able to reverse the alteration in the O-glycosylation due to stress. Under the influence of stress, hydrophobic domains of the mucus were found to be self-condensed, leading to the formation of mucin cables of three-fold thickness. Such interaction downregulated the electrostatic interaction among the glycosylated domain, altering its profile towards the replacement by more neutral or negatively charged sugars. These physical and chemical alterations and the formation of thick cable-like structures favored the development of large pore-sized structures, leading to an increase in the permeability and translocation of bacteria. However, the entire alteration was reversible if treated with *L. farciminis*, which stopped visceral hypersensitivity and stress-induced damage to the epithelial barrier. *L. farciminis* was also observed to adhere to muc2 via cross-links with o-glycan receptors, which hypothesize its function in glycosylation pattern. Experimental analysis has also verified the production of nitric oxide by the probiotic in the intestinal lumen, that declined the phosphorylation of the myosin light chain and which in turn encouraged the production of mucin in certain cell lines [27]. Most of the species of *Lactobacillus* are probiotic in nature, however few of them like *L. acidophilus* negatively regulate level of AMPs produced by Goblet cells, such as RELMβ, TFF3, and AGR2. However, no negative effect was seen on mucin, as MUC-2 expression was found to be elevated. Hence, most of the species of the *Lactobacillus* are probiotic species. Thus, data indicate that this strain is only involved in MUC2 production but does not have a role in maintaining the quality of the epithelial barrier [19].

3.3 Application of Probiotics

International organizations like United Nations Food and Agriculture Organization (FAO), and the World Health Organization (WHO) defined the term probiotics in 2001 for the microorganism that improved the individuals' health when consumed at optimum concentration. As we know, many microorganisms occupy the human intestine, and various clinical research have appreciated their contribution in maintaining a healthy gut. Those microbes which are expected to be immensely beneficial are selected to be probiotics [28]. Many clinical studies have indicated the beneficial effects of probiotics when consumed or applied to any part of the tissue. Their valuable properties are increasing their demands of being used as therapeutic agents [29]. The current article reviews the previous studies, which explained the activity of numerous probiotics in healing mucus-related gastrointestinal and respiratory disorders, such as IBS, cystic fibrosis, Asthma, etc. (summarized in Table 3.2). It also discusses how any alteration in the mucus or mucin expression causes progression of the disease and the impact of probiotics in combating them.

3.3.1 Probiotics for Gastrointestinal Disorders

3.3.1.1 Inflammatory Bowel Syndrome

Inflammatory bowel syndrome (IBS) occurs due to disruption in the balance of immune cells associated with the gut mucosa. After analyzing the disease by conducting multiple tests, IBS was categorized into three types—Crohn's disease, ulcerative colitis (UC), and unclassified IBD [30]. Alpha-defensin is one of the AMPs released by the Paneth cells whose downregulation is associated with Crohn's disease. A peptidoglycan Microbe-associated Molecular Pattern (MAMP) receptor, NOD2, regulates the expression of a-defensins. Thus, the loss of function mutation of the receptor elevates the susceptibility to the disease. Other conditions, such as malnutrition, can also dysregulate the antimicrobial property of the Paneth cells [31]. Patients afflicted with Ulcerative Colitis have defective mucus with increased permeability. Few pathogenic bacteria take advantage and invade the inner layer of mucus, hence, contributing to the progression of the disease. An increase in the bacterial load triggers the activation of adaptive immunity, which in turn increases the inflammatory mediators, as well as elevates the expression of mucus, ultimately leading to a weariness of mucus [11]. Upon tissue examination from the colitis patients, a low amount of goblet cells was also witnessed in the epithelial lining of the colon. The inflammation of the mucosal layer in this disease is associated with MUC-2 depleted activity. This was confirmed in the MUC-2 knockout mice which resulted in a lack of goblet cells. Impairment, such as an increase in mucosal thickness, reduced differentiation in the colon was also observed [32]. It is reported that some alteration in the O-glycosylation of the mucus is evident in the inflamed human

Table 3.2 Use of probiotics in ameliorating gastrointestinal and respiratory disease.

S. no.	Disease	Abnormality in mucus	Suggested probiotics	References
1.	Ulcerative Colitis	MUC-2 Depletion, Low Goblet Cells	*L. acidophilus,* *L. rhamnosus, B. bifidum, B. lactis, L. casei CRL 431,* *L. paracasei CNCM I-1518* *L. fermentum* *Bifidobacterium quadruple viable tablet (B. infantis, L. acidophilus, E. faecalis, and Bacillus cereus)*	[1, 36] [37] [42]
2.	Colon Cancer	Disruption in the mucosal barrier (Hyperactive Notch and Wnt Signaling)	*Clostridium butyricum*	[43]

(Continued)

Table 3.2 Use of probiotics in ameliorating gastrointestinal and respiratory disease. (*Continued*)

S. no.	Disease	Abnormality in mucus	Suggested probiotics	References
3.	Gastric Ulcers	Damage to mucous barrier, Low MUC5AC Alteration in O-Glycosylation	VSL#3 (Cocktail of Probiotics) *B. bifidum BF-1, Streptococcus thermophilus YIT 2021 ST*	[50, 51]
4.	Acute Gastroenteritis	Low expression of MUC5A, Increase Necrosis and Apoptosis	*Bacillus clausii (strains O/C, T, SIN, and N/R)* *Lactobacillus casei*	[53, 56]

(*Continued*)

Table 3.2 Use of probiotics in ameliorating gastrointestinal and respiratory disease. (*Continued*)

S. no.	Disease	Abnormality in mucus	Suggested probiotics	References
5.	Asthma	Hypersecretion of MUC5AC	*Cocktail of Lactobacillus Species* *Bifidobacterium lactis Probio-M8 Powder* *Lactobacillus rhamnosus GG* *Bifidobacterium longum spp. infantis S12*	[61] [62] [67]
6.	Cerebral ischemia/ reperfusion injury	Hypersecretion of Mucus (MUC5AC)	*C. butyricum*	[68]

(*Continued*)

Table 3.2 Use of probiotics in ameliorating gastrointestinal and respiratory disease. (*Continued*)

S. no.	Disease	Abnormality in mucus	Suggested probiotics	References
7.	Cystic Fibrosis and COPD	Dehydrated Mucus Upregulated expression of MUC5AC and MUC5B	*Lactobacillus species* *(L. acidophilus, L. plantarum (ATCC 8014),* *L. rhamnosus Strains of Lactobacillus Plantarum (KCC-25, KCC-26, KCC-27, and KCC-28)* *B. breve*	[76–79]

(*Continued*)

Table 3.2 Use of probiotics in ameliorating gastrointestinal and respiratory disease. (*Continued*)

S. no.	Disease	Abnormality in mucus	Suggested probiotics	References
8.	Viral infection (mainly SARS-CoV-2)	Elevated level of MUC5AC, MUC5B, MUC-1/2/4	*Lactobacillus and Bifidobacterium*	[80, 87]

colon when compared with healthy individuals. Moreover, mice suffering from severe colitis had shorter O-glycans in MUC-2. Further analysis revealed that the reason for severe colitis is due to the lack of enzyme core 1 glycosyltransferase [33, 34]. In addition, short chain fatty acids (SCFAs), especially propionic acid from the probiotics, have been shown to possess goblet cells restoring properties. They increase the goblet cell production by upregulating the MUC-2 production. While conducting experiments on animal models to understand the efficacy of the probiotic, a propionic acid-producing *Propionibacterium freudenreichii* was noticed to improve the MUC-2 production in dextran sodium sulphate (DSS)-induced acute colitis afflicted rat models [35]. A cocktail of probiotics *Lactobacillus acidophilus, Lactobacillus rhamnosus, Bifidobacterium bifidum*, and *Bifidobacterium lactis* showed a reduction in the risk associated with recurrence of UTI Infection. *Lactobacillus* strains have demonstrated significant activity in ameliorating the diseases [1, 36]. In their experiments, the role of probiotic lactic acid bacteria (*Lactobacillus casei CRL 431* and *Lactobacillus paracasei CNCM I- 1518*) in the enhancement of the antimicrobial property have also been verified. Moreover, the probiotics revived the intestinal epithelial barrier by focusing on the upregulation of AMP and mucus-producing activity of the cell. Probiotics also lessened the inflammatory mediators by secreting an important cytokine IL-10, which maintains the homeostasis in the intestinal environment. Cytokine reduces the mucosal barrier damages associated with the release of Reactive Oxygen Species (ROS) and Nitric Oxide (NO) by macrophages. In another experiment 42-day-old mice were fed with *L. paracasei CNCM I-1518, L. casei CRL 431 (Lc 431)* and *L. fermentum.* A significant increase in the crypts of Paneth cells was observed in the case of *L. paracasei* and *L. casei,* in contrast to that of *L. fermentum.* Their results were similar to that of conventional mice as it is a part of the commensal microbiome. These probiotics also exerted their competitive exclusion activity by eliminating the pathogens *Staphylococcus aureus* and *Salmonella typhimurium* [37]. The lactic acid and hydrogen peroxide production from the *Lactobacillus* makes it a potent probiotic candidate. They also secrete bacteriocins against uropathogens like E. coli, thereby declining the virulence genes [38]. Hence, it is likely that *Lactobacillus* from the mother's vagina and breast milk can be a potent probiotic in preventing urinary diseases. *Lactobacillus salivarus,* originally isolated from the mother's milk, regulate various vaginal parameters such as an increase in TGF-β 1 and TGF-β 2 concentrations and downregulates the pH of the vagina during pregnancy. Its activity hinders the colonization of few invading microbes, such as *Candida* spp, *Streptococcus agalactiae.* This characteristic feature of *L. salivarius* can be exploited to comprehend its role in inhibiting urinary infections [39]. IBS is also associated with stress, which leads to hypersensitivity in visceral organs, changes the membrane permeability, as well as downregulate the expression of Nuclear Oligomerization Domain Receptor (NOD-like Receptos)-like receptors NLRP6. This receptor imparts various beneficial effects like reducing the mucosal damage, heightening mucus production, inhibition of inflammatory cytokine IL-18 and IL-1β. However, studies indicate the role of *Clostridium butyricum* in provoking NLRP6 expression and suppression of inflammation. Thus, this bacterium can also be considered as one of the probiotics for IBS due to its immunomodulatory feature [40, 41]. Recently, Hangzhou Grand Biologic Pharmaceutical has produced a *Bifidobacterium* quadruple viable tablet to treat patients suffering from IBS. The tablet is composed of four probiotics—*Bifidobacterium infantis, Lactobacillus acidophilus, Enterococcus faecalis, and Bacillus cereus.* Clinical studies have ensured the health benefits of these tablets. Bacillus in this group has been observed to colonize the intestine and generate an anaerobic ambiance for supporting the growth of anaerobic microbes, such as *Bifidobacterium.* The placebo study trials have demonstrated the effectiveness of tablets in lowering the severity of IBS [42].

3.3.1.2 Colon Cancer

Wingless (Wnt) and Notch pathways are quite essential for maintaining intestinal homeostasis as any dysregulation in the signaling causes disruption in the mucosal barrier. Patients suffering from colon cancer showed hyperactivated signaling as it contributed to the progression of the tumor. Probiotics *Clostridium butyricum* downregulated the beta-catenin expression in cancerous cells, which restores the functionality of the Wnt signaling [43]. The anti-tumor activity of the probiotic includes elevation of fecal short chain fatty acids (SCFA) butyrate, downregulation of bile acids and activation of few GPCR [44]. SCFA butyrate regulates histone deacetylase activity (HDAC), which further regulates the MUC-2 promoter. Hence, it is hypothesized that the butyrate affects the *MUC-2* expression [45]. The HDAC inhibition activity of butyrate hyperacetylated the histones, ultimately intervening in the activity of colon carcinoma cells. Excess of acetyl groups inactivates the genes responsible for the continuity of the cell cycle, leading to a halt in the proliferation of oncogenic cells. It is reported that the butyrate upregulates the p21 expression impairing the cell cycle. Similar epigenetic control of probiotics, especially their metabolites like SCFA, can pave the opportunity in treating a wide array of cancer in the future [46].

3.3.1.3 Gastric Ulcers

Gastric ulcers penetrate the gastric mucosa and bring about an alteration in the defense system of the host. They intervene in the integrity of the mucosal barrier and allow the growth of the pathogen. There are two reasons behind the growth of ulcers. One of them is destructive action of *Heliobacter pylori* on the mucosa, which triggers gastric secretion by somatostatin activation. Another factor is the employment of nonsteroidal anti-inflammatory (NSAID) drugs. This drug, when it comes across the acidity of the gastric juice, being a weak acid, increases the permeability of the cell, thereby making the mucosa susceptible to injury [47]. The clinical finding suggests involvement of *H. pylori* in altering the glycosylation of mucin, interfering with the integrity of mucus [48]. The pathogen interacts with the host via binding of outer membrane protein BabA with the receptors on MUC5AC. O-glycosylation of mucin is by the enzyme FUT-2, which is nonfunctional in the presence of the microbe. There is a significant reduction in α1,2-fucosylated terminal structures in the infected mucins [49]. A cocktail of eight probiotics has been recommended to treat patients with Gastric Ulcers. Combination of probiotics include four species of *Lactobacillus (acidophilus, bulgaricus, casei, plantarum)*, among the species of *Bifidobacteria*, three species (*breve, infantis, longum*) and one *Streptococcus* species collectively known as VSL#3 was administered. Although some changes could be observed in the level of MUC5AC the results were not that significant. However, the probiotic elevated the growth factors and exhibited dose-dependent healing of the mucus layer. The efficacy of probiotics in the case of gastric ulcers is low as the gastric mucosal lining is too damaged to support the growth of microorganisms [50]. *Bifidobacterium*-1 (*B. bifidum* BF-1), when administered in the mouse having gastric ulcers, it demonstrated its protective activity by increasing the *muc5ac* gene expression. Similar activity was also noticed in *Streptococcus thermophilus* YIT 2021 ST [51]. Among the SCFAs, acetate and propionate were orally administered to mice to assay their beneficial effect against gastric mucosa damage. The findings reveal antioxidant, anti-inflammatory, and anti-apoptotic effects of the acetate. It also upregulated the expression of *MUC5AC*. Hence this finding can help in the designing of probiotics in which acetate can be a prominent metabolite [52].

3.3.1.4 Acute Gastroenteritis

Acute gastroenteritis is one of the gastrointestinal disorders commonly evident in young children. This gastric disorder occurs due to rotavirus infection.

Probiotic *Bacillus clausii* (*B. clausii*) has been beneficial in ameliorating the progression of the disease. A cocktail of its strains, i.e., O/C, T, SIN, and N/R has been suggested for the treatment. The curing mechanism involves the protection of enterocytes by normalizing the trans-epithelial electrical resistance, as well as escalating the expression of *MUC5A* and tight junction proteins. Infected cells showed reduced necrosis and apoptosis when treated with *B. clausii*. Moreover, an increase in ROS due to infection was also normalized. It has been reported in previous studies that *B. clausii* O/C strain produces few bacteriocins and antimicrobial compounds, which further enhance their protective power [53]. Sialic acid residues on the mucin prevent the adherence of Rotavirus by interacting with its outer shell. The viral infection in the cell line HT-29 was prevented by a protein isolated from the milk named Lactoferrin [54]. Lactoferrin has also been reported to reduce the effect of pollen grain-induced oxidative stress in the mucosal surface, thereby restoring its integrity in animal models [55]. Many clinical studies have reported the involvement of *Lactobacillus casei* in the production of human Lactoferrin, hence making it a promising probiotic candidate. In one of the experiments, mice were infected with pathogenic microbes, such as *E. coli*, which led to abnormalities in the intestine such as drastic deprivation of mucosa and villi. However, no abnormality could be identified in the mice treated with *L. casei* before the infection [56].

3.3.2 Probiotics for Respiratory Disorders

Although we inhale several bacteria, lungs are completely kept free of microbes. The reason lies in the beating of cilia and the movement of mucus to the larynx, which help in their clearance. Presence of Submucosal Gland releases mucus (prominently MUC-5B mucin), chloride, and bicarbonate-rich fluid. These bundles are coated with two mucin proteins, mucin 5B and mucin 5AC. Both of these mucin proteins make up the mucociliary clearance system (MCC). In the case of Cystic Fibrosis and Chronic Obstructive Pulmonary Disease (COPD), MUC5AC remains abnormally high [11, 57].

3.3.2.1 Asthma

Hypersecretion of mucus and narrowing of air passage is associated with death due to Asthma. A significantly elevated amount of MUC5AC has been reported in airway narrowing. The inflammatory cytokine IL-16 causes activation of *muc5ac* gene promoter leading to downregulation of a negative regulator Forkhead box a2 (Foxa2) by the stimulation of STAT6 transcription factor. This fact is supported by the studies suggesting about the overexpression of *muc5ac* gene, i.e., excess amount of MUC5AC protein in the organism lacking *Foxa2*. Moreover, EGFR signaling pathway has also been associated with defective mucus secretion in asthmatic conditions as it also downregulated *Foxa2*. Like EGFR signaling, the pathway driven by b2-adrenoceptor has proven to upregulate MUC5AC expression as well as boosted mucin accumulation within cell and this activity was reversed using inverse agonist of b2-adrenoceptor [58]. Different glycoforms of MUC5B contribute to different stages of asthma. Clinical studies on children below age 16 were conducted, and their sputum was analyzed. A mixture of high and low charge glycoforms was found in the sputum of healthy controls, whereas variable glycoforms were seen in children with stable asthma. A high number of low glycoforms of MUC5B was found among people living with acute asthma. An increase in MUC5AC and low charge glycoforms of MUC5B leads to airway obstruction [59]. Many studies have tried to evaluate the Notch Signaling and its isoform in the progression of the disease. Among all isoforms, Notch 3 has been reported to regulate the production of MUC5AC. It is overexpressed in asthmatic patients if compared to non–asthmatics patients. Earlier findings have also confirmed the involvement of Notch signaling in the differentiation of mucus-producing goblet cells located in the airway epithelium. In contrast to Notch 3, Notch 1 was found to be downregulated in diseased individuals [60]. To combat the allergic disease, probiotic supplementation has been suggested. In one of the clinical studies, a mixed strain of *Lactobacillus* was administered to an asthmatic mouse model, and the response was assessed. Six strains of *Lactobacillus*, i.e., *L. gasseri, LK001, L. salivarius, LK002; L. johnsonii, LK003; L. paracasei, LK004; L. reuteri, LK005;* and *Bifidobacterium animals, LK011* was introduced in both low and high doses. A significant amount of depletion was observed in neutrophils and eosinophils, as well as inflammatory cytokines present in the lungs, i.e., IL-4, IL-13, and IL-17A, were also reduced. Probiotic action included the increase in the differentiation of Treg cells which downregulated the allergic inflammation. The action of probiotic strains expanded to the beneficial intestinal microbiota as the cocktail of strains led to an increased bacteroidetes/firmicutes (B/F) ratio, thereby restoring the homeostasis [61]. Currently, various human trials are carried out to examine the efficacy of adjuvant probiotic theory on asthmatic patients. One of the trials was conducted using *Bifidobacterium lactis* Probio-M8 powder and Symbicort Turbuhaler against placebo. The administration of probiotic cause decrease in the nitric oxide in the alveolar region [62]. Nitric oxide is produced by the enzyme nitric-oxide synthase (NOS). The two isoforms—constitutive and inducible of the enzyme are found in the airways. Constitutive NOS possesses a protective function, whereas the inducible NOS contributes to inflammation [63]. Drastic pulmonary inflammation and infection are a few symptoms associated with the disease. In extreme cases, it causes death due to respiratory failure. Colonization of *Pseudomonas aeruginosa* is observed, which contributes to inflammation and infection [64]. Biofilms of this pathogen are highly distributed in the mucus layer, limiting the permeability of beneficial bacteria and antibiotics [65, 66]. It is hypothesized that mucin fermentation led to the release of SCFAs, which aid in the propagation of colonizers such as *P. aeruginosa*. These colonizers have been reported to escalate the level of IL-8 and human beta-defensin 2 (hBD-2) in the intestinal epithelial cells indicating about importance of Gut-Lung axis. *Lactobacillus rhamnosus* GG and *Bifidobacterium longum spp. infantis* S12 have been reported to be find a use as a probiotic against the infection by *P. aeruginosa*. Upon the analysis of the transcripts, the probiotic-treated cells showed an increase in human beta-defensin-2 (hBD-2) mRNA, whereas a low level of IL-8 was reported indicating its suppressive activity [67]. Also, administration of *Lactobacillus reuteri* (LR) ATCC55730 with the diet resulted in lowering of upper respiratory tract infection [64].

3.3.2.2 Cerebral Ischemia/Reperfusion Injury

Few neurological disorders are observed to be associated with pulmonary exacerbation. One of them is Cerebral Ischemia which, when induced, showed high expression of *MUC5AC* in the pulmonary regions. This increase was directly proportional to the severity of dysfunction in neurons. Hypersecretion of Mucus led to upregulation of sputum production, as explained in this neurological disorder. Cytokine IL-13 and NF-κB signaling pathway which is believed to control the mucus production, is found to be highly upregulated hence causing narrowing of the airway passage [68, 69]. Sun *et al.* have tried to explain the probiotic action of *C. butyricum* in the injury due to ischemia stroke. The microbe has shown to downregulate apoptotic factors such as caspase-3, which restored the histopathological alterations. The neuroprotective activity was also seen with the rise of butyrate, a metabolite from *C. butyricum* [68]. Few recent studies have demonstrated the function of sodium butyrate, a SCFA in ameliorating apoptosis in the neurons. This was the result of increased expression of G-coupled protein receptor—GPR41 and GP43 [70]. However, an excess amount of butyrate displayed adverse effects on neurons such as obstruction of metabolism (TCA cycle, glycolysis, pentose phosphate pathway) in the mitochondria of the hypothalamic region [71]. It is reported that hyperglycemic conditions in Diabetes help in the progression of the disease. To combat this condition, *C. butyricum* was supplemented, which not only lowered the glucose concentration in the blood but also activated PI3K/Akt pathway, a neuronal regulatory pathway [72].

3.3.2.3 Cystic Fibrosis and Chronic Obstructive Pulmonary Disease (COPD)

A thin covering of mucus protects the respiratory tract by trapping the harmful microorganisms, which are later removed by the mucociliary clearance system. However, an increase in the mucus thickness causes resistance to the airflow. This provides an opportunity for the growth of entrapped microbes leading to inflammation. This condition causes the emergence of diseases, such as cystic fibrosis and chronic obstructive pulmonary disease. Many studies have mentioned the role of proper hydration, finely tuned CFTR, and chloride channels as crucial component for maintaining a healthy mucus layer, as any mutation in the regulator or channel causes the development of disease. In diseased conditions, mucus is found to be hyper dehydrated because of upregulated expression of *MUC5AC* and *MUC5B*. This causes an increase in the osmotic pressure, which exceeds the osmotic pressure of MUC-1 and MUC-4 generated in the periciliary region. As a result, the cilia are compressed, leading to a slowdown of the activity of mucociliary clearance system. The plugged mucus in the airways is rich in the pathogens like *Pseudomonas aeruginosa* and *Haemophilus influenzae* [73]. The progression of both diseases is linked to the abnormalities in both airway and alveolar epithelium. Defective bicarbonate secretion by CFTR causes modulation in the pH posing deleterious effects on mucus [74]. MUC5AC activity is elevated in the diseased state, whereas MUC5B is active in maintaining the MCC functionality. Many studies have stated the role of various proteases in upregulating the expression of MUC5AC through a different mechanism. The main aim of proteases is to cause degranulation of goblet cells inducing mucus secretion. One of the serine proteases, neutrophil elastase (from neutrophils), is observed to increase MUC5AC mRNA in COPD. Proteases from the fungus *Aspergillus fumigatus* are notably found in the lungs of cystic fibrosis patients, which can also be targeted by probiotics. Viscoelastic properties of mucus are highly disrupted in the diseased condition. Normal subjects account for up to 3% solid in their mucus however, 15% solid is observed in patients. It is reported that proteases from pathogenic *P. aeruginosa* possess the ability to degrade the mucin (MUC5AC) which tends to harm the integrity of the barrier. Moreover, the protease of pathogenic fungus uses the mucin degrading strategy for deriving nutrition and energy. Hence, designing the probiotics having a strong ability to inhibit the protease or completely remove the pathogen will be beneficial in improving the condition of COPD [75]. *Lactobacillus* species *(L. acidophilus, Lactobacillus plantarum* (ATCC 8014), *and L.* rhamnosus*)* employed in the clinical studies have demonstrated their antimicrobial effect against *P. aeruginosa* by the releases of bacteriocin [76, 77]. Many strains of *Lactobacillus Plantarum* (KCC-25, KCC-26, KCC-27, and KCC-28) isolated from the animal manure are found to be effective against the fungus, mainly *Aspergillus fumigatus.* These strains are observed to tolerate different parameters such as pH, bile acids, etc., which indicate about their probiotic property [78]. Moreover, many clinical studies have suggested the use of *B. breve* and *L. rhmanosus* as a probiotic treatment for COPD patients [79].

3.3.2.4 Viral Infection (Mainly SARS-CoV-2)

Previous studies have already shown the influence of viral infection on the expression of different mucin proteins, especially MUC5AC, MUC5B, MUC1, MUC2, and MUC4, however there is difference in their level of expression. Many researchers have demonstrated the involvement of JAK, NF-κB and MAPK signaling pathway behind the overstimulation of mucin [80]. The basic mechanism against the viral attack involves activation of cytokines like IFN-β and IFN-γ, which further stimulate the aryl-hydrogen receptor, thereby inducing the expression of MUC-5AC. The mucus traps the invading viruses, and cilia aid in the transport of mucus, ultimately eliminating the pathogen. However, in the case of SARS-CoV-2. it is reported that these cytokines are overly elevated leading to excess secretion of mucus, which eventually generates hypoxia [81]. Findings have reported the presence of mucus plug and dysfunction of macrophages in alveolar cells to be a marked feature in most of the COVID-19–related abnormalities [82]. Some reports have mentioned about the hyperactive state of tracheal goblet cells in acute COVID-19 patients leading to the formation of mucus plugs in the respiratory tract [83]. Almost 33% of COVID-19 autopsies showed swelling of the mucus membrane in the trachea and bronchi. This results in respiratory failure due to blockage in the air passage. Many clinical studies have verified the variation in the Gut microbiota in COVID-19 patients, depicting the role of the gut microbiome in the progression of the disease. Some of the pathogenic bacteria such as *Coprobacillus, Clostridium ramosum*, and *Clostridium hathewayi* were observed to be highly populated. In contrast, there was a low abundance of *Lactobacillus, Bifidobacterium, Streptococcus,*

Clostridium in the fecal matter of patients [84]. Therefore, scientists believe that usage of probiotics can bring an early end to COVID-19 infection as many of them have proven to be effective against viral infection. For example, *L. rhamnosus* administered to H1N1 afflicted mice exhibited higher survivability. Whereas *Bifidobacterium longum* BB536 exhibited anti-viral activity against H1N1 flu soaring up the level of IFNγ and IL-6. Several studies claim the immunomodulatory effects of probiotic administration, which help in the reduction of influenza-like symptoms [85, 86]. Owing to such experimental results, many researchers suggest the use of probiotics, especially *Lactobacillus and Bifidobacterial,* as well as their metabolites as a remedy for COVID-19 infection [87].

3.3.3 Application of Probiotics on Ageing-Related Mucus Impairment

The mucus layer was found damaged in aged mice. The most dominant mucin-MUC-2 was also lessened. MUC-1 was found to be downregulated in old male mice if compared to that of younger ones. Whereas elevated levels of MUC-6 were notable in old female mice. Several genes associated with the regulation of Goblet cells and mucous production were suppressed. Age-related intervention in mucous production causes a disturbance in the intestinal microbiota as it paves way for the increased growth of pathogens [88]. One of the studies on the aged animal model showed absence or highly diminished colon mucus in 19-month-old mice if compared to 10-week-old. Another experiment verified the loss of up to 5-μm-thick mucus in 38 weeks old rats. Depleted mucus increases the susceptibility to colitis. Especially the loss of mucin, *MUC-2* led to the development of diseases [89]. Ageing-induced mucosal barrier impairment was not only restricted to the intestinal mucus layer. Rather its effect was also evident on the mucus layer covering the respiratory tract. Reduced mucin *MUC5b* and impaired mucociliary clearance system were perceived in the older mice. Hence, it indicates that aged organisms are prone to respiratory tract infections also [90]. Moreover, many researchers in their study on humans above 60 years, confirmed the depletion of glycosylation and sialylation in salivary mucin (*MUC-7*) in the older adults stating it as one of the reasons behind the taste loss [91]. To understand the role of probiotics on ageing, one of the clinical studies of probiotics (*Lactobacillus plantarum* WCFS1, *Lactobacillus casei* BL23, or *Bifidobacterium breve*) was administered to aged mice. *L. plantarum* showed positive results and reduced the depletion of colonic Mucus.

In contrast, *B. breve* and *L. casei* deteriorated the condition 6 [92]. Another research reveals the increase of mucin (*MUC-2*) production in duodenum, ileum, and colon when *Lactobacillus paracasei D3-5* was administered to elderly obese mice. High Goblet cell mass was also noticed. MUC-2 production was also stimulated when the mice were fed with a microbe derived acidic substance, named lipoteichoic acid [93].

3.4 Conclusion

Nowadays, other than just limiting the focus to nutritional status, researchers have started to acknowledge the impact of probiotics from various aspects. For the last few years, intensive research has been carried out to evaluate its health benefits. As a consequence, huge omics data at multiple levels are created, which require necessary homogenization. Integrating this information would be very helpful and perhaps can lead to the increased commercialization of probiotics in the health sector. Hence, future studies demand the attention on in-depth analysis of these data to characterize the underlying mechanism behind the probiotic action. In this review, we have tried to highlight the efficacy of probiotic supplements on the mucosal barrier to strengthen the host defense system against pathogenic agents. The safety of the mucosal layer is foremost as their damage increases susceptibility to life-threatening diseases. The study throws light on the effect of probiotic supplementation on mucin expression, which is one of the primary factors responsible for the mucosal protective properties. However, advanced technologies must ensure that the probiotics are free of any associated pathogenic factors. Exploring the benefit-risk ratio of each of the strains would also be advantageous. Widening our knowledge about Gut microbiome would further enhance in designing nonvirulent and effective probiotics. Isolating the most appropriate strains of microbe would be an important step for deciding its therapeutic application. Additional investigation on the metabolites and their epigenetic role would help in comprehending the probiotic properties. Moreover, there is a need for awareness about the protocol to gain the optimum expertise for excellent outcomes.

Acknowledgment

This work is supported by Science and Engineering Research Board (SERB), Department of Science and Technology (DST), Government of India for the research grants (YSS/2014/000896 and CRG/2018/003725) to UN.

References

1. Monteros, M., Galdeano, C.M., Balcells, M.F., Weill, R., De Paula, J.A., Perdigón, G., Cazorla, S. I., Probiotic lactobacilli as a promising strategy to ameliorate disorders associated with intestinal inflammation induced by a non-steroidal anti-inflammatory drug. *Sci. Rep.*, 11, 1, 1–15, 2021.
2. Wang, L., Cao, H., Liu, L., Wang, B., Walker, W. A., Acra, S. A., Yan, F., Activation of epidermal growth factor receptor mediates mucin production stimulated by p40, a Lactobacillus rhamnosus GG-derived protein. *J. Biol. Chem.*, 289, 29, 20234–20244, 2014.
3. Derrien, M., van Passel, M.W.J., van de Bovenkamp, J.H.B., Schipper, R., de Vos, W., Dekker, J., Mucin-bacterial interactions in the human oral cavity and digestive tract. *Gut Microbes*, 1, 4, 254–268, 2010.
4. González-Morelo, K.J., Vega-Sagardía, M., Garrido, D., Molecular insights into O-linked glycan utilization by gut microbes. *Front. Microbiol.*, 11, 591568, 2020.
5. Johansson, M.E.V., Sjövall, H., Hansson, G.C., The gastrointestinal mucus system in health and disease. *Nat. Rev. Gastroenterol. Hepatol.*, 10, 6, 352–361, 201.
6. Kim, Y.S. and Ho, S.B., Intestinal goblet cells and mucins in health and disease: recent insights and progress. *Curr. Gastroenterol. Rep.*, 12, 5, 319–330, 2010.
7. Ohland, C.L. and Macnaughton, W.K., Probiotic bacteria and intestinal epithelial barrier function. *Am. J. Physiol. Gastrointest. Liver Physiol.*, 298, 6, G807–19, Jun. 2010.
8. Wan, L.Y.M., Chen, Z.J., Shah, N.P., El-Nezami, H., Modulation of intestinal epithelial defense responses by probiotic bacteria. *Crit. Rev. Food Sci. Nutr.*, 56, 16, 2628–2641, 2016.
9. Howarth, G.S. and Wang, H., Role of endogenous microbiota, probiotics and their biological products in human health. *Nutrients*, 5, 1, 58–81, 2013.
10. Milani, C., Duranti, S., Bottacini, F., Casey, E., Turroni, F., Mahony, J., Belzer, C., Delgado Palacio, S., Arboleya Montes, S., Mancabelli, L., Lugli, G. A., Rodriguez, J. M., Bode, L., de Vos, W., Gueimonde, M., Margolles, A., van Sinderen, D., & Ventura, M.,The first microbial colonizers of the human gut: composition, activities, and health implications of the infant gut microbiota. *Microbiol. Mol. Biol. Rev.*, 81, 4, e00036–17, 2017.
11. Hansson, G.C., Mucus and mucins in diseases of the intestinal and respiratory tracts. *J. Intern. Med.*, 285, 5, 479–490, 2019.
12. Ashaolu, T.J. and Fernández-Tomé, S., Gut mucosal and adipose tissues as health targets of the immunomodulatory mechanisms of probiotics. *Trends Food Sci. Technol.*, 112, 764–779, 2021.

13. Gupta, V. and Garg, R., Probiotics. *Indian J. Med. Microbiol.*, 27, 3, 202–209, 2009.
14. Di Gioia, D., Aloisio, I., Mazzola, G., Biavati, B., Bifidobacteria: their impact on gut microbiota composition and their applications as probiotics in infants. *Appl. Microbiol. Biotechnol.*, 98, 2, 563–577, 2014.
15. Engevik, M.A., Luk, B., Chang-Graham, A.L., Hall, A., Herrmann, B., Ruan, W., Endres, B.T., Shi, Z., Garey, K.W., Hyser, J.M., Versalovic, J., Bifidobacterium dentium fortifies the intestinal mucus layer via autophagy and calcium signaling pathways. *MBio*, 10, 3, e01087-19, 2019.
16. Sarkar, A. and Mandal, S., Bifidobacteria—Insight into clinical outcomes and mechanisms of its probiotic action. *Microbiol. Res.*, 192, 159–171, 2016.
17. Gomi, A., Harima-Mizusawa, N., Shibahara-Sone, H., Kano, M., Miyazaki, K., Ishikawa, F., Effect of Bifidobacterium bifidum BF-1 on gastric protection and mucin production in an acute gastric injury rat model. *J. Dairy Sci.*, 96, 2, 832–837, 2013.
18. Fernandez, N., Wrzosek, L., Radziwill-Bienkowska, J.M., Ringot-Destrez, B., Duviau, M.P., Noordine, M.L., Laroute, V., Robert, V., Cherbuy, C., Daveran-Mingot, M.L., Cocaign-Bousquet, M., Léonard, R., Robbe-Masselot, C., Rul, F., Ogier-Denis, E., Thomas, M., Mercier-Bonin, M., Characterization of mucus-related properties of streptococcus thermophilus: From adhesion to induction. *Front. Physiol.*, 9, 980, 2018.
19. Shastri, M.D., Chong, W.C., Vemuri, R., Martoni, C.J., Adhikari, S., Bhullar, H., Kunde, D., Tristram, S.G., Eri, R.D., Streptococcus thermophilus UASt-09 upregulates goblet cell activity in colonic epithelial cells to a greater degree than other probiotic strains. *Microorganisms*, 8, 11, 1758, 2020.
20. Plaisancié, P., Claustre, J., Estienne, M., Henry, G., Boutrou, R., Paquet, A., Léonil, J., A novel bioactive peptide from yoghurts modulates expression of the gel-forming MUC2 mucin as well as population of goblet cells and Paneth cells along the small intestine. *J. Nutr. Biochem.*, 24, 1, 213–221, 2013.
21. Bergonzelli, G.E., Granato, D., Pridmore, R.D., Marvin-Guy, L.F., Donnicola, D., Corthésy-Theulaz, I.E., GroEL of Lactobacillus johnsonii La1 (NCC 533) is cell surface associated: Potential role in interactions with the host and the gastric pathogen Helicobacter pylori. *Infect. Immun.*, 74, 1, 425–434, 2006.
22. Hodges, R.R., Bair, J.A., Carozza, R.B., Li, D., Shatos, M.A., Dartt, D.A., Signaling pathways used by EGF to stimulate conjunctival goblet cell secretion. *Exp. Eye Res.*, 103, 99–113, 2012.
23. Seth, A., Yan, F., Polk, D.B., Rao, R.K., Probiotics ameliorate the hydrogen peroxide-induced epithelial barrier disruption by a PKC-and MAP kinase-dependent mechanism. *Am. J. Physiol. Liver Physiol.*, 294, 4, G1060–G1069, 2008.
24. Valan Arasu, M., Jung, M. W., Ilavenil, S., Jane, M., Kim, D.H., Lee, K.D., Park, H.S., Hur, T.Y., Choi, G.J., Lim, Y.C., Al-Dhabi, N.A., Choi, K.C.,

Isolation and characterization of antifungal compound from Lactobacillus plantarum KCC-10 from forage silage with potential beneficial properties. *J. Appl. Microbiol.*, v115, 5, 1172–1185, Nov. 2013.
25. Li, C., Li, Y., Sui, L., Wang, J., Li, F., Phenyllactic acid promotes cell migration and invasion in cervical cancer via IKK/NF-κB-mediated MMP-9 activation. *Cancer Cell Int.*, 19, 241, 2019.
26. Ohshima, M., Sugahara, K., Kasahara, K., Katakura, A., Metabolomic analysis of the saliva of Japanese patients with oral squamous cell carcinoma. *Oncol. Rep.*, 37, 5, 2727–2734, May 2017.
27. Da Silva, S., Robbe-Masselot, C., Ait-Belgnaoui, A., Mancuso, A., Mercade-Loubière, M., Salvador-Cartier, C., Gillet, M., Ferrier, L., Loubière, P., Dague, E., Theodorou, V., Mercier-Bonin, M., Stress disrupts intestinal mucus barrier in rats via mucin O-glycosylation shift: Prevention by a probiotic treatment. *Am. J. Physiol. Liver Physiol.*, 307, 4, G420–G429, 2014.
28. Shi, L.H., Balakrishnan, K., Thiagarajah, K., Ismail, N.I.M., Yin, O.S., Beneficial properties of probiotics. *Trop. Life Sci. Res.*, 27, 2, 73, 2016.
29. Dhillon, P. and Singh, K., Therapeutic applications of probiotics in ulcerative colitis: An updated review. *PharmaNutrition*, 13, 100194, 2020.
30. Nemati, S. and Teimourian, S., An overview of inflammatory bowel disease: General consideration and genetic screening approach in diagnosis of early onset subsets. *Middle East J. Dig. Dis.*, 9, 2, 69, 2017.
31. Mergaert, P., Role of antimicrobial peptides in controlling symbiotic bacterial populations. *Nat. Prod. Rep.*, 35, 4, 336–356, 2018.
32. Van der Sluis, M., De Koning, B.A., De Bruijn, A.C., Velcich, A., Meijerink, J.P., Van Goudoever, J.B., Büller, H.A., Dekker, J., Van Seuningen, I., Renes, I.B., Einerhand, A. W., Muc2-deficient mice spontaneously develop colitis, indicating that MUC2 is critical for colonic protection. *Gastroenterology*, 131, 1, 117–129, 2006.
33. Paone, P. and Cani, P.D., Mucus barrier, mucins and gut microbiota: The expected slimy partners? *Gut*, 69, 12, 2232–2243, 2020.
34. Bergstrom, K., Fu, J., Johansson, M.E., Liu, X., Gao, N., Wu, Q., Song, J., McDaniel, J.M., McGee, S., Chen, W., Braun, J., Hansson, G.C., Xia, L., Core 1- and 3-derived O-glycans collectively maintain the colonic mucus barrier and protect against spontaneous colitis in mice. *Mucosal Immunol.*, 10, 1, 91–103, 2017.
35. Ma, S., Yeom, J., Lim, Y.-H., Dairy Propionibacterium freudenreichii ameliorates acute colitis by stimulating MUC2 expression in intestinal goblet cell in a DSS-induced colitis rat model. *Sci. Rep.*, 10, 1, 1–13, 2020.
36. Sadeghi-Bojd, S., Naghshizadian, R., Mazaheri, M., Ghane Sharbaf, F., Assadi, F., Efficacy of probiotic prophylaxis after the first febrile urinary tract infection in children with normal urinary tracts. *J. Pediatr. Infect. Dis. Soc.*, 9, 3, 305–310, 2020.

37. Cazorla, S.I., Maldonado-Galdeano, C., Weill, R., De Paula, J., Perdigón, G.D.V., Oral administration of probiotics increases paneth cells and intestinal antimicrobial activity. *Front. Microbiol.*, 9, 736, Apr. 2018.
38. Loubet, P., Ranfaing, J., Dinh, A., Dunyach-Remy, C., Bernard, L., Bruyère, F., Lavigne, J. P., & Sotto, A., Alternative therapeutic options to antibiotics for the treatment of urinary tract infections. *Front. Microbiol.*, 11, 1509, 2020.
39. Fernández, L., Castro, I., Arroyo, R., Alba, C., Beltrán, D., Rodríguez, J.M., Application of Ligilactobacillus salivarius CECT5713 to achieve term pregnancies in women with repetitive abortion or infertility of unknown origin by microbiological and immunological modulation of the vaginal ecosystem. *Nutrients*, 13, 1, 162, 2021.
40. Zhao, K., Yu, L., Wang, X., He, Y., Lu, B., Clostridium butyricum regulates visceral hypersensitivity of irritable bowel syndrome by inhibiting colonic mucous low grade inflammation through its action on NLRP6. *Acta Biochim. Biophys. Sin. (Shanghai)*, 50, 2, 216–223, 2018.
41. Sun, Y., Zhang, M., Chen, C. C., Gillilland, M., 3rd, Sun, X., El-Zaatari, M., Huffnagle, G.B., Young, V.B., Zhang, J., Hong, S.C., Chang, Y.M., Gumucio, D.L., Owyang, C., Kao, J.Y., Stress-induced corticotropin-releasing hormone-mediated NLRP6 inflammasome inhibition and transmissible enteritis in mice. *Gastroenterology*, 144, 7, 1478–1487.e14878, 2013.
42. Bai, T., Zeng, H., Long, Y., Li, X., Sun, X., Lan, Y., Gao, L., Zhang, L., Feng, Z., Hou, X., The efficacy of Bifidobacterium quadruple viable tablet in the treatment of diarrhea predominant irritable bowel syndrome: Protocol for a randomized, double-blind, placebo-controlled, multicenter trial. *Trials*, 21, 1, 1–13, 2020.
43. Pu, Z., Yang, F., Wang, L., Diao, Y., Chen, D., Advancements of compounds targeting Wnt and Notch signalling pathways in the treatment of inflammatory bowel disease and colon cancer. *J. Drug Targeting*, 29, 5, 507–519, 2021.
44. Chen, D., Jin, D., Huang, S., Wu, J., Xu, M., Liu, T., Dong, W., Liu, X., Wang, S., Zhong, W., Liu, Y., Jiang, R., Piao, M., Wang, B., Cao, H., Clostridium butyricum, a butyrate-producing probiotic, inhibits intestinal tumor development through modulating Wnt signaling and gut microbiota. *Cancer Lett.*, 469, 456–467, 2020.
45. Burger-van Paassen, N., Vincent, A., Puiman, P. J., van der Sluis, M., Bouma, J., Boehm, G., van Goudoever, J.B., van Seuningen, I., & Renes, I. B., The regulation of intestinal mucin MUC2 expression by short-chain fatty acids: Implications for epithelial protection. *Biochem. J.*, 420, 2, 211–219, 2009.
46. Kumar, M. *et al.*, Epigenetics, probiotic metabolites and colon cancer prevention: An overview of progress, opportunities and challenges. *Med. Epigenet.*, 1, 1, 60–69, 2013.
47. Woolf, A. and Rose, R., *Gastric Ulcer*, Treasure Island (FL), USA, 2021.

48. Ota, H., Nakayama, J., Momose, M., Hayama, M., Akamatsu, T., Katsuyama, T., Graham, D.Y., Genta, R.M., Helicobacter pylori infection produces reversible glycosylation changes to gastric mucins. *Virchows Arch.*, 433, 5, 419–426, 1998.
49. Magalhães, A., Rossez, Y., Robbe-Masselot, C., Maes, E., Gomes, J., Shevtsova, A., Bugaytsova, J., Borén, T., Reis, C.A., Muc5ac gastric mucin glycosylation is shaped by FUT2 activity and functionally impacts Helicobacter pylori binding. *Sci. Rep.*, 6, 1, 1–13, 2016.
50. Dharmani, P., De Simone, C., Chadee, K., The probiotic mixture VSL# 3 accelerates gastric ulcer healing by stimulating vascular endothelial growth factor. *PLoS One*, 8, 3, e58671, 2013.
51. Russo, F., Linsalata, M., Orlando, A., Probiotics against neoplastic transformation of gastric mucosa: Effects on cell proliferation and polyamine metabolism. *World J. Gastroenterol. WJG*, 20, 37, 13258, 2014.
52. Liu, J., Wang, J., Shi, Y., Su, W., Chen, J., Zhang, Z., Wang, G., Wang, F., Short chain fatty acid acetate protects against ethanol-induced acute gastric mucosal lesion in mice. *Biol. Pharm. Bull.*, 40, 9, 1439–1446, 2017.
53. Paparo, L., Tripodi, L., Bruno, C., Pisapia, L., Damiano, C., Pastore, L., Berni Canani, R., Protective action of Bacillus clausii probiotic strains in an *in vitro* model of Rotavirus infection. *Sci. Rep.*, 10, 1, 1–10, 2020.
54. Superti, F., Ammendolia, M.G., Valenti, P., Seganti, L., Antirotaviral activity of milk proteins: lactoferrin prevents rotavirus infection in the enterocyte-like cell line HT-29. *Med. Microbiol. Immunol.*, 186, 2, 83–91, 1997.
55. Kruzel, M.L., Bacsi, A., Choudhury, B., Sur, S., Boldogh, I., Lactoferrin decreases pollen antigen-induced allergic airway inflammation in a murine model of asthma. *Immunology*, 119, 2, 159–166, 2006.
56. Chen, H.L., Lai, Y.W., Chen, C.S., Chu, T.W., Lin, W., Yen, C.C., Lin, M.F., Tu, M.Y., Chen, C.M., Probiotic Lactobacillus casei expressing human lactoferrin elevates antibacterial activity in the gastrointestinal tract. *Biometals*, 23, 3, 543–554, 2010.
57. Ermund, A., Meiss, L.N., Rodriguez-Pineiro, A.M., Bähr, A., Nilsson, H.E., Trillo-Muyo, S., Ridley, C., Thornton, D.J., Wine, J.J., Hebert, H., Klymiuk, N., Hansson, G.C., The normal trachea is cleaned by MUC5B mucin bundles from the submucosal glands coated with the MUC5AC mucin. *Biochem. Biophys. Res. Commun.*, 492, 3, 331–337, 2017.
58. Welsh, K.G., Rousseau, K., Fisher, G., Bonser, L. R., Bradding, P., Brightling, C.E., Thornton, D.J., & Gaillard, E.A., Tuvim, M.J., Dickey, B.F., Mucus hypersecretion in asthma: causes and effects. *Curr. Opin. Pulm. Med.*, 15, 1, 4, 2009.
59. Welsh, K.G., Rousseau, K., Fisher, G., Bonser, L.R., Bradding, P., Brightling, C.E., Thornton, D.J., Gaillard, E.A., MUC5AC and a glycosylated variant of

MUC5B alter mucin composition in children with acute asthma. *Chest*, 152, 4, 771–779, 2017.
60. Reid, A.T., Nichol, K.S., Chander Veerati, P., Moheimani, F., Kicic, A., Stick, S.M., Bartlett, N.W., Grainge, C.L., Wark, P., Hansbro, P.M., Knight, D.A., Blocking Notch3 signaling abolishes MUC5AC production in airway epithelial cells from individuals with asthma. *Am. J. Respir. Cell Mol. Biol.*, 62, 4, 513–523, Apr. 2020.
61. Zhang, J., Ma, J., Li, Q., Su, H., Sun, X., Exploration of the effect of mixed probiotics on microbiota of allergic asthma mice. *Cell. Immunol.*, 367, 104399, Sep. 2021.
62. Liu, A., Ma, T., Xu, N., Jin, H., Zhao, F., Kwok, L. Y., Zhang, H., Zhang, S., Sun, Z., Adjunctive Probiotics Alleviates Asthmatic Symptoms via modulating the gut microbiome and serum metabolome. *Microbiol. Spectr.*, 9, 2, e0085921, Oct. 2021.
63. Ricciardolo, F.L.M., Multiple roles of nitric oxide in the airways. *Thorax*, 58, 2, 175–182, 2003.
64. Di Nardo, G., Oliva, S., Menichella, A., Pistelli, R., De Biase, R.V., Patriarchi, F., Cucchiara, S., Stronati, L., Lactobacillus reuteri ATCC55730 in cystic fibrosis. *J. Pediatr. Gastroenterol. Nutr.*, 58, 1, 81–86, 2014.
65. Cho, D.Y., Skinner, D., Hunter, R.C., Weeks, C., Lim, D.J., Thompson, H., Walz, C.R., Zhang, S., Grayson, J.W., Swords, W.E., Rowe, S.M., Woodworth, B.A., Contribution of short chain fatty acids to the growth of Pseudomonas aeruginosa in rhinosinusitis. *Front. Cell. Infect. Microbiol.*, 10, 412, 2020.
66. Frisch, S., Boese, A., Huck, B., Horstmann, J.C., Ho, D.K., Schwarzkopf, K., Murgia, X., Loretz, B., de Souza Carvalho-Wodarz, C., Lehr, C. M., A pulmonary mucus surrogate for investigating antibiotic permeation and activity against Pseudomonas aeruginosa biofilms.*J. Antimicrob. Chemother.*, 76, 6, 1472–1479, 2021.
67. Huang, F.-C., Lu, Y.-T., Liao, Y.-H., Beneficial effect of probiotics on Pseudomonas aeruginosa–infected intestinal epithelial cells through inflammatory IL-8 and antimicrobial peptide human beta-defensin-2 modulation. *Innate Immun.*, 26, 7, 592–600, 2020.
68. Sun, J., Ling, Z., Wang, F., Chen, W., Li, H., Jin, J., Zhang, H., Pang, M., Yu, J., Liu, J., Clostridium butyricum pretreatment attenuates cerebral ischemia/reperfusion injury in mice via anti-oxidation and anti-apoptosis. *Neurosci. Lett.*, 613, 30–35, 2016.
69. Xu, B., Zhang, L., Che, Y., Song, C., Jiang, W., Fan, J., Tian, D., Cerebral ischemia/reperfusion injury induces airway mucus hypersecretion in rats and activates IL13associated inflammatory mechanisms. *Mol. Med. Rep.*, 16, 5, 7577–7584, 2017.
70. Zhou, Z., Xu, N., Matei, N., McBride, D.W., Ding, Y., Liang, H., Tang, J., Zhang, J.H., Sodium butyrate attenuated neuronal apoptosis via GPR41/

Gβγ/PI3K/Akt pathway after MCAO in rats. *J. Cereb. Blood Flow Metab.*, 41, 2, 267–281, 2021.

71. Xu, Y., Peng, S., Cao, X., Qian, S., Shen, S., Luo, J., Zhang, X., Sun, H., Shen, W.L., Jia, W., Ye, J., High doses of butyrate induce a reversible body temperature drop through transient proton leak in mitochondria of brain neurons. *Life Sci.*, 278, 119614, 2021.
72. Sun, J., Wang, F., Ling, Z., Yu, X., Chen, W., Li, H., Jin, J., Pang, M., Zhang, H., Yu, J., Liu, J., Clostridium butyricum attenuates cerebral ischemia/reperfusion injury in diabetic mice via modulation of gut microbiota. *Brain Res.*, 1642, 180–188, 2016.
73. Mall, M.A., Unplugging mucus in cystic fibrosis and chronic obstructive pulmonary disease. *Ann. Am. Thorac. Soc.*, 13, Supplement 2, S177–S185, 2016.
74. De Rose, V., Molloy, K., Gohy, S., Pilette, C., Greene, C.M., Airway epithelium dysfunction in cystic fibrosis and COPD. *Mediators Inflamm.*, 2018, 1309746, 2018
75. McKelvey, M.C., Brown, R., Ryan, S., Mall, M.A., Weldon, S., Taggart, C.C., Proteases, Mucus, and Mucosal Immunity in Chronic Lung Disease. *Int. J. Mol. Sci.*, 22, 9, 5018, 2021.
76. Al-Malkey, M.K., Ismeeal, M.C., Al-Hur, F.J.A., Mohammed, S.W., Nayyef, H.J., Antimicrobial effect of probiotic Lactobacillus spp. on Pseudomonas aeruginosa. *J. Contemp. Med. Sci.*, 3, 10, 218–223, 2017.
77. Lash, B.W., Mysliwiec, T.H., Gourama, H., Detection and partial characterization of a broad-range bacteriocin produced by Lactobacillus plantarum (ATCC 8014). *Food Microbiol.*, 22, 2–3, 199–204, 2005.
78. Ilavenil, S., Park, H. S., Vijayakumar, M., Arasu, M. V., Kim, D. H., Ravikumar, S., & Choi, K. C., Probiotic potential of Lactobacillus strains with antifungal activity isolated from animal manure. *Sci. World J.*, 2015, 802570, 2015.
79. Aimbire, F., Costa Carvalho, J., Fialho, A., Miranda, M., Albertini, R., Keller, A., Role of probiotics Bfidobacterium breve and Lactobacillus rhmanosus on lung inflammation and airway remodeling in an experimental model of chronic obstructive pulmonary disease, *The FASEB Journal.,* 33, S1, 516.4-516.4, 2019.
80. Khan, M.A., Khan, Z.A., Charles, M., Pratap, P., Naeem, A., Siddiqui, Z., Naqvi, N., Srivastava, S., Cytokine storm and mucus hypersecretion in COVID-19: Review of mechanisms. *J. Inflamm. Res.*, 14, 175, 2021.
81. Liu, Y., Lv, J., Liu, J., Li, M., Xie, J., Lv, Q., Deng, W., Zhou, N., Zhou, Y., Song, J., Wang, P., Qin, C., Tong, W.M., Huang, B., Mucus production stimulated by IFN-AhR signaling triggers hypoxia of COVID-19. *Cell Res.*, 30, 12, 1078–1087, 2020.

82. Wang, C., Xie, J., Zhao, L., Fei, X., Zhang, H., Tan, Y., Nie, X., Zhou, L., Liu, Z., Ren, Y., Yuan, L., Zhang, Y., Zhang, J., Liang, L., Chen, X., Liu, X., Wang, P., Han, X., Weng, X., Chen, Y., … Bian, X.W., Alveolar macrophage dysfunction and cytokine storm in the pathogenesis of two severe COVID-19 patients. *EBioMedicine*, 57, 102833, 2020.
83. Manckoundia, P. and Franon, E., Is persistent thick copious mucus a long-term symptom of COVID-19? *Eur. J. Case Rep. Intern. Med.*, 7, 12, 002145, 2020.
84. Zuo, T., Zhang, F., Lui, G., Yeoh, Y. K., Li, A., Zhan, H., Wan, Y., Chung, A., Cheung, C. P., Chen, N., Lai, C., Chen, Z., Tso, E., Fung, K., Chan, V., Ling, L., Joynt, G., Hui, D., Chan, F., Chan, P., … Ng, S. C., Alterations in gut microbiota of patients with COVID-19 during time of hospitalization. *Gastroenterology*, 159, 3, 944–955, 2020.
85. Gohil, K., Samson, R., Dastager, S., Dharne, M., Probiotics in the prophylaxis of COVID-19: Something is better than nothing. *3 Biotech.*, 11, 1, 1–10, 2021.
86. Olaimat, A. N., Aolymat, I., Al-Holy, M., Ayyash, M., Abu Ghoush, M., Al-Nabulsi, A. A., Osaili, T., Apostolopoulos, V., Liu, S. Q., Shah, N. P., The potential application of probiotics and prebiotics for the prevention and treatment of COVID-19. *NPJ Sci. Food*, 4, 1, 1–7, 2020.
87. Santacroce, L. *et al.*, Potential beneficial role of probiotics on the outcome of COVID-19 patients: An evolving perspective. *Diabetes Metab. Syndr. Clin. Res. Rev.*, 15, 1, 295–301, 2021.
88. Elderman, M., Sovran, B., Hugenholtz, F., Graversen, K., Huijskes, M., Houtsma, E., Belzer, C., Boekschoten, M., de Vos, P., Dekker, J., Wells, J., Faas, M., The effect of age on the intestinal mucus thickness, microbiota composition and immunity in relation to sex in mice. *PLoS One*, 12, 9, e0184274, 2017.
89. Sovran, B., Hugenholtz, F., Elderman, M., Van Beek, A. A., Graversen, K., Huijskes, M., Boekschoten, M.V., Savelkoul, H., De Vos, P., Dekker, J., Wells, J. M., Age-associated impairment of the mucus barrier function is associated with profound changes in microbiota and immunity. *Sci. Rep.*, 9, 1, 1–13, 2019.
90. Grubb, B.R., Livraghi-Butrico, A., Rogers, T.D., Yin, W., Button, B., Ostrowski, L.E., Reduced mucociliary clearance in old mice is associated with a decrease in Muc5b mucin. *Am. J. Physiol. Cell Mol. Physiol.*, 310, 9, L860–L867, 2016.
91. Pushpass, R.-A.G., Pellicciotta, N., Kelly, C., Proctor, G., Carpenter, G.H., Reduced salivary mucin binding and glycosylation in older adults influences taste in an *in vitro* cell model. *Nutrients*, 11, 10, 2280, 2019.

92. van Beek, A.A. *et al.*, Supplementation with Lactobacillus plantarum WCFS1 prevents decline of mucus barrier in colon of accelerated aging Ercc1(-/Δ7) mice. *Front. Immunol.*, 7, 408, 2016.
93. Wang, S., Ahmadi, S., Nagpal, R., Jain, S., Mishra, S.P., Kavanagh, K., Zhu, X., Wang, Z., McClain, D.A., Kritchevsky, S.B., Kitzman, D.W., Yadav, H., Lipoteichoic acid from the cell wall of a heat killed Lactobacillus paracasei D3-5 ameliorates aging-related leaky gut, inflammation and improves physical and cognitive functions: From C. elegans to mice. *Geroscience*, 42, 1, 333–352, 2020.

4

Prebiotics and Probiotics as Anticancer Therapeutics

Dixita Chettri, Ashwani Kumar Verma and Anil Kumar Verma*

Department of Microbiology, Sikkim University, Gangtok, Sikkim, India

Abstract
The use of prebiotics and probiotics as functional food has various health benefits from maintaining a healthy microbial composition of the human body to immunomodulation for fighting various diseases. They do so via influencing the gut microbiome which is directly associated with proper function of the overall human health and also the central nervous system. Their metabolic activities are directly associated with production of compounds that promote the growth and proliferation of beneficial microorganism while eliminating pathogenic organisms, thus improving the overall well-being. Their market demand and consumption as food supplement has seen a rapid increase with some of the formulations mixing them together as a synbiotic, which has a synergistic effect. These functional foods have also been shown to have potential as treatment methods for various disorders with cancer being one of the prominent illnesses. The chapter discusses the various sources, criteria for identification of prospective prebiotic and probiotic, their implications on human health and safety assessment with cancer as the theme.

***Keywords*:** Cancer, carcinogens, *Lactobacillus*, prebiotic, probiotic and symbiotic

Abbreviations

ADH	Atypical ductal hyperplasia
AOM/DSS	Azoxymethane/dextran sodium sulphate

**Corresponding author*: akverma@cus.ac.in

Rajesh K. Kesharwani, Tingirikari Jagan Mohan Rao and Raj K. Keservani (eds.) Prebiotics and Probiotics in Disease Regulation and Management, (95–132) © 2022 Scrivener Publishing LLC

AR	Androgen receptor activation
BCC	Basal cell carcinoma
CRC	Colorectal cancer
DEHP	di-(2-ethylhexyl) phthalate
DMN	Dimethyl-nitrosamine
DPN	Diphenyl-nitrosamine
FDA	Food & Drug Association
FEA	Flat epithelial atypia
FOS	Fructooligosaccharides
GABA	Gamma-Aminobutyric acid
GI	Gastrointestinal tract
GOS	Galacto-oligosaccharides
GPCRs	G protein-coupled receptors
GpS	Gp saponins
IARC	International Agency for Research on Cancer
IPMNs	Intraductal papillary mucinous neoplasms
MAP	Mitogen-associated protein kinase
MDSCs	Myeloid-derived suppressor cells
NCI	National Cancer Institute
PanINs	Pancreatic intraepithelial neoplasms
PFOA	Perfluorooctanoic acid
SASP	Senescence-associated secretory phenotype
SCC	Squamous cell carcinoma
SCFAs	Short Chain Fatty Acids
TCDD	2,3,7,8-tetrachlorodibenzo-p-dioxin
TOS	Trans-galacto-oligosaccharides
TPA	Tetradecanoylphorbol acetate (12-O-tetradecanoylphorbol-13-acetate)
WHO	World Health Organization

4.1 Introduction

Cancer is a genetic disorder caused by multiple factors, both genomic and environmental, that interact with each other and lead to abnormal cell division [1]. The National Cancer Institute (NCI) in the US defines cancer as "a disease in which some cells of the body grow uncontrollably and spread to other parts of the body." It is caused by mutations (chemical and natural) and defects in the DNA repair mechanism [2]. Uncontrolled DNA replication and cell division, lack of response to signals that control cell division, evasion of apoptosis, and invasion of other tissues (metastasis) are the characteristics of a cancer cell [3]. Cancer is one of the leading diseases with a high mortality rate (8.7 million per year) and ranked second in the number of deaths in 2015, followed by cardiovascular disease [4]. Developing countries are at higher risk. A survey found that 63% of the total cancer-related mortality was reported from these countries [5]. For the year 2020, the International Agency for Research on Cancer (IARC) reported 19.29 million new cancer cases, with breast, lung, colorectal, prostate, stomach, and liver cancers as the major cancers with high mortality rates [6]. The incidence and mortality rates are constantly increasing. A report from the World Health Organization (WHO) estimates that by 2040, approximately 37 million new cases of cancer will be added as a global burden [7].

Common treatment approaches for cancer include radiation, chemotherapy, immunotherapy, gene therapy, stem cell therapy, and surgery used in combination to increase the effectiveness of the drugs [1]. However, the prolonged use of these chemicals, drugs, and radiation can have serious side effects, such as the development of resistance to the drugs and also attack the neighboring noncancerous cells. They also affect the quality of life and are very expensive and unaffordable for the weaker sections of the society [8]. Therefore, the development of an efficient treatment method that effectively removes metastatic cells and reduces mortality has still not been achieved. Based on the understanding of the signaling pathways, the biomolecules involved, and the unique characteristics of different types of cancer, various approaches have been developed to develop drugs and cures that target the neoplastic cells [1]. Recently, scientists have focused on developing treatments with minimal or no side effects and high efficacy. One such approach is the use of probiotic cells and prebiotics. Several studies have shown that they have the potential to fight cancer, both preventively and curatively. Given their influence on the gut microbiome, which regulates the uptake of essential chemical compounds associated with cancer treatment, as well as their own release of some of these compounds and their biocompatibility, they are suitable for use as adjuvants in cancer medicine [9]. Moreover, they perform immunomodulation, affect metabolism, maintain intestinal barrier and prevent proliferation of human host cells, thereby suppressing cancer cell development [10]. The chapter provides a basic understanding of prebiotics and probiotics, their differences, properties and their role in cancer treatment.

4.2 Prebiotic vs Probiotic

Since ancient times, there have been numerous theories and studies on the role of microorganisms in human health. In this context, prebiotics and probiotics are common terminology. These are functional foods used as dietary supplements to influence the microbial composition of the gut (Figure 4.1). They have been found to have a positive influence on the gut and overall human health. However, the different usage of these terms along with synbiotics requires a clear understanding of their meaning and how they differ from each other.

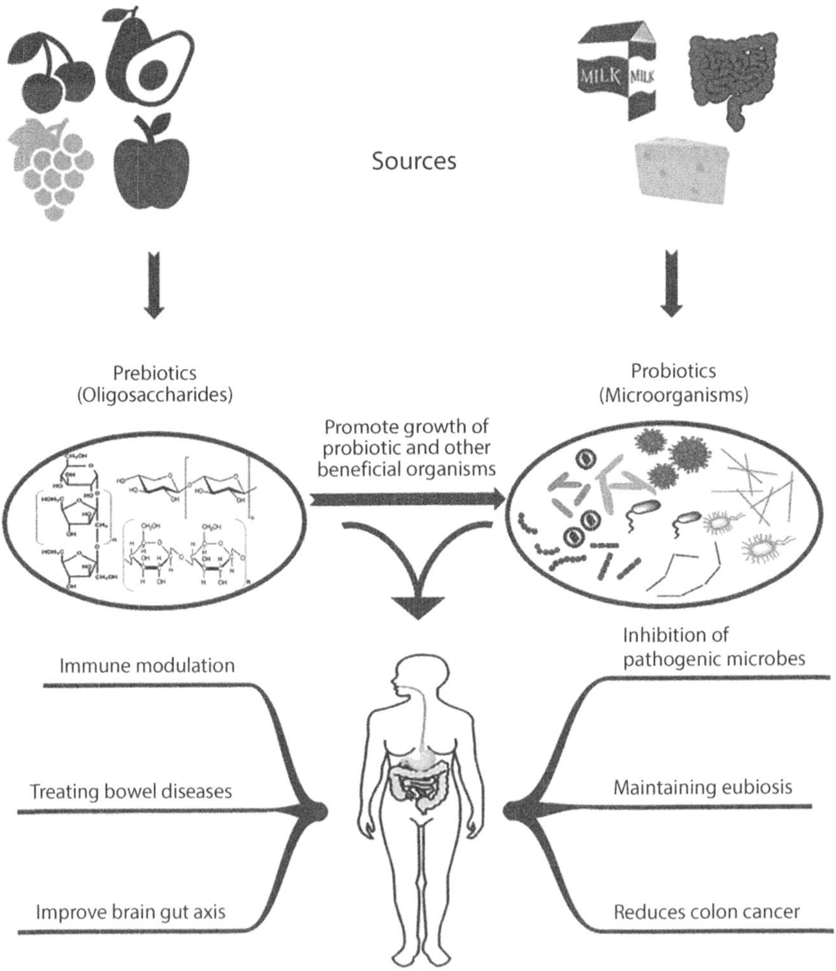

Figure 4.1 Sources, association and human health benefits of the functional food prebiotic and probiotics.

4.2.1 Definition and Difference

The term probiotic refers to nonpathogenic organisms that, when colonize a human body, have positive effects on the health of the host. The Food & Drug Association (FDA), along with the WHO, has defined probiotics as "live microorganisms that, when administered in appropriate amounts, have health benefits for the host." The commonly used probiotic organisms belong to the genera of Lactobacilli and Bifidobacteria, such as *Lactobacillus reuteri*, *Lactobacillus casei*, *Lactobacillus rhamnosus*, although other microorganisms such as *Enterococcus faecium* SF68, *Saccharomyces boulardii*, *Bacillus coagulans*, and *Escherichia coli* strain Nissle 1917 are also used as probiotics. They are used as monocultures or combined and added to various foods consumed by humans, especially fermented foods.

Prebiotics are the indigestible food components that modulate the growth of probiotic microorganisms to confer health benefits to the corresponding host body. Although there is a lack of accurate understanding of prebiotics in terms of their dosage and fermentation profiles, the commonly used prebiotics are of carbohydrate origin, such as inulin, oligosaccharides, and low molecular weight polysaccharides, although other prebiotic sources exist.

When the prebiotics and probiotics are used in combination, it is called synbiotics. The approach is designed to increase the effectiveness of the probiotic supplement by increasing the establishment, survival, and growth rate of these organisms in the gut. However, the term is limited to the formulation where the use of prebiotics selectively stimulates the survival and growth of the health-promoting probiotic organisms, making it different from the term synergism, which can support the growth of any organism regardless of its effects on human health [11]. Table 4.1 lists some of the commercially available symbiotic food supplements.

4.2.2 Criteria for Use as a Dietary Supplement

Although numerous microorganisms and dietary fibers can positively impact host health under certain conditions, there are specific criteria for an organism or dietary fiber to be considered a probiotic/prebiotic.

Probiotics: There are four major areas that have been used for decades to analyze an organism before it can be used as a probiotic strain in dietary supplements. The first criterion is to properly identify the microorganism in terms of genus, species, subspecies, and strain, and to assign a name

Table 4.1 Commercial synbiotics used as dietary supplements.

Product	Brand name	Prebiotic	Probiotic
Bactisubtil complex	Klosterfrau	Trägerstoffe Cellulose,Maltodextrin, Accharose	*Lactobacillus acidophilus* LA-5, *Bifidobacterium lactis* BB-12
Daily Probiotic + Prebiotic	Wellbeing Nutrition	Apple Pomace, and Chicory root	*Lactobacillus acidophilus, Lactobacillus casei, Lactobacillus rhamnosus, Bifidobacterium lactis, Bifidobacterium bifidum, Streptococcus thermophilus.*
Synbiotics Probiotics+Prebiotics	Exerfit	Inulin, Glucomannan, spirulina, fructooligosaccharides	*L.acidophilus, L. plantarum, L. rhamnosus, L. salivarius, L. gasseri, B. infantis, B. bifidum, S. thermophilus, L. fermentum, L. casei, L. reuteri, L. paracasei, B. lactis, B. longum, B. breve, S. boulardii*
Probiotics & Prebiotics - Lactobacillus Acidophilus & FOS Complex	Innopure	Fructoligosaccharides	*Lactobacillus acidophilus*

(*Continued*)

Table 4.1 Commercial synbiotics used as dietary supplements. (*Continued*)

Product	**Brand name**	**Prebiotic**	**Probiotic**
Digestive Enzymes Probiotic and Prebiotic	Healthmonde	Fructoligosaccharides,	*Lactobacillus acidophilus.*
ASEA VIA Biome	Probiotic and prebiotic complex	Fructooligosaccharide,Xylooligosaccharide, Galactooligosaccharide, Red elm (Ulmus rubra)	*Bifidobacterium bifidum, L. plantarum, L. bulgaricus, L. rhamnosus, B. breve, L. salivarius, L. casei, L. helveticus, B. longum, Streptococcus thermophilus, Lactococcus lactis, L. brevis, L.acidophilus, B. lactis, L. gasseri*
Enzyme Probiotic Complex Plus	American Health	Vegetable Cellulose,Maltodextrin	*L. plantarum*

(*Continued*)

Table 4.1 Commercial synbiotics used as dietary supplements. (*Continued*)

Product	**Brand name**	**Prebiotic**	**Probiotic**
Biom Probiotics 3-in-1 precision Formula	Biom Probiotics®	Oligosaccharide blend, fiber from yellow pea, pomegranate, mango, beetroot, blueberry; green-tea extract	*Lactobacillus acidophilus* UBLA 34, *L. plantarum* UBLP 40, *L. fermentum* UBLF 31, *L. bacillus rhamnosus*UBLR 58, *L.reuteri* UBLRu 87, *L. casei* UBLC 42, *L. lactis* UBLL 36, *Bifidobacterium bifidum* UBBF 55, *Bi. lactis* UBBLa 70, *Bi. longum* UBBL-64, *Bacillus coagulans* IS-2, *B. subtilis* UBBS-13, *B. clausii* UBBC-07, *Streptococcus thermophilus* UBST 50, *Saccharomyces boulardii*-Unique 28
Biopron junior	Valosun	Inulin, Fructooligosaccharide	*Bifidobacterium bifidum, Bifidobacterium infantis, Lactobacillus acidophilus*

based on International Code nomenclature. Since some of the probiotic activities are very specific to a particular strain, the organism must be identified in order to assign it to the different strains. There are several phenotypic and molecular approaches to characterize the microorganism, with whole genome sequencing considered the "gold standard." Further characterization of the microorganism's properties indicative of its probiotic potential should also be performed, such as the ability to be the source of lactic acid and other Short Chain Fatty Acids (SCFAs), the ability to adhere to epithelial cells, survive bile, digestive enzymes and acid, and thus colonize the intestine and other relevant body sites, antagonistic activity against pathogenic organisms through the production of bacteriocins, and exclusion of competition. The second criterion is to evaluate the safety of the selected strain for its intended use. Since probiotics are intended for human consumption, risk assessment is a fundamental obligation for the probiotics industry. Various organizations/nations have regulatory authority that has established a list of organisms that are considered "safe for use" based on historical and clinical evidence. Thus, once an organism is properly identified, this catalog can be used to evaluate the safety of the organism. Finally, *in vivo* safety testing must be conducted to confirm the information obtained for this historical evidence. The third step involves a human clinical trial in which a proper protocol is designed, the results are reported, and the reliability of the study results is evaluated based on the risk of bias. If possible, this is followed by a confirmatory study, which must be conducted according to scientifically accepted and government-approved regulations. The final criterion is that the probiotic strain with health-promoting effects should be able to remain alive during the shelf life of the product at an effective dosage to provide the purported health benefits of the food [12].

Prebiotics: In the case of prebiotics, there are five major criteria for their classification as prebiotics. The first criterion is that the prebiotics should be able to withstand gastric acid and should not be hydrolyzed by the mammal's digestive enzymes or absorbed in the gastrointestinal tract so that they remain available to the probiotic microorganisms in the colon. Second, the probiotic microorganisms or the intestinal microflora should be able to ferment these fibers. The third factor for the prebiotic status of a fiber is that it should be able to selectively stimulate the growth and activity of intestinal microorganisms, thus conferring a positive impact on human health via production of SCFAs, control of pH to inhibit pathogenic organisms, and enhancement of immunity. The final criterion is that the fibers must be able to withstand food processing conditions and remain intact, undegraded, and chemically unaltered in order to be utilized by gut microflora. Prebiotics should have a well-documented structure, and components used in pharmaceutical formulations, food or feed additives should be relatively easy to produce on a large scale [13].

4.2.3 Source/Method of Administration

Probiotics should be of human origin and isolated from the gastrointestinal tract of a healthy person or from naturally fermented foods, while prebiotics are obtained from fruits, vegetables, and whole grain products, such as Jerusalem artichokes, chicory roots, barley, asparagus, bananas, etc. Breast milk is also a source of prebiotics [14]. For oligosaccharide-based prebiotics, such as fructo-oligosaccharides (FOS), trans-galacto-oligosaccharides (TOS), and galacto-oligosaccharides (GOS), enzymes of microbial origin, such as fructosyl transferase, β-fructofuranosidase and β-galactosidase from various microbial strains, such as *Aspergillus oryzae*, *Bacillus macerans*, *Fusarium*sp, *Aspergillus* sp., are used for their commercial production [15]. Prebiotics and probiotics are consumed by humans as dietary supplements, where they are added individually or in combination as synbiotics. The formulation is added to various foods, such as dairy products (yoghurt, cottage cheese) and fermented pickles, but they can also be consumed from natural sources, such as rhubarb fruits and vegetables [13].

4.3 Prebiotics and Probiotics Association with Gut Microbiota and Human Health

The human body harbors a multitude of microorganisms whose number far exceeds the number of host cells (100 trillion for microbes and quadrillions for viruses). These organisms, which reside in various parts of our bodies, include bacteria, viruses, archaea, and some eukaryotes, which form a community called the microbiota, and the microbiota, along with its entire genomic content, is called the microbiome. The microbiota interacts with each other and with the human host and shapes human health and physiology [16]. The microbiota present in the human body has various roles, from absorbing nutrients to inhibiting the growth of pathogens and protecting against other environmental factors. Given their importance, the great interest in the composition of the microbiota and its role in human health is an interesting area for food and medical research, with a particular focus on the gut microbiota [17]. Diet is an important extrinsic factor affecting the gut microbiome, and functional foods such as prebiotics and probiotics interact with the gut microbiota, with probiotics increasing the microbial diversity of the gut microflora, while prebiotics are taken up by this microflora to maintain the gut and overall human health [18]. In this section, we discuss the importance of the gut microbiota and the influence of functional foods on its composition and function.

4.3.1 Role of the Gut Microbiota in Overall Human Health

The gastrointestinal tract (GI) of humans begins at the mouth and includes the digestive organs of the body such as the oesophagus, stomach, small intestine, large intestine, and appendix, finally ending at the anus. The GI tract is associated with a diverse group of organisms (~1000 species), with bacteria forming the majority and Bacteroidetes and Firmicutes being the major phyla [19]. Each part of the GI tract has a characteristic environment with a different microbial composition at each site, and the microbial load is comparatively greater in the colon than in the stomach and intestine [20]. Since the environment in the intestine is anaerobic, the microbial composition includes obligate and facultative anaerobes, such as *Bacteroides, Lactobacilli, Eubacterium, Bifidobacterium, Enterococci, Fusobacterium, Streptococci, Peptostreptococcus,* and *Atopobium,* with the obligate microbes dominating the facultative ones in a ratio of 1000:1 [19]. Some rare microbial taxa, such as *Oxalobacter formigenes,* which play an essential role in oxalate homeostasis, are also present along with the pathogenic species *Vibrio cholera, Campylobacter jejuni, Salmonella enteric,* etc. Archaea, such as *Methanomassiliicoccusluminyensis, Nitrososphaera, Methanobrevibacter smithii,* and eukaryotes, such as *Saccharomyces boulardii,* are also found in the gut [20]. These organisms form a reciprocal relationship and have co-evolved with their host, which is why they are also known as symbiotic microorganisms [21].

The composition of microorganisms in the gut is influenced by dietary habits, age, physical condition, gender, geographical conditions, etc., and any imbalance can lead to the development of diseases as the gut microflora is associated with various functions, such as immunity, metabolism, and energy. Moreover, gut microflora has been found to be associated with various diseases, such as obesity, diabetes, allergies, various mental disorders, and even cancer [19]. The most important function of the gut microflora is to aid digestion and extract energy and nutrients from ingested food, especially from dietary carbohydrates. The human digestive system lack various enzymes for digestion of polysaccharides, such as cellulose and hemicellulose, and the gut microbiota secretes various enzymes, such as glycosyltransferases, carbohydrate esterases, polysaccharide lyases, and amino acid decarboxylases with metabolic activity that help in digestion and fermentation of various indigestible carbohydrate molecules, which account for about 10% of daily energy requirements [22]. Microbial fermentation of carbohydrates, which usually occurs in the proximal colon, is an important source of short-chain fatty acids such as acetate, butyrate, and propionate, with acetate being the chief energy source for epithelial cells. In addition, acetate is used in the metabolic pathway of lipogenesis and gluconeogenesis, while butyrate and propionate are important for maintaining gut physiology and immune modulation. Fermentation also lowers pH, which, along with SCFAs, inhibits the growth of pathogenic Enterobacteriaceae organisms, such as *Salmonella* sp. and *E. coli.* In the distal colon, the microorganisms utilize other nutrients, such as proteins and amino acids, which can lead to the production of ammonia, amines, phenols, hydrogen sulphide, etc., which are harmful to the gut and can also be associated with various diseases such as cancer [23].

In addition to modulating the immune response of the gut to regulate immune homeostasis, the microbiota also provides physical protection from invading pathogens by competing for food and space. The microflora can recognize and trigger the activity of immune cells and proteins, such as dendritic cells, cytokines, and NF-κB, while the tryptophan metabolites and the SCFAs they produce induce the lymphoid system to produce innate immune cells such as IL -17, IL -22, IgA, and so on. In addition, the intestinal microflora also contributes to the differentiation of $CD8^+$ and $CD4^+$ T cells, thus activating the adaptive immune system.

An important function of the gut microflora is its antitumor and anticancer activity. While a number of pathogenic microorganisms in the gut have been found to have carcinogenic properties (*Helicobacter pylori*, *Enterococcus faecalis*, *Fusobacterium nucleatum*), other microorganisms (*Lactobacillus* and *Bifidobacterium*) inhibit carcinogenesis by stimulating the antitumor immune response. The microbes have also been shown to produce various neurochemicals and analogs of human hormones that help regulate various hormones and thus can be used to treat various hormone-related diseases, etc. Further gut microflora modulates gut-brain interaction through the production of serotonin, gamma-Aminobutyric acid (GABA), SCFAs, and catecholamines, which may influence the microbiome-gut-brain axis through various mechanisms to regulate central nervous system function and have been associated with various mental disorders. Metabolic and growth abnormalities, blood pressure regulation, and obesity are other important functions of the gut microbiota, which is regulated by the gut microbiota via the production of various metabolites, and whose dysbiosis is associated with the development of a pathological condition [19].

4.3.2 Prebiotic and Probiotic Influence on Gut Microbiome Composition

Considering the importance of the intestinal microflora and the influence of dietary intake on its species distribution, diversity and activity, the consumption of probiotics and prebiotics is becoming increasingly important. Probiotic microorganisms added to the diet are usually isolated from the GI tract of humans and have health-promoting activities. Their importance to human health has already been discussed in the previous section. When added in sufficient quantity, probiotic microorganisms provide a competitive environment for the pathogenic microorganisms while they interact commensally with the harmless or beneficial microbes in the gut. They do this by producing antimicrobial compounds, competing for nutrients, binding sites and receptors in the intestinal mucosa. They also increase the integrity of the epithelial barrier, modulate the gut immune response to microbes and during the inflammatory response, and restrict bacterial translocation, reducing GI infections. Probiotics stabilize the gut microbiome and also release various secretory factors that influence the function of immune cells and epithelial cells in the gut [24] (Figure 4.2).

However, in order for probiotics to exert all of these beneficial effects, they must be consumed in sufficient doses and be able to self-colonize and stabilize in the gut, which is greatly aided by prebiotics. Prebiotics influence the gut microbiome by selectively growing a specific group of microorganisms with beneficial activities and by reducing the number of pathogenic microorganisms in the gut. In this way, the prebiotic can help change the gut microbiota by increasing the number of beneficial microbes and eliminating potential pathogens. The beneficial microbes with saccharolytic activity use the prebiotics to produce SCFAs and lower the pH of the gut, making it unfavorable for other pathogenic microbes, such as *Bacteroides* and *Clostridium*, forcing them out of the GI tract [25].

However, the proper classification and identification of beneficial microbes and their selective stimulation by prebiotics is a critical detail that requires a clear understanding. Several mechanisms have been proposed for the selective stimulation of beneficial microbes by the prebiotic, including substrate-specificity and the presence of genes encoding enzymes that hydrolyze the prebiotic to release metabolites that stimulate the growth of a specific group of microorganisms, structural properties of the prebiotic, cross-feeding, etc. [25]. Experimental studies show that

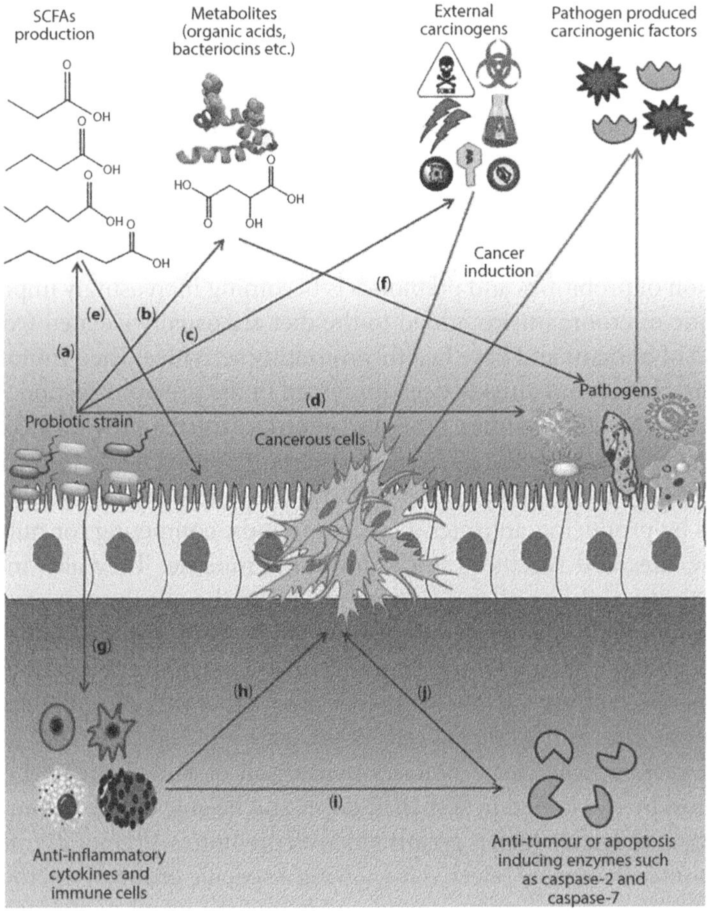

Figure 4.2 Mechanisms of anticancer potential of probiotics: (a) Production of SCFAs (b) Production of organic acids and metabolites (c) Binding and degradation of carcinogenic substances (DMN, DPN, etc) in the intestinal environment, (d) Modulation in microbial composition in gut environment and modification in enzymatic activities of intestinal pathogenic microflora. via competitive exclusion of pathogenic microflora and mediating changes in metabolic activities of pathogenic enzymes with carcinogenic potential, (e) SCFAs helps in improving intestinal barrier, mediates acidosis, inhibits formations of secondary bile, etc., thus preventing risks of carcinogenesis, (f) Organic acids, bacteriocins and other metabolites kills the pathogens by creating a pH change, disruption of proton gradient, neutralization of electrochemical potential across cytoplasm and pore formation, (g) Stimulate the immune system by NK cell and lymphocytes activation and production of anti-inflammatory cytokines such as IL-6, 8, 1β, 12, 17 etc., (h) Antitumor functions such as restriction of TNF-α into blood mononuclear cells, Lowering TLR expression, inhibition expression of NF-kB signaling, etc., (i) Activation and regulation of apoptotic proteins, such as Bcl-2, B-cell lymphoma protein, Bak protein, caspase-2 and caspase-7, and (j) Apoptosis in cancerous cells via induction of apoptotic pathways.

the structure and chain length of the prebiotic is an important factor contributing to the selective stimulation of the probiotic and other beneficial microorganisms. The structural monomers and their glycosidic linkage also influence the microbial species capable of fermenting the added prebiotics [26]. Cross-feeding and substrate selection are the main factors responsible for the selectivity of the gut microflora or probiotic in digesting prebiotics. The probiotic organisms encode a large number of enzymes related to the hydrolysis and metabolism of the complex carbohydrates in the prebiotics, which are absent in the nonhabitants of the GI tract. They are also tolerant to the bile and acidic environment of the gut microflora where the prebiotics are degraded and readily available for microbial consumption, or have a mechanism for transporting these prebiotics to these environments for degradation. Another approach for selective utilization of prebiotics by these microbes is cross-feeding, in which the final metabolite of one group of microorganisms is utilized by the other microbial community, thus stimulating the growth of the other. It has been reported that numerous probiotic organisms such as *Eubacterium*, *Bacteroides*, *Roseburia*, *Faecalibacterium*, *Ruminococcus*, etc., exhibit this cross-feeding activity in addition to the commonly used probiotics, i.e., *Bifidobacterium* and *Lactobacillus*, thus expanding the range of probiotic strains. These microbes probably coevolved with the host to better utilize the various dietary fibers and maintain the intestinal health of the human host [25].

4.4 Cancer

Cancer is among the deadliest chronic diseases in recent times in the world. The International Agency for Research on Cancer (IARC) released updated Globocan 2020 on December 14 with new estimates of global cancer burden, showing that it has increased to 19.3 million cases and 10 million cancer deaths in 2020 (https://www.uicc.org/). Breast cancer is very common in middle-aged women and is estimated to cause about 571,000 deaths [27]. Men are more prone to this disease compared to women. Men are 20% much likely to develop cancer and have 40% higher rate of mortality. Carcinogen exposure leads to abnormal proliferation of neoplastic cells due to genetic alterations in proto-oncogenes or tumor suppressive genes. The altered clonal cells may develop into an active cancerous tumor that continues to spread, invade tissues, or metastasize and interfere with normal body functions [28]. Carcinogens include physical carcinogens (UV and ionizing radiation), chemical carcinogens (constituents of tobacco smoke, pollutants such arsenic, aflatoxin, asbestos, etc.), and biological carcinogens (infections by specific bacteria and viruses). A single genetic change in a cell rarely leads to a full-blown tumor; in most cases, it is a series of mutations in multiple genes that lead to oncogenesis. Age is an important factor contributing to cancer progression. The incidence of this chronic disease increases with age, most likely due to an accumulation of cancer associated risk factors over time [29]. Therefore, continued research dedicated to exploring sharp treatment options is essential to reduce the global cancer burden.

4.4.1 Procarcinogens and Carcinogens

Cancer is caused by substances that cause alteration, mutation, or damage to DNA. Carcinogens are substances that initiate carcinogenesis, while procarcinogens are all substances that are transformed into potential carcinogens after metabolism. Procarcinogens or proximal carcinogens are defined as the parent carcinogens or the metabolites that eventually give rise to the final carcinogens capable of reacting with nuclear DNA. The final carcinogens formed are highly reactive electrophiles that form strong covalent bonds with nucleophilic adducts. Carcinogens are generally classified into two types: genotoxic carcinogens and nongenotoxic carcinogens. Genotoxic carcinogens include those carcinogens that physically interact with DNA and induce DNA modification or damage. Such carcinogens have irreversible effects after binding to DNA. Genotoxic carcinogens can be divided into two types: direct-acting and indirect-acting genotoxic carcinogens. Direct-acting genotoxic carcinogens interact directly with DNA and are independent of prior metabolism. Direct-acting genotoxins are usually reactive electrophilic substance that binds DNA as nucleophiles. Examples of such substances are chemical substances, such as nitrogen mustard, sulphur mustard, N-nitroso-N-methylurea (NMU), methyl methanesulfonate, bis-(chloromethyl) ether, β-propiolactone, etc. Indirectly acting genotoxic carcinogens require metabolism before they bind to genomic DNA. Examples of such substances are polycyclic aromatic hydrocarbons, heterocyclic aromatic compounds, hydrazine, aflatoxins B1, bracken fern, safrole, azo dyes, N-nitrosoamines, etc. [30]. Certain biological carcinogens, such as viruses, also interact with DNA and induce carcinogenesis. Most genotoxic carcinogens induce carcinogenicity through indirect acting mechanisms. The indirectly acting genotoxic agents are often affected by the cytochrome P450 enzyme complex and metabolized to specific products that can bind and disrupt nuclear DNA function and structure.

Nongenotoxic carcinogens do not physically interact with DNA but cause alteration of DNA expression pathways via indirect methods.

Such carcinogens disrupt the normal cell cycle, stimulating uncontrolled cell proliferation and tumor development. These substances include heavy metals, hormones, arsenic, etc. [31]. Studies have shown that certain substances can trigger tumor formation even without these substances and their metabolites interacting with genomic DNA. Nongenotoxic substances exhibit a nonlinear dose-response pattern that is crucial for regulating their carcinogenicity. This type of carcinogenesis induced by nongenotoxic carcinogens requires prolonged exposure of the cell to such substances. Nongenotoxic agents induce cancer through various mechanisms, including methylation, immunosuppression, receptor-mediated oncogenesis, oxidative stress, gap junctional intercellular communication, cytotoxicity, etc. Examples of such substances include radiation, choline deficiency, chloroform, transplant organ drugs, di-(2-ethylhexyl) phthalate (DEHP), tetradecanoylphorbol acetate (12-O-tetradecanoylphorbol-13-acetate) (TPA), perfluorooctanoic acid (PFOA), 2,3,7,8-tetrachlorodibenzo-p-dioxin (TCDD), etc. [32].

4.4.2 Types of Cancer

Cancer represents a strain of disease that affects almost all parts of the human body. Colorectal cancer (CRC), breast cancer, prostate cancer, tongue cancer, pancreatic cancer, leukemia, skin cancer, liver cancer, kidney cancer (renal cell or renal pelvic cancer), uterine cancer, non-Hodgkin's lymphoma, bladder cancer, etc. are among the common types of cancer that affect large populations. Some types of cancer have already been discussed:

4.4.2.1 Colorectal Cancer (CRC)

Abnormal and uncontrolled proliferation of cells under the crypts leads to colorectal cancer, also called colon carcinoma or rectal carcinoma. This type of cancer begins as a polyp, a type of noncancerous cell growth that develops in inner lining of the colon and/or rectum. The most common type of polyp is the adenomatous polyp. The adenoma develops from glandular cells that play an important role in producing mucus to lubricate the wall of the colon. These adenomas are usually localized, but 10% of them can metastasize. Adenocarcinoma is the cancer of glandular cells, and 96% of colorectal cancers are adenocarcinomas [33]. Cancer cells once formed in inner lining of the colon, they migrate and invade nearby tissues by entering the lymphatics or bloodstream. Through the lymphatic vessels, cancer cells travel to the lymph nodes and through the bloodstream, they can travel to major organs of the body, such as the liver or lungs [34]. The bloodstream also causes the cancer cells to travel to other parts of the body, such as the abdominal cavity, pelvis, peritoneum, and ovaries. This type of cancer is usually caused by a carcinogenic mutation of DNA by mutagens, for example, oxygen-free radicals. Identifying the stage of cancer spread is important for prognosis and assigning an appropriate treatment approach for CRC.

4.4.2.2 Gastric Cancer

Gastric cancer is the sixth most common cancer, and third leading cause of cancer-related deaths worldwide. It is a heterogeneous and multifactorial disease. Gastric cancer development is triggered by a number of factors, such as lifestyle, health, diet and *Helicobacter pylori* infection. Several studies concluded that the spiral bacilli are important in the development of gastric ulcers and gastric cancer, which is why WHO classifies *H. pylori* as a type I carcinogen [35]. Several virulence factors are expressed by *H. pylori*, but two proteins: vacuolating cytotoxin (*VacA*) and cytotoxin-associated gene A (*CagA*) play key role in development of gastric cancer. *VacA* secretes toxins that form large vacuoles in the host cell. It also reduces mitochondrial transmembrane potential, activates mitogen-associated protein kinase (MAP), and inhibits T lymphocyte activation [36]. *VacA* gene has s1/s2 alleles encoding signal peptides, m1/m2 alleles encoding intermediate regions, and i1/i2/i3 encoding intermediate locations. s1 and i1 alleles cause aggressive clinical symptoms. *H. pylori* strains containing s1 with *VacA* usually contain another gene called *cagA*, which remains in the cag pathogenicity island and contributes to a greater extent to severe diseases, such as adenocarcinomas. The *cagA* gene encodes EPIYA motifs that are phosphorylated after translocation of cagA into host cells. Phosphorylated cagA associates and deregulates SHP -2 protein, ultimately leading to cancer [37].

4.4.2.3 Pancreatic Cancer

One of the most common cancers leading to high mortality and morbidity rates is pancreatic cancer. Pancreatic cancer is a genetic disease caused by acquired mutations in cancer-associated genes and inherited germline cells. The precursor lesions of pancreatic cancer cells or pancreatic intraepithelial neoplasms (PanINs) have been classified into four stages depending on the histological grade the invasive neoplasm has reached. These four grades are PanIN-1A (flat lesion), 1B (papillary lesion), 2 (micropapillary features), and 3 (loss of polarity, nuclear atypia, and mitosis) [38].

In addition to PanINs, mucinous cystic neoplasms and intraductal papillary mucinous neoplasms (IPMNs) includes cystic precursor lesion of pancreatic adenocarcinoma. Carcinogenesis of pancreatic cancer is triggered by alterations in genome maintenance genes, oncogenes, tumor suppressive genes, etc. The tumor suppressor gene that is most common in pancreatic cancer is *p16INK4A/CDKN2A*. Homozygous mutation, hypermethylation, and intragenic mutation affecting the second allele in the promoter of the *p16INK4A/CDKN2A* gene trigger pancreatic cancer. Pancreatic ductal carcinoma, which is 90% fatal, is caused by a mutation in the *KRAS2* oncogene, located on chromosome 12p. Genome maintenance genes associated with the development of pancreatic cancer include *FANCC* and *FANCG*, which also play a role in Fanconi anemia [39]. Pancreatic cancer is a fatal disease with a high mortality rate in the late stages. Therefore, a better understanding of the molecular basis of this cancer may provide new targets for drug development and improved treatment efficacy.

4.4.2.4 Prostate Cancer

One of the leading causes of cancer-related morbidity and mortality in men is prostate cancer. The development of prostate cancer is triggered by various risk factors, such as chemical injury, diet, obesity, bacterial or viral infections, and most importantly, intraprostatic inflammation. Contributing to these inflammatory storms are genomic, environmental, and immunologic factors that lead to the development of prostate cancer cells. Neoplastic and malignant prostate cancer cells have shown that chronic inflammation is present and, together with other risk factors, initiates carcinogenesis [40]. Inflammation is maintained and extended by the co-expression of luminal and basal cell markers by tumor progenitor cells with an intermediate phenotype. Such intraprostatic inflammation recruits various leukocytes, such as lymphocytes, macrophages, and myeloid cells. Interleukin (IL)-23 is secreted by myeloid-derived suppressor cells (MDSCs), which eventually activate IL-23 receptors on cancer cells. This function then controls gene targeting of the downstream androgen receptor via the STAT3-RORγ pathway. MDSCs produce a large number of free radicals that target DNA. This recruitment and expansion, which is triggered by inflammation, results in single-stranded and double-stranded DNA breaks along with androgen receptor activation (AR) and senescence-associated secretory phenotype (SASP). Following such events, mutagenic insults are triggered by overexpression of tumor suppressive genes and DNA repair systems. Germline DNA repair defects then further accelerate prostate cancer carcinogenesis [41]. Recent advances in treatment approaches have resulted in prostate cancer being less lethal in early stages, but advanced stages often develop resistance to castration treatment for metastases.

4.4.2.5 *Breast Cancer*

One of the most common chronic diseases that occur in middle-aged women is breast cancer. Alessandro Bombonati *et al.* have proposed a developmental model of breast cancer in humans that involves a linear, multistep process. Progression begins with flat epithelial atypia (FEA), which then develops into atypical ductal hyperplasia (ADH). ADH eventually progresses to ductal carcinomona in situ (DCIS) and develops into potentially fatal stage of invasive ductal carcinoma [42].

4.4.2.6 *Skin Cancer*

Two most common types of nonmelanoma skin cancer are squamous cell carcinoma (SCC) and basal cell carcinoma (BCC). BCC develops *de novo*, while SCC formation occurs in a multistep process. Exposure to UV radiation, especially UV-B, and mutations in p53 are the main causes of SCC development. Sun-induced precancerous skin lesions include actinic ketosis, and 10% of these lesions eventually develop SCC [43]. Keratocanthoma is another sun-induced skin tumor, a benign cutaneous squamous neoplasm. Skin cancer is among common cancers worldwide, but new treatment techniques show a significant reduction in mortality rates [44].

4.5 Anticancer Potential of Probiotics and Prebiotics

Global cancer burden has increased exponentially over the last decades encouraging much research works dedicated toward the development of more effective and less deleterious methods for its treatment. Relevant evidences derived from large number of nutritional and medicinal studies conclude the importance of probiotics and prebiotic compounds in the fields of human benefits. Such positive role of probiotics and prebiotics and their anticarcinogenic potential forms a solid ground in the field of future anticancer applications. The anticarcinogenic potential of such probiotics and prebiotic compound is mediated through various anti-inflammatory and immunomodulating effects and works significantly against various types of cancers, such as colorectal cancer (CRC), gastrointestinal cancer, breast cancer, tongue cancer, skin cancer, etc [45]. Hence, a profound knowledge can establish a sharp significance of probiotics and prebiotics in medicinal applications with an effective edge towards prevention of paramount disease like cancer.

4.5.1 Clinical Evidences

A number of experiments have been conducted to evaluate effects of probiotics and prebiotics as future cancer therapeutics (Table 4.2). The mechanism of anticancer activity of probiotics and prebiotics has been discussed in section 4.3. Medical evidence is necessary to assess the suitability and applicability of probiotics and prebiotics in cancer treatment. Such clinical trials demonstrate the relative efficacy of different prebiotic cultures, thus measuring the best efficacy for probiotic cancer therapies. Similarly, clinical evidence provides a comparative analysis of different types of prebiotics, allowing the most appropriate agents to be used [46].

4.5.1.1 Clinical Evidence for the Anticancer Potential of Probiotics

The health benefiting and anticancer potential of probiotics is based on several mechanisms, which act against anticancer activity through different pathways induced by probiotic microorganisms. Modulation of gut microbial composition by probiotic bacteria is an important aspect that prevents dysbiosis-mediated inflammation and carcinogenesis. Dysbiosis has been considered as one of the most important causes of the production of carcinogenic substances in the intestinal environment and thus the development of CRC. In one study, the microbial composition in fecal samples from colorectal cancer patients and healthy individuals was compared. It was concluded that stool samples from CRC patients showed higher composition of pathogenic microbial genera, such as *Bacteroides, Fusobacterium, Prevotella, Eubacterium, Salmonella, Clostridium*, and lower number of *Lactobacillus* spp., whereas samples from healthy individuals showed significant composition of *Lactobacillus* spp [47]. Similarly, the effects of a probiotic strain on the inhibition of pathogenic microbes that can trigger carcinogenesis were investigated in a clinical study by Ohara *et al.* The intestinal microflora of CRC patients and healthy subjects were compared and the effects induced by ingestion of *L. gasseri* OLL2716: LG21 were analyzed. Study showed an increase in the composition of Lactobacillus and a very significant decrease in pathogenic microbes, such as *C. perfringens* in the intestinal environment. The results also showed a higher production of SCFAs and inhibition of acidosis and synthesis of fecal putrefactive products [48]. Probiotic strains have shown promising results in altering the metabolic activities of the gut microbiota, thereby

Table 4.2 Clinical evidence for anticancer potential of probiotics and prebiotics.

Types of cancer	Probiotics cultures involved	Source of probiotic isolation	Results obtained	Ref.
Colorectal cancer (CRC)	*Lactobacillus, Lactococcus, Leuconostoc, Saccharomyces, Pichia, Candida* and *Kluyveromyces*	Kefir, a fermented milk product	1. Increase in cecal concentration of short chain fatty acids (SCFAs). 2. Increase in concentration of IL-1β and TNF-α in the colon. 3. Increase in catalase enzyme activity 4. Decrease in intestinal permeability 5. Reduced lactulose/mannitol ratio 6. Inhibited the lesion development	[71]
	L. brevis, L. plantarum, Lactococcus lactis	Kimchi, a fermented vegetable product	1. Reduction in the expression of Bcl-2 protein 2. Increase in the expression of caspase-3 and caspase-9 3. Decreased mRNA expression of pro-inflammatory factors 4. Promotion in expression of Bax	[72]

(*Continued*)

Table 4.2 Clinical evidence for anticancer potential of probiotics and prebiotics. (*Continued*)

Types of cancer	Probiotics cultures involved	Source of probiotic isolation	Results obtained	Ref.
	L. acidophilus, L. lactis, L. delbruekii subsp. *Bulgaricus*	Yoghurt	1. Increase in IgA+ antibody (P<0.01) 2. Induction of IFN-γ and TNF-α cytokine release 3. Increase in IL-10 (P<0.001) 4. Increase in the number of apoptotic cells	[73]
	L. pentosus B281 and *L. plantarum* B282	Olive microbiota	1. High adherence capability to Caco-2 cells, which are human colonic epithelial cell lines. 2. Treatment with conditioned media showed high reduction in cellular proliferation demonstrated by clonogenic assay and sulforhodamine B assay. 3. Induction of cell arrest at G1 phase. 4. Downregulation of cyclin genes	[74]

(*Continued*)

Table 4.2 Clinical evidence for anticancer potential of probiotics and prebiotics. (*Continued*)

Types of cancer	Probiotics cultures involved	Source of probiotic isolation	Results obtained	Ref.
Gastric cancer	*Propionibacterium freudenreichii*	Fermented milk	1. Induction of apoptosis of HGT-1 gastric cancer cell line by chromatin condensation, apoptotic bodies formation, DNA laddering, arrest of cell cycle 2. Mitochondrial disruption, activation of caspase and cytochrome C release was observed 3. Increased activity of camptothecin drug	[75]
	L. kefir	Kefir PFT, a fermented milk product	1. Dose dependent apoptosis of AGS gastric cancer cells. Apoptosis increased by 5% when the dose increased from 0.3 mg/ml to 0.6 mg/ml. 2. Decreased polarization of MMP 3. Reduction in Bcl2 protein expression	[76]

(*Continued*)

Table 4.2 Clinical evidence for anticancer potential of probiotics and prebiotics. (*Continued*)

Types of cancer	Probiotics cultures involved	Source of probiotic isolation	Results obtained	Ref.
Breast cancer	*L. acidophilus, L. bulgaricus, Streptococcus lactis, Bifidobacteria*	Fermented soy milk product	1. A dose dependent cytotoxic effect was shown. Significant inhibition at >0.32 mg/ml of FSP 2. Higher apoptosis in FSP treated MCF-7 breast cancer cell lines with 34.11% of cells in gated region	[77]
	L. casei, L. hilgardii, L. nagelii	Kefir water	1. Cytotoxicity towards 4T1 cells at IC_{50} of 12.5 and 8.33 mg/ml. 2. Reduction in tumor size and weight (0.9132+/-0.219 g) 3. 5 fold increase in helperT cells 4. 7 fold increase in cytotoxic T cells. 5. Reduction in proangiogenic and proinflammatory markers.	[78]

(*Continued*)

Table 4.2 Clinical evidence for anticancer potential of probiotics and prebiotics. (*Continued*)

Types of cancer	Probiotics cultures involved	Source of probiotic isolation	Results obtained	Ref.
Acute erythroleukemia	*L. kefir*	Kefir, a fermented milk product	1. MTT assay on KG-1 acute erythroleukemia cell lines showed apoptosis induced by kefir treatment in dose and time dependent manner. 2. Necrosis was observed on KG-1 cells 3. High antiproliferation activity against KG-1, with least viability at 300 micro litres of kefir ($P<0.05$)	[79]
Tongue cancer	*L. fermentum* CQPC08	Fermented brine pickle	1. Increased superoxide dismutase activity 2. Reduction in levels of IL-12, IL-4, IgG, G-CSF, GM-CSF, IFN-γ and TNF-α	[80]

(*Continued*)

Table 4.2 Clinical evidence for anticancer potential of probiotics and prebiotics. (*Continued*)

Types of cancer	Probiotics cultures involved	Source of probiotic isolation	Results obtained	Ref.
Colorectal cancer (CRC)	Mushroom polysaccharide and Gp saponins	Mushroom *Genoderma lucindum* (Lingzi) and an herbal tea, *Gynostemma petaphyllum* (Gp)	1. Colonic M1 and M2 macrophage shifting, polyps reduction, converting E-cadherin/N-cadherin ratio and oncogenic signal molecules down-regulation, hence improving inflamed intestinal barrier in $Apc^{Min/+}$ mice model. 2. Enhanced production of SCFAs by promoting SCFAs producing bacteria. 3. Stimulation of G-protein coupled receptors. 4. Modulated expression of anticancer hormones in gut such as PYY and PPAPγ.	[81]

(*Continued*)

Table 4.2 Clinical evidence for anticancer potential of probiotics and prebiotics. (*Continued*)

Types of cancer	Probiotics cultures involved	Source of probiotic isolation	Results obtained	Ref.
	Phenolic compounds such as anthocyanin and ellagic acid	*Myrciariajaboticaba* seeds	1. Decreased number of *Firmecutes* and higher *Bacteroidetes* abundance. 2. Reduction in β-glucosidase, β-glucoronidase, nitroreductase, mucinase, β-galactosidase and other tumor-inducing pathogenic enzymes. 3. Decreased activity of inflammatory cytokines in the gut.	[81]
	NV polysaccharides	*Nostoc commune* Vaucher (NV)	1. Immunostimulation 2. Decreased CRC marker expression and reduction in tumor number. 3. Stimulation of SCFAs producing bacterial growth. 4. Activation of macrophages.	[82]
	Galacto-oligosaccharides	Lactulose	1. Increase in abundance of Bifidobacterium and inhibition of bacteria inducing pro-inflammatory functions. 2. Induced production of SCFAs in gut. 3. Apoptosis of tumor cells and decrease in tumor area and number.	[64]

reducing the production of carcinogenic metabolites. *L. acidophilus* N-2 and NCFM, a probiotic bacterium, has shown significant effect against the activities of three enzymes: nitroreductase, azoreductase, and β-glucoronidase. These enzymes are very harmful and can convert procarcinogens into active carcinogens. *Lactobacillus* N-2 strain showed significant reduction in the activities of these enzymes [49]. Probiotics also produce various metabolites that are inhibitory to pathogens, such as organic acids, bacteriocins, etc. Lievin *et al.* showed that bifidocin B, a bacteriocin produced by *Bifidobacterium bifidum* NCFB 1454, has significant antimicrobial effect against the pathogen *S. typhimurium* SL1344 [50].

Probiotic bacteria may play an important role in binding and degrading various carcinogenic factors that contribute to CRC or other cancers. Studies have shown that various probiotic bacteria, such as *Streptococcus salivarius, Lactobacillus acidophilus,* and *Bifidobacterium longum* can bind and eliminate different types of carcinogenic mutagens and heterocyclic amines, such as 2-amino3-methyl-3H-imidazole [4,5-f]-quinoline, 2-amino-3,4-dimethylimidazo [4,5-f]-quinoline, 3-amino-1-methyl-5-h-pyrido [4,3-b]indole acetate and 5-phenyl-2-amino-1-methylimidazo [4,5-f]pyridine, etc. [51, 52]. Similarly, a study investigated the ability of *Streptococcus, Lactobacillus,* and *Bifidobacterium* to degrade dimethyl-nitrosamine (DMN) and diphenyl-nitrosamine (DPN). Nitrosamines are potent carcinogens and certain foods for human consumption contain this chemical carcinogen. Nitrosamines are also formed in the gastrointestinal tract from secondary amines and nitrites. Gastric acid causes nitrosation of dimethylamine, resulting in the carcinogen DMN. Strain *Lactobacillus* 33 performed DPN degradation both in the presence and absence of glucose and the amount of nitrite produced in μmol/ml per 20 hours was 0.16, 0.18 (in the absence of glucose) and 0.17, 0.18 (in the presence of glucose). *Lactobacillus* showed the maximum DPN degradation rate of 0.1 μmol/ml per 20 hours when the initial DPN concentration reached 0.5 μmol/ml. At this DPN concentration, almost 20% of the substrate was completely degraded by the test bacterium [53].

Most studies evaluating anticancer effects of probiotics are conducted in animal models. Such results derived from animal models are considered promising for anticancer application in humans. Mouse models injected with 1,2-dimethylhydrazine (chemical carcinogen) were treated with probiotic strains such as *L. plantarum, L. acidophilus, L. rhamnosus, L. salivarius, L. casei, L. lactis, Bacillus polyfermenticus, B. longum,* and *B. infantum.* The study showed degradation of carcinogens and effective inhibition of colon carcinogenesis [54, 55]. Similarly, a study conducted by Dubey *et al.* demonstrated the antitumor and azoxymethane degrading ability of *Pediococcus pentosaceus* GS4 strain in mouse model [56]. Studies have shown that probiotic cultures can prevent gastric cancer by inhibiting *H. pylori*. In one study, probiotic strains of *L. reuteri* were subjected to competitive binding to gangliotetraosylceramides and sulfatides, putative glycolipid receptors of *H. pylori*. The study demonstrated the presence of a possible sulfatide-binding protein in *Lactobacillus* strains. Thin layer chromatography overlay assay using biotin-labeled microbial cells demonstrated the ability of *L. reuteri* strains (JCM1081 AND TM105) to inhibit *H. pylori* infection by binding to sulfatide and Asialo-GM1 receptors. Due to the glycolipid specificity of *L. reuteri* for *H. pylori*, they are able to inhibit the colonization of spiral bacilli in the early stages and are therefore suitable for a probiotic approach [57]. The probiotic strains help in improving the intestinal barrier through various mechanisms including mucin production. Probiotics increase mucin production by upregulating the MUC gene. Franco *et al.* conducted an experiment to demonstrate increased mucin production by consuming probiotics in Wister rats. The probiotic strains used were *L. casei, L. plantarum, L. delbruekii subsp. bulgaricus, L. acidophilus, B. longum, B. infantis, B. breve*, and *Streptococcus salivarius* subsp *thermophilus*. The model rats showed 5-fold increased expression of the MUC2 gene for mucin production with slightly increased expression of MUC3 and MUC1 [58]. Various clinical studies and the satisfactory results suggest that probiotics represent a solid field for future cancer therapies.

4.5.1.2 Clinical Evidences for Anticancer Potential of Prebiotics

The efficacy of prebiotics in future cancer therapies needs to be proven by various clinical trials, and studies have shown a positive inhibitory effect on different types of cancer, especially CRC. The anticancer effect of prebiotics is due to several mechanisms that are somewhat related to those of probiotics. Prebiotic compounds help to increase the composition of health-promoting bacteria in the gut. Inulin has been studied to help prevent inflammatory diseases such as diabetes and obesity by promoting the growth of propionate-producing bacteria from the *Porphyromonadaceae, Bacteroidaceae*, and *Prevotellaceae* families, while inhibiting the proliferation of Firmicutes. A higher ratio of *Fermicutes/Bacteroidetes* contributes to such diseases. Therefore, the role of inulin in maintaining a low ratio of these bacterial members in the intestinal environment is highlighted [59]. Most of these studies evaluating the effects of prebiotics on cancer treatment have been conducted in animal models. Liao *et al.* conducted a study to demonstrate the reciprocal relationship between probiotics and prebiotics in CRC prevention in the APC Min/+ mouse model. They first demonstrated the ability of a plant food, *Gynostemma pentaphyllum* saponins (GpS), to prevent the formation of CRC polyps in the GpS-treated APC Min/+ mouse model. They also isolated 16 bacterial species from APC Min/+ mice feces treated with Gp saponins (GpS) and demonstrated the involvement of *B. animalis* as the major growth stimulus of GpS by RNA sequencing and biochemical analysis. GpS were shown to play the key role in the expression of genes encoding metabolic pathways and biogenesis in *B. animalis* culture [60]. Similarly, the anticancer potential of another prebiotic, jujube polysaccharide, was investigated in C57BL/6 mice. The mouse models were first treated with the carcinogenic agent CRC, azoxymethane/dextran sodium sulphate (AOM/DSS), and then treated with jujube polysaccharide. The result showed the ability of the prebiotic to interact with the gut microbiota and exert a protective effect against CRC carcinogenesis [61].

Prebiotics have the ability to inhibit the production of pre-inflammatory cytokines by binding to G protein-coupled receptors (GPCRs) and modulating signaling pathways in various immune cells and colonocytes. Many GPCRs, such as GPCR109A, GPCR43, GPCR41, etc., bind specifically to SCFAs and cause modulation in carcinogenic inflammation. A study was conducted to investigate the relationship between prebiotics and the expression of GPCRs in polyposis mice. The prebiotics administered contained 50% raw potato starch and 50% chitin-glucan substrates. The result showed higher GPCR109A expression and tumor cell inhibition in the mouse models [62]. Several studies were conducted on mice treated with CRC AOM/DSS to analyze the anti-CRC potential of various prebiotics, such as ellagic acid and anthocyanin from *Myrciariajaboticaba* seeds [63], galacto-oligosaccharides derived from lactulose [64], *Chenopodium formosanum*(a cereal) [65] etc., with positive and promising results. Thus, it is proved that prebiotics will play important role in future anticancer activities.

4.5.2 Safety and Quality Control Assurance

The use of probiotics and prebiotics for human benefit requires an assessment of their safety and quality in different categories of people. Various clinical evidences and previous findings on safe consumption form the branches of the safety profile of probiotics and prebiotics. The safety and quality of probiotic and prebiotic therapy is of critical importance when used in neonates and immunocompromised adults. The importance of safety and quality assessment in this type of therapy is justified by the potential sepsis, bacteremia, or endocarditis that can be caused by certain probiotic strains. There are few reports of such infections in *L. casei* and *L. rhamnosus* GG strains [66]. Bifidobacterium is sometimes associated with certain infections but is rare. Several studies and clinical trials have been conducted to evaluate the safety and efficacy of probiotic therapy, especially in hospitalized or intensive care unit patients. Several clinical trials have demonstrated that hospitalized patients with regular antibiotic administration experienced probiotic-induced long-term dysbiosis after probiotic therapy [67]. Dysbiosis causes a delay in the reconstitution of mucosal and faecal microbial composition, as mentioned previously. Antibiotic resistance of lactobacilli and bifidobacterial must be reviewed and subjected to safety evaluation before use in therapy. Clinical studies have shown atypical resistance of various probiotic strains to some clinically important antibiotics such as nalidixic acid, polymyxin B, neomycin, streptomycin, gentamycin, vancomycin, etc. Therefore, probiotic strains must be tested for antibiotic suitability before therapeutic use [68]. The various organic acids and metabolites produced by probiotic strains can inhibit the healthy gut microbiota and reduce its composition in the gastrointestinal environment. In a clinical study by Parekh *et al.*, it was demonstrated that the administration of probiotics in patients receiving antibiotics resulted in a significant reduction in composition of the gut microbiome compared to control patients who did not receive probiotics [69]. Similar to probiotics, the safety and quality of prebiotics must be evaluated before they are used in the medical treatment of serious diseases such as cancer. Most studies evaluating the anticancer potential of prebiotics have been conducted in animal models, so the efficacy and applicability of such cancer therapy in humans is sometimes questionable. Most clinical trials have yielded promising results with no side effects with respect to prebiotic cancer therapy. Overall, the use of probiotic and prebiotic supplements is very effective in healthy individuals and has little or no effect in patients with compromised immune systems. Therefore, further research and investigation into the safety and quality of probiotic and prebiotic cancer therapy may expand its use to more areas and expand the possibilities of eliminating this dangerous disease in a less harmful way.

Several criteria determine the selection and assurance of the quality of probiotic supplements. Several tests that determine the adequate and satisfactory number of probiotic bacteria in a specific sample throughout the sample shelf life gives an assurance of quality of probiotic supplement. The probiotic strain must always retain the desired functions with promising efficacy for its selection as supplement. Besides retaining the proper function, the selected probiotic strain must show stability against the acid and bile conditions, thus maintaining its survival in the gastrointestinal environment. The probiotics must adhere strongly and colonize on the gastrointestinal cell linings. Characterization of adhesion property contributes toward another quality assurance aspect. Adhesion properties of probiotic strains are analyzed on human intestinal mucus and intestinal epithelial cell cultures (example: Caco-2 cells) to evaluate their efficacy as probiotic supplement. A strong adhesion of probiotic strain makes them more viable and more active in pathogenic competitive exclusion, immune stimulation, diarrhoea prevention, etc [70]. Hence, quality assurance beholds high significance in probiotic selection for human supplementation.

4.6 Conclusion and Future Prospect

The recent past has seen a growing demand for the use of prebiotic and probiotic as food supplement for improving the gut and overall health. These functional foods have various health benefiting effects from production of various metabolites, modification of the gut microbiome to competitive elimination of pathogens. They also modulate the immune system of the human host, thus their study for the treatment of cancer has shown some potential. There have been clinical evidences that showed their capability to inhibit the growth of tumorous cells via binding and degradation of potential carcinogens to induction of apoptosis. Further scope on identification of potential microbial strains and dietary fiber, and their formulations for use as medication along with their safety evaluation have future scope for treatment of cancer, which is currently considered one of the diseases with high mortality.

Acknowledgment

The authors would like to thank the Department of Microbiology, Sikkim University for providing the computational infrastructure and central library facilities for procuring references.

References

1. Abbas, Z. and Rehman, S., An overview of cancer treatment modalities, in: *Neoplasm*, vol. 1, pp. 139–57, 2018.

2. Anand, P. *et al.*, Cancer is a preventable disease that requires major lifestyle changes. *Pharm. Res.*, 25, 9, 2097–2116, 2008.
3. Hanahan, D. and Weinberg, R.A., Hallmarks of cancer: The next generation. *Cell*, 144, 5, 646–674, 2011.
4. Wang, H. *et al.*, Global, regional, and national life expectancy, all-cause mortality, and cause-specific mortality for 249 causes of death, 1980–2015: A systematic analysis for the Global Burden of Disease Study 2015. *Lancet*, 388, 10053, 1459–1544, 2016.
5. Ferlay, J. *et al.*, Estimates of worldwide burden of cancer in 2008: GLOBOCAN 2008. *Int. J. Cancer*, 127, 12, 2893–2917, 2010.
6. Wild, C., Weiderpass, E., Stewart, B.W., *World cancer report: Cancer research for cancer prevention*, IARC Press, Lyon, France, 2020.
7. World Health Organization, *WHO report on cancer: Setting priorities, investing wisely and providing care for all*, World Health Organization, Geneva, Switzerland, WHO Press, 2020.
8. Bedada, T.L. *et al.*, Probiotics for cancer alternative prevention and treatment. *Biomed. Pharmacother.*, 129, 110409, 2020.
9. Thilakarathna, W.W., Langille, M.G., Rupasinghe, H.V., Polyphenol-based prebiotics and synbiotics: Potential for cancer chemoprevention. *Curr. Opin. Food Sci.*, 20, 51–57, 2018.
10. Scott, A.J. *et al.*, Pre-, pro-and synbiotics in cancer prevention and treatment—A review of basic and clinical research. *Ecancermedicalscience*, 12, 869, 2018.
11. Pandey, K.R., Naik, S.R., Vakil, B.V., Probiotics, prebiotics and synbiotics-A review. *J. Food Sci. Technol.*, 52, 12, 7577–7587, 2015.
12. Binda, S. *et al.*, Criteria to qualify microorganisms as "probiotic" in foods and dietary supplements. *Front. Microbiol.*, 11, 1662, 2020.
13. Markowiak, P. and Śliżewska, K., Effects of probiotics, prebiotics, and synbiotics on human health. *Nutrients*, 9, 9, 1021, 2017.
14. Pokusaeva, K., Fitzgerald, G.F., van Sinderen, D., Carbohydrate metabolism in Bifidobacteria. *Genes Nutr.*, 6, 3, 285–306, 2011.
15. Davani-Davari, D. *et al.*, Prebiotics: Definition, types, sources, mechanisms, and clinical applications. *Foods*, 8, 3, 92, 2019.
16. Clemente, J.C. *et al.*, The impact of the gut microbiota on human health: An integrative view. *Cell*, 148, 6, 1258–1270, 2012.
17. Jayachandran, M. *et al.*, A critical review on the impacts of β-glucans on gut microbiota and human health. *J. Nutr. Biochem.*, 61, 101–110, 2018.
18. Ballan, R. *et al.*, Interactions of probiotics and prebiotics with the gut microbiota. *Prog. Mol. Biol. Transl. Sci.*, 171, 265–300, 2020.
19. Nie, Y., Luo, F., Lin, Q., Dietary nutrition and gut microflora: A promising target for treating diseases. *Trends Food Sci. Technol.*, 75, 72–80, 2018.
20. Dekaboruah, E. *et al.*, Human microbiome: An academic update on human body site specific surveillance and its possible role. *Arch. Microbiol.*, 202, 8, 2147–2167, 2020.

21. Neish, A.S., Microbes in gastrointestinal health and disease. *Gastroenterology*, 136, 1, 65–80, 2009.
22. Shankar, V. *et al.*, Differences in gut metabolites and microbial composition and functions between Egyptian and US children are consistent with their diets. *Msystems*, 2, 1, e00169–16, 2017.
23. Andoh, A., Physiological role of gut microbiota for maintaining human health. *Digestion*, 93, 3, 176–181, 2016.
24. Hemarajata, P. and Versalovic, J., Effects of probiotics on gut microbiota: mechanisms of intestinal immunomodulation and neuromodulation. *Therap. Adv. Gastroenterol.*, 6, 1, 39–51, 2013.
25. Wang, S. *et al.*, Rational use of prebiotics for gut microbiota alterations: Specific bacterial phylotypes and related mechanisms. *J. Funct. Foods*, 66, 103838, 2020.
26. Ferreira-Lazarte, A. *et al.*, *In vitro* digestibility of galactooligosaccharides: effect of the structural features on their intestinal degradation. *J. Agric. Food Chem.*, 67, 16, 4662–4670, 2019.
27. World Health Organization, *World health statistics 2016: Monitoring health for the SDGs sustainable development goals*, World Health Organization, Geneva, Switzerland, WHO Press, 2016.
28. Shishodia, S. *et al.*, Ursolic acid inhibits nuclear factor-κB activation induced by carcinogenic agents through suppression of IκBα kinase and p65 phosphorylation: Correlation with down-regulation of cyclooxygenase 2, matrix metalloproteinase 9, and cyclin D1. *Cancer Res.*, 63, 15, 4375–4383, 2003.
29. DePinho, R.A., The age of cancer. *Nature*, 408, 6809, 248–254, 2000.
30. Hayashi, Y., Overview of genotoxic carcinogens and non-genotoxic carcinogens. *Exp. Toxicol. Pathol.*, 44, 8, 465–471, 1992.
31. Klaunig, J.E., Chemical carcinogenesis, in: *Principles of Toxicology: Environmental and Industrial Applications*, 3rd edition, pp. 259–281, 2014.
32. Nohmi, T., Thresholds of genotoxic and non-genotoxic carcinogens. *Toxicol. Res.*, 34, 4, 281–290, 2018.
33. Hilimire, M.R., DeVylder, J.E., Forestell, C.A., Fermented foods, neuroticism, and social anxiety: An interaction model. *Psychiatry Res.*, 228, 2, 203–208, 2015.
34. Siegel, R.L. *et al.*, Colorectal cancer statistics, 2020. *CA: Cancer J. Clin.*, 70, 3, 145–164, 2020.
35. Schulz, C., Schütte, K., Malfertheiner, P., Does, H., pylori eradication therapy benefit patients with hepatic encephalopathy?: Systematic review. *J. Clin. Gastroenterol.*, 48, 6, 491–499, 2014.
36. Torres, V.J. *et al.*, Helicobacter pylori vacuolating cytotoxin inhibits activation-induced proliferation of human T and B lymphocyte subsets. *J. Immunol.*, 179, 8, 5433–5440, 2007.
37. Hatakeyama, M., Helicobacter pylori CagA and gastric cancer: a paradigm for hit-and-run carcinogenesis. *Cell Host Microbe*, 15, 3, 306–316, 2014.

38. Sreedhar, U.L. *et al.*, A systematic review of intra-pancreatic fat deposition and pancreatic carcinogenesis. *J. Gastrointest. Surg.*, 24, 11, 2560–2569, 2020.
39. Reiter, J.G. and Iacobuzio-Donahue, C.A., Pancreatic carcinogenesis—Several small steps or one giant leap? *Nat. Rev. Gastroenterol. Hepatol.*, 14, 1, 7–8, 2017.
40. Aird, J. *et al.*, Carcinogenesis in prostate cancer: The role of long non-coding RNAs. *Non-coding RNA Res.*, 3, 1, 29–38, 2018.
41. de Bono, J.S. *et al.*, Prostate carcinogenesis: Inflammatory storms. *Nat. Rev. Cancer*, 20, 455–469, 2020.
42. Bombonati, A. and Sgroi, D.C., The molecular pathology of breast cancer progression. *J. Pathol.*, 223, 2, 308–318, 2011.
43. Liu-Smith, F., Jia, J., Zheng, Y., UV-induced molecular signaling differences in melanoma and non-melanoma skin cancer. Ultraviolet Light in Human Health, Diseases and Environment. Advances in Experimental Medicine and Biology, 996, 27–40, Springer, Cham, 2017.
44. Cullen, J.K. *et al.*, Topical treatments for skin cancer. *Adv. Drug Delivery Rev.*, 153, 54–64, 2020.
45. Sehrawat, N. *et al.*, Probiotics in microbiome ecological balance providing a therapeutic window against cancer. *Semin. Cancer Biol.*, 70, 24-36, Academic Press, 2021.
46. Taper, H.S. and Roberfroid, M.B., Prebiotics and cancer therapy, in: *Handbook of prebiotics*, pp. 347–358, CRC Press, Boca Raton, 2008.
47. Kahouli, I., Tomaro-Duchesneau, C., Prakash, S., Probiotics in colorectal cancer (CRC) with emphasis on mechanisms of action and current perspectives. *J. Med. Microbiol.*, 62, 8, 1107–1123, 2013.
48. Ohara, T., Yoshino, K., Kitajima, M., Possibility of preventing colorectal carcinogenesis with probiotics. *Hepato-gastroenterology*, 57, 104, 1411–1415, 2010.
49. Goldin, B.R. and Gorbach, S.L., The effect of milk and lactobacillus feeding on human intestinal bacterial enzyme activity. *Am. J. Clin. Nutr.*, 39, 5, 756–761, 1984.
50. Lievin, V. *et al.*, Bifidobacterium strains from resident infant human gastrointestinal microflora exert antimicrobial activity. *Gut*, 47, 5, 646–652, 2000.
51. Bolognani, F., Rumney, C., Rowland, I., Influence of carcinogen binding by lactic acid-producing bacteria on tissue distribution and *in vivo* mutagenicity of dietary carcinogens. *Food Chem. Toxicol.*, 35, 6, 535–545, 1997.
52. Orrhage, K. *et al.*, Binding of mutagenic heterocyclic amines by intestinal and lactic acid bacteria. *Mutat. Res./Fundam. Mol. Mech. Mutagen.*, 311, 2, 239–248, 1994.
53. Rowland, I. and Grasso, P., Degradation of N-nitrosamines by intestinal bacteria. *Appl. Microbiol.*, 29, 1, 7–12, 1975.
54. Lee, N.-K. *et al.*, The prophylactic effect of probiotic Bacillus polyfermenticus KU3 against cancer cells. *J. Funct. Foods*, 14, 513–518, 2015.

55. Śliżewska, K., Markowiak-Kopeć, P., Śliżewska, W., The role of probiotics in cancer prevention. *Cancers*, 13, 1, 20, 2021.
56. Dubey, V. *et al.*, Appraisal of the anti-cancer potential of probiotic Pediococcus pentosaceus GS4 against colon cancer: *In vitro* and *in vivo* approaches. *J. Funct. Foods*, 23, 66–79, 2016.
57. Mukai, T. *et al.*, Inhibition of binding of Helicobacter pylori to the glycolipid receptors by probiotic Lactobacillus reuteri. *FEMS Immunol. Med. Microbiol.*, 32, 2, 105–110, 2002.
58. Caballero-Franco, C. *et al.*, The VSL# 3 probiotic formula induces mucin gene expression and secretion in colonic epithelial cells. *Am. J. Physiol.-Gastrointest. Liver Physiol.*, 292, 1, G315–G322, 2007.
59. Fernández, J. *et al.*, traditional processed meat products re-designed towards inulin-rich functional foods reduce polyps in two colorectal cancer Animal Models. *Sci. Rep.*, 9, 1, 1–17, 2019.
60. Liao, W. *et al.*, Bifidobacterium animalis: the missing link for the cancer-preventive effect of Gynostemma pentaphyllum. *Gut Microbes*, 13, 1, 1847629, 2021.
61. Ji, X. *et al.*, Metagenomic analysis of gut microbiota modulatory effects of jujube (Ziziphus jujuba Mill.) polysaccharides in a colorectal cancer mouse model. *Food Funct.*, 11, 1, 163–173, 2020.
62. Bishehsari, F. *et al.*, Dietary fiber treatment corrects the composition of gut microbiota, promotes SCFA production, and suppresses colon carcinogenesis. *Genes*, 9, 2, 102, 2018.
63. Fidelis, M. *et al.*, Polyphenols of jabuticaba [Myrciaria jaboticaba (Vell.) O. Berg] seeds incorporated in a yogurt model exert antioxidant activity and modulate gut microbiota of 1, 2-dimethylhydrazine-induced colon cancer in rats. *Food Chem.*, 334, 127565, 2021.
64. Fernández, J. *et al.*, A galacto-oligosaccharides preparation derived from lactulose protects against colorectal cancer development in an animal model. *Front. Microbiol.*, 9, 2004, 2018.
65. Lee, C.-W. *et al.*, Synbiotic combination of Djulis (Chenopodium formosanum) and Lactobacillus acidophilus inhibits colon carcinogenesis in rats. *Nutrients*, 12, 1, 103, 2020.
66. Boyle, R.J., Robins-Browne, R.M., Tang, M.L., Probiotic use in clinical practice: what are the risks? *Am. J. Clin. Nutr.*, 83, 6, 1256–1264, 2006.
67. Suez, J. *et al.*, Post-antibiotic gut mucosal microbiome reconstitution is impaired by probiotics and improved by autologous FMT. *Cell*, 174, 6, 1406–1423. e16, 2018.
68. Li, T. *et al.*, A critical review of antibiotic resistance in probiotic bacteria. *Food Res. Int.*, 109571, 136, 2020.
69. Parekh, P.J. *et al.*, The role and influence of gut microbiota in pathogenesis and management of obesity and metabolic syndrome. *Front. Endocrinol.*, 5, 47, 2014.

70. Tuomola, E. *et al.*, Quality assurance criteria for probiotic bacteria. *Am. J. Clin. Nutr.*, 73, 2, 393s–398s, 2001.
71. dos Reis, S.A. *et al.*, Kefir reduces the incidence of pre-neoplastic lesions in an animal model for colorectal cancer. *J. Funct. Foods*, 53, 1–6, 2019.
72. Kim, B. *et al.*, Anticancer effects of kimchi fermented for different times and with added ingredients in human HT-29 colon cancer cells. *Food Sci. Biotechnol.*, 24, 2, 629–633, 2015.
73. Perdigon, G. *et al.*, Role of yoghurt in the prevention of colon cancer. *Eur. J. Clin. Nutr.*, 56, 3, S65–S68, 2002.
74. Saxami, G. *et al.*, Two potential probiotic lactobacillus strains isolated from olive microbiota exhibit adhesion and anti-proliferative effects in cancer cell lines. *J. Funct. Foods*, 24, 461–471, 2016.
75. Cousin, F.J. *et al.*, Milk fermented by Propionibacterium freudenreichii induces apoptosis of HGT-1 human gastric cancer cells. *PLoS One*, **7**, 3, e31892, 2012.
76. Ghoneum, M. and Felo, N., Selective induction of apoptosis in human gastric cancer cells by Lactobacillus kefiri (PFT), a novel kefir product. *Oncol. Rep.*, 34, 4, 1659–1666, 2015.
77. Chang, W.-H. *et al.*, Growth inhibition and induction of apoptosis in MCF-7 breast cancer cells by fermented soy milk. *Nutr. Cancer*, 43, 2, 214–226, 2002.
78. Zamberi, N.R. *et al.*, The antimetastatic and antiangiogenesis effects of kefir water on murine breast cancer cells. *Integr. Cancer Ther.*, 15, 4, NP53–NP66, 2016.
79. Jalali, F., Sharifi, M., Salehi, R., Kefir induces apoptosis and inhibits cell proliferation in human acute erythroleukemia. *Med. Oncol.*, 33, 1, 7, 2016.
80. Liu, B. *et al.*, Preventive effect of lactobacillus fermentum CQPC08 on 4-nitroquineline-1-oxide induced tongue cancer in C57BL/6 mice. *Foods*, 8, 3, 93, 2019.
81. Khan, I. *et al.*, Mushroom polysaccharides and jiaogulan saponins exert cancer preventive effects by shaping the gut microbiota and microenvironment in ApcMin/+ mice. *Pharmacol. Res.*, 148, 104448, 2019.
82. Guo, M. and Li, Z., Polysaccharides isolated from Nostoc commune Vaucher inhibit colitis-associated colon tumorigenesis in mice and modulate gut microbiota. *Food Funct.*, 10, 10, 6873–6881, 2019.

5

Application of Nanotechnology in Formulation of Nutraceuticals

Pradnya Jadhav, Sakshi Kor and Shadab Ahmed*

Institute of Bioinformatics and Biotechnology (Merged with Department of Biotechnology), Savitribai Phule Pune University, Pune, India

Abstract

Nutraceuticals is the term derived from "nutrition" and "pharmaceuticals," thus, having nutritional, as well as medicinal importance, with therapeutic efficacy. Nutraceuticals are products obtained from food sources, which are known to improve health, cause antiaging, prevent chronic diseases, and increase life expectancy. Due to today's lifestyle and eating habits, there is a need to maintain healthy living. There are various strategies designed to combat diseases using pharmaceuticals, but there is an alternative known as nutraceuticals, which is a diet-based strategy to prevent diseases. Driven by the increasing demand for new food products and to strengthen the qualitative ingredients, the functional food market needs to administer these nutraceuticals to the consumers with specific and selective target delivery and minimum side effects. This can be improvised using nanotechnology. The nanoparticle delivery system is a system in which nanocarriers are used to encapsulate bioactive compounds and delivery these compounds to specific target. But this nanoprocessing does not affect the chemical structure or nutritional value of the food. The various applications of nanotechnology in food and nutrition are to design and develop the novel functional food ingredients with improved water solubility, thermal stability, oral bioavailability, sensory attributes, and physiological performance.

Keywords: Nutraceuticals, nanotechnology, nano-delivery systems, nanoprocessing, challenges, nanoparticles, micelles, nanomaterials

**Corresponding author*: sahmed@unipune.ac.in; shadabghazi@gmail.com

Rajesh K. Kesharwani, Tingirikari Jagan Mohan Rao and Raj K. Keservani (eds.) Prebiotics and Probiotics in Disease Regulation and Management, (133–160) © 2022 Scrivener Publishing LLC

5.1 Introduction

People nowadays recognize the value of a well-balanced diet and intake of nutrients. The ideology stated by Hippocrates 2,500 years ago, that is "Let food be the medicine and medicine be the food" has come to major importance. Unhealthy eating habits of consumption of junk food have led to a decrease in nutritional aspects. Nutraceuticals are seen as a promising approach as they are known to prevent and cure various diseases. Nutraceuticals are the arising class of medicine, which are being preferred by the people as an alternative to costly treatments, modern medicines, and side effects of drugs. Nutraceuticals are essentially diet supplements. Stephen De Felice, chairman of the Foundation for Innovation in Medicine, coined the term nutraceutical made up of nutrition and pharmaceutical [1]. The idea of nutraceuticals was first observed in a study conducted in France, Germany, and the UK, where the people preferred a healthy diet [2]. Nutraceuticals have various bioactive compounds like amino acids, probiotics, antioxidants, fatty acids, polyphenols, carotenoids, phytosterols, and essential oils. Functional foods can be made by adding these substances in the ingredients, to provide extra health benefits [3]. Sometimes people confuse nutraceuticals with functional foods. However, the parameters like mass of consumption and volume, the boundary between a nutraceutical and functional food are not very clear. The three main components of the nutraceutical industry comprise dietary supplements, natural products, and functional foods [4, 5]. A nutraceutical can be sold in powder, pill, capsule; the bioactive component in it can be in a single or mixture of components. Nutritionally rich foods like omega-3 oil, soya, and spirulina can also be used as nutraceuticals. Mainly nutraceuticals are classified into two major groups—potential nutraceuticals and established nutraceuticals [6]. The potential nutraceutical is the one that promises to provide a specific medical or health benefit. Once enough research is conducted, and clinical data are gathered on the specific health benefit provided, then the potential nutraceutical becomes an established one. The oral route is generally the much more preferable approach for drug and nutraceutical administration since it is noninvasive and requires no specific technique or complicated instructions [7]. When it comes to adding nutraceuticals to foods, there are many restrictions. Some active substances in nutraceuticals may interact with the chemical components that may be other nutraceutical products or other drugs. The interaction could either raise or diminish the desired therapeutic impact, or it could produce a new outcome that is potentially harmful and undesirable. A few foods and therapeutic drugs, when consumed jointly, can affect the body's ability to use a drug or specific food, or induce major side effects [8]. Many other physiochemical properties and physiological mechanisms, like, restrained release from the food matrix, formation of insoluble complexes with some other elements in the gastrointestinal tract (GIT), biotransformation in the GIT, also may result in low nutraceutical bioavailability [9–12]. Most of the compounds that are used as active pharmaceutical ingredients have poor oral bioavailability due to their various characteristics. Some of these include degradability, limited permeability, high melting point, and high lipophilicity, which limit their therapeutic advantages. Various formulations have been developed for the efficient delivery of nutraceuticals. The objective of these is to enhance their solubility, improve their bioavailability, and enhance their biological activity. Nanotechnology has the potential to resolve the problem of nutraceutical delivery [13]. Nanotechnology can be defined as a growing field of interdisciplinary research focused on 1 to 100 nm particles with the goal of designing, improving, and using nanoscale structures in advanced learning [12]. There has been a growing interest in food nanotechnology since its first featured article was published back in 2003. Nanotechnology applications have also begun to have an impact on several parts of the nutraceutical, food, and pharmaceutical industries, as evidenced by a variety of papers, evaluations, patent filings, and corporate goods [14]. Governments, academia, and the private sector in the United States, Europe, Japan, and other countries around the world have launched numerous nanotechnology initiatives, commissions, or establishments to ensure rapid development and implementation of nanotechnology, to stimulate economic development, maintain global competitiveness, and work on improving innovative capability [15, 16]. The food industry suffers from significant losses due to food wastage. A major cause of food wastage is microbial contamination and food spoilage, which affects the quality and security of food, causes food products to lose shelf life and increases the risks of foodborne illness. There are many applications of nanotechnology for the food industry in food production, processing, storage, and distribution [17]. Nanomaterials' unique qualities open up lots of new possibilities for the food industry [18, 19]. Various forms of functional nanostructures can be used as building blocks to develop innovative structures and add new functions to foods. The term "nanoceuticals" is becoming more popular, and commercial dairy/food and food supplements that contain nanoparticles are now available. Carotenoids nanoparticles can be diffused in water that improves its bioavailability, and nanotechnology systems protect the B- carotene from degradation [20].

And some other examples of nanofoods are nanotea (Shenzhen Become Industry Trading Co. Guangdong, China), fortified fruit juice (High Vive.com, USA), oat nutritional drink (assorted flavors, Toddler Health, Los Angeles, USA), nanocapsules containing tuna fish oil (a source of omega 3 fatty acids), NanoSlim beverage (NanoSlim), Nanoceuticals Slim Shake (assorted flavors, RBC Lifesciences, Irving, USA), "Daily Vitamin Boost" fortified fruit juice (Jamba Juice Hawaii, USA), "Tip-Top" Up bread (Enfield, Australia) [21].

Inorganic and organic types of substances are employed as nanomaterials in food products. The type of nanomaterial has various sizes for specific molecules or crystallites, constellations. quantum dots, nanoparticles, and nanoclusters, nanorods or nanotubes, nanothin films, and nanomaterials, are some examples of zero; one, two, and three dimensions of range limit 1 to 100 nm [22–24]. Various delivery systems are developed by applying nanotechnology—polymer nanoparticles, nanostructured lipid carriers, nanoemulsions, nanoliposomes, solid lipid nanoparticles, and nanosuspension.

Nutraceuticals are administered orally. They having a target-specific effect, they need to be delivered to that target without any change in the formulation of the bioactive component. Solubility of nutraceuticals and their efficient delivery are the main target to use nanotechnology delivery systems. If these bioactive components are not successfully delivered, it can affect in various ways:

1) Poor water solubility can limit the range of formulations available for a bioactive compound.
2) Poorly soluble compounds are likely to have limited bioavailability because they do not remain in solution at the site of action, once in the body. This leads to lower absorption and decreased efficiency.
3) Thus, to overcome this, high dosages of nutraceuticals are administered, which can have adverse side effects. Thus, there is a change in the formulation, which increases the cost and nutrients for both manufacturer and consumer.

To overcome these problems, we use nanodelivery targets which increase bioavailability, solubility and longer storage protection, and shelf life [6].

Nanomaterials provide a larger surface/volume ratio because of their smaller size. This leads to an increase in bioavailability, solubility, encapsulation efficiency, stability, sustained and site-specific drug delivery, protection against degradation and microbial contamination, and improved pharmacological activity, like pharmacodynamics, pharmacokinetics, site-specific delivery, and controlled release of these bioactive compounds [25, 26].

The main mechanisms involved in the enhanced bioactive molecules absorption by polymeric nanoparticles are:

1) provide security to the bioactive molecule from the harsh environment of the gastrointestinal tract,
2) longer retention in the gut by mucoadhesion,
3) endocytosis of the particles,
4) permeabilizing effect of the polymer [27].

5.2 Delivery System

The nanotechnology platforms are mostly employed to create delivery systems for nutraceuticals that have a low solubility in water. The use of nanoscale delivery systems could help nutraceuticals increase and improve their functionality as the delivery systems mentioned in Figure 5.1. The fundamental concepts of nanotechnology are used for nanoformulations of nutraceuticals. The nanotechnology platforms are mostly employed to create delivery systems for nutraceuticals that have a low solubility in water. This technology has a great future for the commercialization of nutraceuticals with important bioactive compounds by addressing the restrictions connected with them due to this multifold growth for this technology is expected [28]. The nanodelivery system should be regarded as safe before using it in nutraceuticals to avoid any possible side effects. The preferred delivery method should be both physically and chemically stable to

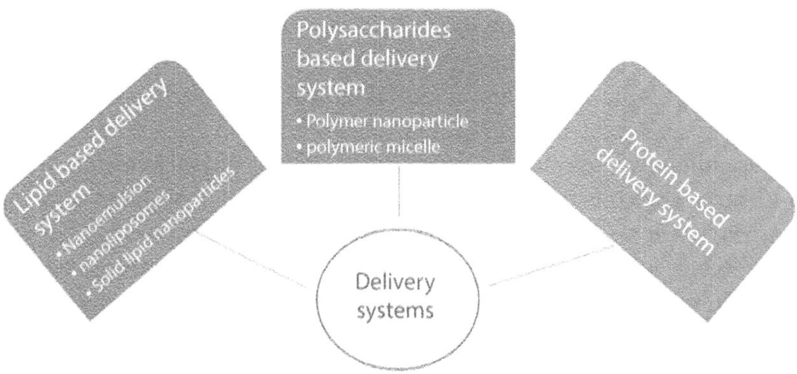

Figure 5.1 Different nanodelivery systems for neutraceuticals.

environmental stresses while serving its main purpose [29]. Gastric retention time should be increased by the preferred delivery method [30]. The gastric stability of the liable bioactive compound should be improved by the use of the preferred delivery method.

5.2.1 Lipid-Based Delivery System

5.2.1.1 Nanoemulsions

Nanoemulsion is made up of two words nano and emulsion, that is emulsions contain particles of nanosize approximately 50 to 200 nm [31]. Nanoemulsions are kinetically and thermodynamically stable systems [32]. They are transparent in nature [33]. It is a biphasic system, comprised of two immiscible liquids. If the droplet added is oil to water, then a hydrophilic emulsifier stabilizes these droplets [34]. If the water droplet is dispersed in oil, then a hydrophobic emulsifier stabilizes this droplet. Generally, the size estimated of surfactant and micelle is 2 nm and 5 nm (or more) respectively. Sometimes, the addition of the oil phase in the micellar core may lead to an increase in size. Nanoemulsions are preferable options for delivering poorly soluble weakly soluble nutraceuticals in the matrix of food. The hydrophobic bioactive component can be dissolved in the organic phase of oil-water emulsion. Double emulsions can be used for hydrophilic bioactive compounds [35].

Two types of methods can be used to produce nanoemulsifiers, high-energy process, and low energy process. The mechanical or high-energy processes are sonication, microfluidizers, and homogenizers. In addition, chemical or low energy processes are spontaneous emulsification and phase inversion temperature [34]. Freeze-drying or spray drying techniques can be used to convert nanoemulsion liquid form to powder form. Surfactants or some stabilizing agents are used to stabilize emulsions, like polysaccharides, lipids, and amphiphilic proteins [36].

These are some examples of nutraceuticals to which nanoemulsion technology was applied:Curcumin (1,7-bis(4-hydroxy-3-methoxyphenyl)-1,6-heptadiene-3,5-dione) a natural polyphenolic phytochemical, known for its large amounts of beneficial activities. The major problem with curcumin is that at acidic or neutral pH, it is not soluble in water [37]. To solve this problem, a large number of studies were conducted. Encapsulation of curcumin in oil in water emulsion resulted in increased anti-inflammatory activity. The anti-inflammatory activity was further enhanced when the size of emulsion droplets was brought down below 100 nm in TPA-induced acute mouse ear edema [38, 39]. In the model organism, *Caenorhabditis elegans,* it was observed that by using corn oil in nanoemulsion and in an increase in nanoemulsion droplet size, the accumulation was high [40].

Pterostilbene (trans-3,5-dimethoxy-4-hydroxystilbene), found in blueberries, is known for antioxidation and many more properties. Some polyphenols are susceptible in GIT fluid and the solubility is low. A food grade nanoemulsion was used, carrier oil choice is very important in this process, as they are used for finding out the bioavailability of the bioactive component. By using a food-grade nanoemulsion having olive oil or flaxseed oil (carrier oil) resulted in an increase in bioaccessibility, bioavailability, and metabolism of pterostilbene [41]. Resveratrol (trans3,5,40 -trihydroxystilbene) has many valuable properties. To provide protection against degradation, a spontaneous emulsification method was used, in the oil phase, orange and grade seed oil was used, and surfactant, 10% each, and remaining was the aqueous phase 80% [42].

The same delivery method was applied on β-carotene and tocopherol to increase pharmacological effects, oral bioavailability, and bioaccessibility [43, 44].

5.2.1.2 Nanoliposomes

Liposomes are vesicles made up of lipid bilayers with both hydrophilic and hydrophobic lipid tails as shown in Figure 5.2. If liposomes are used as a delivery system for bioactive components, leakage problems could be faced due to the environmental conditions faced in the gastrointestinal tract. To solve the stability problem, various studies were conducted. Enhancement of stability is done by doing some surface modifications like silica external-layered liposomes [45, 46], poly (ethylene glycol)-surface-conjugated liposomes [47], chitosan-coated liposomes [48], and protein site-specific modified liposomes [49]. Generally, the hydrophobic nutraceuticals are trapped in the lipid bilayer and the hydrophilic nutraceuticals are trapped in the core. Nanoliposomes are nanoscale forms of liposomes [50]. Nanoliposomes have high bioavailability and physical stability as compared with liposomes because of their small size so accordingly larger surface area. Due to the properties like biodegradability and biocompatibility of nanoliposomes, they are numerous applications in the food industry. Nanoliposomes are made up of nontoxic phospholipids. Oral, topical, and parenteral can be the routes of administration of nanoliposomes [51]. Both hydrophilic and hydrophobic types of components can be delivered by the nanoliposomes due to their biocompatibility and bioavailability properties and protect them from enzymatic degradation.

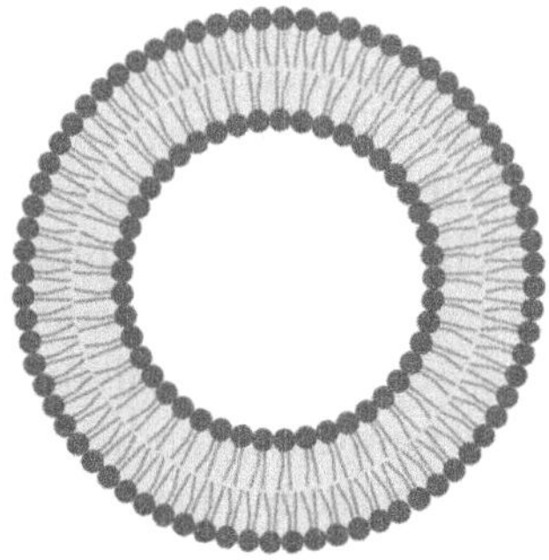

Figure 5.2 Nanoliposome arrangement or assembly.

5.2.1.3 Solid Lipid Nanoparticles (SLN) and Nanostructured Lipid Carriers (NLC)

Solid lipid nanoparticles are frequently made up of synthetic or natural lipid molecules, as shown in Figure 5.3. The synthetic lipid molecules used can be triacylglycerol, glyceryl monostearate, and lecithin. These lipid molecules are used as matrix core to trap the bioactive compounds. These solid lipid nanoparticles are the same as oil in water emulsions, as the lipid matrix core is hydrophobic in nature and the shell is hydrophilic in nature, and they are solid at RT [52]. This system has many advantages like protection of bioactive compounds from the outside environment, stability of the bioactive compound is confirmed, it can encapsulate both types of drugs that are hydrophilic and lipophilic, and controls the release of bioactive compounds. Nevertheless, high water content, aggregation, flocculation, and large particle size and sometimes the bioactive compound may get released while its storage [53]. There are some disadvantages of this method, leakage of bioactive components, aggregation, and low loading capacity [54]. NLC can overcome the disadvantages of SLN [55].

These are some examples of nutraceuticals to which solid lipid nanoparticles delivery system was applied:

Anthocyanin is the class of flavonoids, has antioxidant properties, which makes them a valuable bioactive compound, and is highly in demand as nutraceuticals. This delivery system was used to protect anthocyanin from severe environmental conditions and to increase the stability toward extreme pH [56]. NLCs can be used to increase the bioavailability and water solubility of bioactive.

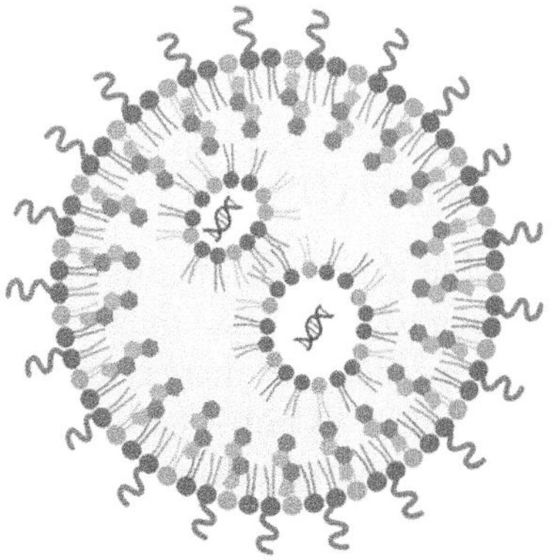

Figure 5.3 Solid lipid nanoparticle.

Caffeine (1,3,7-trimethylxanthine) has various valuable properties like anticancerous properties. And they can also protect skin from skin cancer caused by UV light. This delivery system was used to enhance the permeation of caffeine through the skin [57].

Hesperetin (a 4′-methoxy derivative of eriodictyol), has anti-inflammatory and antioxidant properties. SLN delivery method was used, and which was able to overcome the poor solubility problem, and was also able to efficiently mask the bitter and after taste [58]. This SLN method was also applied for resveratrol to enhance its stability, intestinal permeability, protection, and cytotoxicity against C6 glioma cells [56, 57] and on curcumin to increase its activity of oxygen scavenging [59].

Coenzyme Q10 (ubiquinone) is a powerful bioactive component. But it is not soluble in water. Using a high-pressure homogenizer the CoQ10-NLC, and resulted in increased bioavailability [60].

5.2.2 Polysaccharide-Based Delivery System

For encapsulation of the bioactive compounds, the naturally present polysaccharides are preferred as they are adequate in nature and cheaply available. Polysaccharides can be used to deliver both hydrophilic and hydrophobic bioactive components [61]. They are most preferred due to properties like biocompatibility, stable structure, nontoxic in nature, hydrophilic in nature, and have some reactive sites for chemical modification to take place [62].

5.2.2.1 *Polymeric Nanoparticle*

They are solid carriers able to adsorb the bioactive component, disperse it, encapsulate it and attach to its matrix. They were able to efficiently display some important properties like increased loading efficiency, better stability, and controlled release of nutraceutical's main bioactive components [63]. By modifying the pharmacokinetic parameters, they are able to protect the bioactive compound from degradation and control its release [64]. To encapsulate the bioactive compounds the most commonly used polymers are pectin, poly D, L-lactic-coglycolide, hydroxypropyl methylcellulose, starch, dextran, and chitosan [65, 66].

These are some examples of nutraceuticals to which a polymer nanoparticle delivery system was applied:

Glycyrrhizic acid (triterpentine saponin) isolated from *Glycyrrhiza glabra* having several health benefits like antiulcer, antiviral, antiallergic, anti-inflammatory properties. But, it has problems like less solubility due to which bioavailability also decreases. To overcome such problems, they used polymer nanoparticles as a delivery system. The polymer nanoparticles were made from chitosan-katira gum. This resulted in an increase in oral bioavailability and anti-inflammatory properties [67]. And by using chitosan nanoparticles, the increase in antibacterial activity was observed [68].

Lutein is a natural carotenoid, present in plants naturally. It has anticancer, anti-inflammatory, and antioxidant properties. But the problem with lutein is that it has poor solubility. To overcome this problem of poor solubility, the polymeric nanoparticles were made with chitosan and poly-γ-glutamic acid. By using this method, a significant increase in solubility of lutein was observed [69]. And chitosan and dextran sulphate made nanoparticles were used and an increase in chemical stability was observed [70].

Quercetin is a pigment present in plants, which has antibacterial, anti-inflammatory, and antioxidant properties. However, to use quercetin, there are some problems with it that should be taken into consideration like poor water solubility and lipid solubility due to its hydrophilic phenolic hydroxyl and lipophilic benzene ring. Poly(lactic-co-glycolic acid)-d-α-tocopheryl polyethylene glycol 1000 succinate made nanoparticles were used to overcome this problem, and this resulted in increased therapeutic activity and liver targeting of the liver [71].

The same method was used for melatonin, the polymeric nanoparticles were made up of poly (D, L-lactide-coglycolide), polyvinyl alcohol, lecithin, and chitosan which resulted in controlled release of the melatonin and improved epithelialization of the wound [72, 73].

5.2.2.2 *Polymeric Micelle*

The micellar system is extensively to encapsulate nutraceuticals. In this system, a head region that is hydrophilic, which stabilizes the core region (hydrophobic in nature) on the aqueous solution and in turn increases the water solubility. The drug is trapped in the hydrophobic core region [74]. Critical micelle concentration (CMC) is a concentration above which the micelle is formed. Critical micellization temperature (CMT), above certain temperature micelles, exists [75]. The polymeric micelle is found to have low CMC and stable even below CMC concentrations [76]. The high drug-loading capacity of bioactive compounds enhances water solubility and reduces toxicity. Various types of copolymers are used for polymeric micelle preparation—poly(ethylene glycol)-b-poly(lactide-co-glycolic acid), poly(ethylene glycol)-b-PCL (PEG-PCL), poloxamers, poly(ethylene glycol)-b-poly(lactide-co-glycolic acid), and poly(ethylene glycol)-b-poly(D,L-lactide) [64].

These are some examples of nutraceuticals to which a polymeric micelle delivery system was applied:

Capsaicin (8-methyl-N-vanillyl-6-nonenamide) is an active compound present in chili peppers, which belong to plants of the genus Capsicum. Capsaicin has much therapeutic activity like antioxidant, anti-inflammatory and anticancer. Capsaicin-loaded micelle was prepared by phospholipid, sodium cholate, and PVP K30 to increase oral bioavailability and prolonged plasma circulation [77].

5.2.3 Protein-Based Delivery System

The sources to obtain protein nanoparticles are animal, plant, fungal, and bacteria sources. This delivery system is also applicable to deliver both hydrophilic and hydrophobic nutraceuticals. The commonly used protein carriers from animal sources are casein, gelatin, albumin, and collagen, elastin, from plants wheat gliadin, zein, and soy glycinin [78]. There are some techniques used to make nanoparticles precipitation, desolvation, self-assembly, and thermal gelation [79]. Controlled aggregation of proteins forms nanoparticles and hydrogels can be used for the delivery of hydrophilic compounds. Under certain conditions, some proteins can form fibrils and nanotubes; they also can be used to deliver hydrophilic nutraceuticals. Electrostatic complexation or covalent conjugation between proteins can result in formation of protein-polysaccharide nanoconjugates and can be used to deliver both hydrophilic and hydrophobic bioactive components [79].

5.3 Advantages of Nanotechnology in Nutraceuticals

Advantages of using nanotechnology in nutraceuticals:

i. Enhancement of bioavailability by decreasing the interaction with charged molecules in the gastrointestinal track [80],
ii. Soluble enhancement,
iii. Improved functionality,
iv. Improved sensory attributes like taste and appearance and smell,
v. Environmental protection against light and moisture,
vi. Improved metabolic stability [81],
vii. Sustained action,
viii. Safe for consumption,
ix. Protection against oxidation,
x. Maintenance of volatile ingredients,
xi. Targeted drug delivery,
xii. Lessening in the magnitude of exploited core-shell substantial,
xiii. Fast dissociation and great intracellular endorsement.

5.4 Why are Nanoparticles or Nanomaterials Used?

With increasing efficiency of solubilization, stabilization, encapsulation, and delivery of nutraceuticals or bioactive compounds based on nanotechnology lead to properties, such as the increase in absorption of the bioactive compound at lower dosages, reduction in the frequency of dose administration, and improved therapeutic index.

5.5 Applications and Advantages of Nanotechnology to Improve the Specific Quality

i. The flavanol quercetin is the most commonly found flavonoid in onion, apple, broccoli, tea, and red wine. It has several benefits like antiobesity, antioxidant, anti-inflammatory, and anticancerous products can be obtained. Quercetin encapsulation in cyclodextrins and preservation leads to better protection from UV irradiation, and also, there was an increase in its photostability when encapsulated in drug-in-cyclodextrins-in liposomes [82].

ii. Omega-3 and omega-6 polyunsaturated fatty acids (PUFAs) are important for the maintenance of good health. Thus, to improve its physiochemical characteristics covalent conjugate (sodium caseinate and maltodextrin) and a combination of polyunsaturated lipids protected PUFAs against oxidation and their solubility in an aqueous medium increased [83].

iii. Omega-3 PUFA-rich fish oil was nanoemulsified using natural polymeric proteins isolated from sesame meal (which is a potent nutraceutical) and providing better shelf-life stability, *in vitro* digestibility, and oxidative stability [84].

iv. Phenolic compounds obtained from plant-derived products are health promoters mostly concerning antioxidant properties. But they show poor bioavailability, thus poorly absorbed and rapidly metabolized and eliminated. Thus, the use of solid-liquid nanoparticles was administered to overcome these pharmacokinetic limitations [85].

v. Microvesicles from Gram-positive bacteria with bilayer structure and 10–400 nm diameter can be considered GRAS and thus used as a nanodelivery system for adhesion protein. It also enhances the chance of membrane permeability [86].

vi. Folic acid is a synthetic vitamin added to food and food products to keep the red blood cells healthy. During processing and storage of food, it loses its efficiency, thus higher dosages are administered, which have adverse side effects. Hence, mesoporous silica particles are used to encapsulate folic acid thus, increasing vitamin stability and its bioaccessibility [87].

vii. Beta-carotene is a major carotenoid present in the diet which has pro-vitamin A activity and is also associated with immunity. But it has poor water solubility, thus oil in water nanoemulsion was used which increased bioaccessibility and lipid digestion rate [88].

Specific nutraceuticals and their nano-delivery system and added advantages are mentioned in Table 5.1.

Table 5.1 Typical nanodelivery systems used for specific nutraceuticals and their added advantages for doing so.

Nanodelivery system		Nutraceutical	Advantages
Solid liquid nanoparticles	Anthocyanin SLNs	Palmitic acid, span 85, egg lecithin	Increased stability
	Hesperidin SLNs	Steric acid, glyceryl behenate, oleic acid, Tween 80	Can mask bitter taste and overcome poor solubility of hesperetin
	Resveratrol SLNs	Cetyl palmitate, polysorbate 60, miglyol-812	Validated for trans-resveratrol protection, stabilization and intestinal permeability
	Curcumin SLNs	Tween 80	Effective oxygen scavenging activity
	Caffeine SLNs	Softisan, pluronic F68	Increased permeation through skin
Liposomes	Coenzyme Q10 liposome and SLNs	Lipoid S100 and Compritol® 888 ATO	Enhanced topical delivery
Nanostructured lipid carriers	Green tea extract, nanostructured lipid carrier (NLC)	Cetyl palmitate, glyceryl stearate, grape seed oil, sea buckhorn oil	Increased antioxidant activity
Nanoemulsion	Curcumin nanoemulsion	Tween 20	Controlled lipid digestion rate and free fatty acid adsorption
	Beta carotene-based nanoemulsion	Tween 20	Higher optical clarity and increased bioavailability

(Continued)

Table 5.1 Typical nanodelivery systems used for specific nutraceuticals and their added advantages for doing so. (*Continued*)

Nanodelivery system		Nutraceutical	Advantages
Micelles	Vitamin D3 micelle	Carboxymethyl chitosan-soy protein	Enhanced encapsulation and controlled release
	Capsaicin polymeric micelles	Phospholipid, sodium cholate and PVP K30	Prolonged plasma circulation with increased oral bioavailability
	Reassembled casein micelle and casein nanoparticles	Omega 3-fatty acid	Protection against cardiovascular diseases
Nanohydrogels	Caffeine nanohydrogels	Lactoferrin-glycomacropeptide	Increased permeation through skin
	Curcumin nanohydrogel nanoparticles	Hydrolysed tetramethyl orthosilicate, chitosan, PEG 400	Increased antimicrobial and wound healing
Nanoparticles	Lutein NPs	Zein/soluble soybean polysaccharide	Enhanced *in vitro* bioaccessibility
	Kaempferol NPs	Polyvinylpyrrolidone K-17PF	Improved ocular delivery
	Lycopene NPs	Chitosan	Enhanced cellular accumulation
	Naringenin NPs	Chitosan	Increased nose to brain delivery
	Naringenin NPs	Beta-lactoglobulin	Enhanced bioavailability by supportive crystallization

(*Continued*)

Table 5.1 Typical nanodelivery systems used for specific nutraceuticals and their added advantages for doing so. (*Continued*)

Nanodelivery system		Nutraceutical	Advantages
	5-demethylnobiletin NPs	Unsaturated fatty acids	Enhanced trans-intestinal uptake
	Genistein NPs	Eudragit	Increased bioavailability
	Green tea catechins NPs	Chitosan	Enhanced intestinal absorption and bioavailability
	Caffeine nanoparticles	PLGA	Increase in endurance of dopaminergic neurons, fibre growth and expression of tyrosine hydrolase
	Apigenin NPs	PLGA	Ameliorative potentials in combating skin cancer
	Coenzyme Q10 NPs	PLGA	Increased oral bioavailability and antioxidant property
	Coenzyme Q10 NPs	Brij 78 and/ or Tween 20	Enhanced stability
	Apigenin NPS	Mesoporous silica	Improved solubility and bioavailability
	Thymoquinone NPs	Chitosan	Increased brain targeting through nasal route

(*Continued*)

Table 5.1 Typical nanodelivery systems used for specific nutraceuticals and their added advantages for doing so. (*Continued*)

Nanodelivery system		Nutraceutical	Advantages
	Quercetin NPs	Bovine Serum Albumin (BSA)	Prolonged quercetin release and improved antioxidant properties
	Thymoquinone NPs	Poly(styrene-B-ethylene oxide)	Increased antitumor activity
	Bromelain NPs	Katira gum	Increased anti-inflammatory activity
Polymeric NPs	Lutein polymeric NPs	Poly-γ-glutamic acid, chitosan	Increased solubility
	Melatonin polymeric NPs	Poly (D, L-lactide-coglycolide), polyvinyl alcohol	Sustained release
	Glycyrrhizic acid polymeric NPs	Chitosan, katira gum	Increased anti-inflammatory activity
SNEDDS	Resveratrol SNEDDS	Alpha tocopherol	Improved bioavailability

viii. Enzymes, antibodies, antigens, glycoproteins, polysaccharides encapsulated in nanostructures can be used as biosensors for detecting microbial and chemical spoilage of food [25].

5.6 Challenges Faced During Production of Nutraceuticals Using Nanotechnology

The utilization of nanotechnology in nutraceuticals and food-based products is still in the initial stages of development [89]. The problems can be with respect to:

1) Need for more detailed research
   Although nanotechnology is used to resolve the problems of bioavailability, degradation, and solubility, but these have toxicological perspectives which are serious limitations to the advancement of nanotechnology-based nutraceuticals [81].

   i. Nanoparticles or nanomaterials have a high surface area, thus they will tend to aggregate once delivered to the body;
   ii. Since it is readily observed in the body, the biological half-life is decreased with fast decreasing nanoparticles;
   iii. Higher rates of diffusion due to small size lead to non-targeted delivery, which will lead to acute or chronic toxicity and inflammation.

   The nanomaterials used can be toxic above a certain amount of dosages and its accumulation in a certain organ is of great concern, [90] thus, there is a need for specific research studies of *in vitro, in vivo* studies, and clinical trials for these nanotechnology-based nutraceuticals. For this, much can be learned from the pharmaceutical field [91, 92].

2) Public acceptance
   Although the demand for nutraceuticals has increased with an increasing number of patients, these demands can be satisfied using nanotechnological approaches. But eventually, it depends on society to accept nanotechnology-based food products. Thus, to make these successful, there is a need for *in vitro, in vivo*, and clinical trials to show this technology being harmless [93].
3) Challenges and trends while analyzing nanostructured organic materials (NOMs) [94].
1) Identify analytical method for sampling
   The nanostructured organic material has unique properties. and they do not resemble the characteristics that of normal-sized materials. Thus, while separating the NOMs from biological samples requires specific pretreatment as while separating NOMs may change their composition and size due to their high reactivity in a media [95]. Thus, we cannot access the original NOM for *in vitro* studies since

it will be digested, destroyed, or altered. Hence, there is a necessity for identifying specific analytical treatment methods for its characterization and quantitative analysis [81, 95, 96].

2) Detailed studies and dependable methods:
There is a need for a standard characterization method for NOMs and methods to study its toxicological approaches [97]. Since the NOMs are organic compounds. they are complex and will behave differently in different matrices. Thus, to study them, we will require more than one technique to characterize its type and size so that it matches the European standards of regulations [98].
3) Regulatory framework:
There is no specific international regulatory authority for the application of nanotechnology in the field of food [94]. However, the European Union has strict regulations, which can be more or less similar in the different countries [99]. The NOMs regulatory framework must have the following points:

    a) Nanomaterial definition: clear and single definition of nanomaterial-based drug,
    b) The novel food regulation internationally to make a single platform for trade and economics,
    c) The food/supplements authorization to commercialization process,
    d) Nanolabeling is demanded by European regulations to give the public choice to choose what they want and know the ingredients [94].

The European Union addresses the standardization of NOMs in food, in different parts of legislation like:

a) Regulation Registration, Evaluation, Authorization and Restriction of Chemicals (REACH). Although this regulation does not directly refer to the Nanomaterials, in 2012, the REACH guide was updated using "Safety Information and Assessment Requirements" that directly affect the nanomaterials.
b) Regulation 1169/2011 on the provision of food information provided to the consumer.

c) Regulation (EU) 2283/2015: approved in 2015 by the European Parliament and the European Council, refers to new foods and provides legal security in this area. This regulation contains the definitions of nanomaterials too.
d) Regulation (EC) 1333/2008 for food additives.
e) Directive no. 46/2002/CE for food supplements.
f) Regulation (EC) 1925/2006 for fortified foods
g) Regulation 609/2013 for foods with special purposes, replaced as of July 2016 with Directives 2006/141/EC, 2006/125/EC, 96/8/EC, 1999/21/EC.
h) Regulation 1924/2006 concerning nutrition and health claims in foods
i) Guide to assess the risk of the application of nanoscience and nanotechnology in food and in the food chain (Scientific Committee EFSA, 2011) (not legally binding) [100].

5.7 Conclusion and Future Prospects

There is a need for detailed study of *in vivo, in vitro*, and clinical trials for the characterization of nanomaterials. Then they can be characterized when there are specific pretreatment analytical methods without harming or disturbing the properties of nanostructured organic materials. Also, there is a need for a special regulatory framework for nanomaterials in the food industry at the international level for easy working.

References

1. DeFelice, S.L., The nutraceutical revolution: Its impact on food industry R&D. *Trends Food Sci. Technol.*, *6*, 2, 59–61, 1995.
2. Pandey, M., Verma, R.K., Saraf, S.A., Nutraceuticals: New era of medicine and health. *Asian J. Pharm. Clin. Res.*, *3*, 1, 11–15, 2010.
3. Pateiro, M., Gómez, B., Munekata, P.E., Barba, F.J., Putnik, P., Kovačević, D.B., Lorenzo, J.M., Nanoencapsulation of promising bioactive compounds to improve their absorption, stability, functionality and the appearance of the final food products. *Molecules*, *26*, 6, 1547, 2021.
4. Rishi, R.K., Nutraceutical: Borderline between food and drug. *Pharma Rev.*, 51–53, 2006.
5. Hathcock, J., Dietary supplements: How they are used and regulated. *J. Nutr.*, *131*, 3, 1114S–1117S, 2001.

6. Aklakur, M., Asharf Rather, M., Kumar, N., Nanodelivery: An emerging avenue for nutraceuticals and drug delivery. *Crit. Rev. Food Sci. Nutr.*, 56, 14, 2352–61, 2016.
7. Tomar, D., Singh, P.K., Hoque, S., Modani, S., Sriram, A., Kumar, R., Madan, J., Khatri, D., Dua, K., Amorphous systems for delivery of nutraceuticals: Challenges opportunities. *Crit. Rev. Food Sci. Nutr.* 62, 5, 1204–1221, 2022. https://doi.org/10.1080/10408398.2020.1836607.
8. Bushra, R., Aslam, N., Khan, A.Y., Food-drug interactions. *Oman Med. J.*, *26*, 2, 77, 2011.
9. Moelants, K.R., Lemmens, L., Vandebroeck, M., Van Buggenhout, S., Van Loey, A.M., Hendrickx, M.E., Relation between particle size and carotenoid bioaccessibility in carrot-and tomato-derived suspensions. *J. Agric. Food Chem.*, *60*, 48, 11995–12003, 2012.
10. D'Ambrosio, D.N., Clugston, R.D., Blaner, W.S., Vitamin A metabolism: an update. *Nutrients*, 3, 63–103, 2011.
11. Fernández-García, E., Carvajal-Lérida, I., Jarén-Galán, M., Garrido-Fernández, J., Pérez-Gálvez, A., Hornero-Méndez, D., Carotenoids bioavailability from foods: From plant pigments to efficient biological activities. *Food Res. Int.*, 46, 438–450, 2012.
12. Chen, H., Weiss, J., Shahidi, F., Nanotechnology in nutraceuticals and functional foods. *Food Technol. (Chicago)*, *60*, 3, 30–3, 2006.
13. Ramli, N.A., Ali, N., Hamzah, S., Yatim, N.I., Physicochemical characteristics of liposome encapsulation of stingless bees' propolis. *Heliyon*, *7*, 4, e06649, 2021.
14. Hurst, S., Loi, C.-M., Brodfuehrer, J., El-Kattan, A., Impact of physiological, physicochemical and biopharmaceutical factors in absorption and metabolism mechanisms on the drug oral bioavailability of rats and humans. *Expert Opin. Drug Metab. Toxicol.*, 3, 469–489, 2007.
15. Chen, L., Remondetto, G.E., Subirade, M., Food protein-based materials as nutraceutical delivery systems. *Trends Food Sci. Technol.*, *17*, 5, 272–283, 2006.
16. ETC Group. Action Group on Erosion, Technology and Concentration, *The potential impacts of nano-scale technologies on commodity markets: The implications for commodity dependent developing countries*, 2005.
17. Sperber, W.H., Introduction to the microbiological spoilage of foods and beverages, in: *Compendium of the microbiological spoilage of foods and beverages*, pp. 1–40, Springer, New York, NY, 2009.
18. Sun, Y. and Xia, Y., Shape-controlled synthesis of gold and silver nanoparticles. *Science*, *298*, 5601, 2176–2179, 2002.
19. Cho, Y.J., Kim, C.J., Kim, N. A. M. S. O. O., Kim, C.T., Park, B., Some cases in applications of nanotechnology to food and agricultural systems. *Biochip J.*, *2*, 3, 183–185, 2008.

20. Hejri, A., Khosravi, A., Gharanjig, K., Hejazi, M., Optimisation of the formulation of β-carotene loaded nanostructured lipid carriers prepared by solvent diffusion method. *Food Chem.*, *141*, 1, 117–123, 2013.
21. Sekhon, B.S., Food nanotechnology–An overview. *Nanotechnol. Sci. Appl.*, *3*, 1, 2010.
22. Arivalagan, K., Ravichandran, S., Rangasamy, K., Karthikeyan, E., Nanomaterials and its potential applications. *Int. J. Chemtech Res.*, *3*, 2, 534–538, 2011.
23. Gorain, B., Choudhury, H., Nair, A.B., Dubey, S.K., Kesharwani, P., Theranostic application of nanoemulsions in chemotherapy. *Drug Discovery Today*, *25*, 7, 1174–1188, 2020.
24. Hochella Jr., M.F., Nanoscience and technology: the next revolution in the Earth sciences. *Earth Planet. Sci. Lett.*, *203*, 2, 593–605, 2002.
25. Singh, A.R., Desu, P.K., Nakkala, R.K., Kondi, V., Devi, S., Alam, M.S., Hamid, H., Athawale, R.B., Kesharwani, P., Nanotechnology-based approaches applied to nutraceuticals. *Drug Deliv. Transl. Res.*, 12, 3, 485–499, 2022. https://doi.org/10.1007/s13346-021-00960-3
26. Acosta, E., Bioavailability of nanoparticles in nutrient and nutraceutical delivery. *Curr. Opin. Colloid Interface Sci.*, 14, 1, 3–15, 2009.
27. des Rieux, A., Fievez, V., Garinot, M., Schneider, Y.J., Préat, V., Nanoparticles as potential oral delivery systems of proteins and vaccines: A mechanistic approach. *J. Controlled Release*, 116, 1, 1–27, 2006.
28. Augustin, M.A. and Hemar, Y., Nano-and micro-structured assemblies for encapsulation of food ingredients. *Chem. Soc. Rev.*, *38*, 4, 902–912, 2009.
29. McClements, D.J., Advances in fabrication of emulsions with enhanced functionality using structural design principles. *Curr. Opin. Colloid Interface Sci.*, *17*, 5, 235–245, 2012.
30. Ting, Y.W., Jiang, Y., Ho, C.T., Huang, Q.R., Common delivery systems for enhancing *in vivo* bioavailability and biological efficacy of nutraceuticals. *J. Funct. Foods*, 7, 112–128, 2014.
31. Ali, A., Ansari, V.A., Ahmad, U., Akhtar, J., Jahan, A., Nanoemulsion: An advanced vehicle for efficient drug delivery. *Drug Res.*, *67*, 11, 617–631, 2017.
32. Qadir, A., Faiyazuddin, M.D., Hussain, M.T., Alshammari, T.M., Shakeel, F., Critical steps and energetics involved in a successful development of a stable nanoemulsion. *J. Mol. Liq.*, *214*, 7–18, 2016.
33. Solans, C., Izquierdo, P., Nolla, J., Azemar, N., Garcia-Celma, M.J., Nano-emulsions. *Curr. Opin. Colloid Interface Sci.*, *10*, 3-4, 102–110, 2005.
34. McClements, D.J. and Rao, J., Food-grade nanoemulsions: formulation, fabrication, properties, performance, biological fate, and potential toxicity. *Crit. Rev. Food Sci. Nutr.*, *51*, 4, 285–330, 2011.
35. Sapei, L., Naqvi, M.A., Rousseau, D., Stability and release properties of double emulsions for food applications. *Food Hydrocolloids*, *27*, 2, 316–323, 2012.

36. Guzey, D. and McClements, D.J., Formation, stability and properties of multilayer emulsions for application in the food industry. *Adv. Colloid Interface Sci.*, 128–30, 227–48, 2006.
37. Maiti, K., Mukherjee, K., Gantait, A., Saha, B.P., Mukherjee, P.K., Curcumin–phospholipid complex: Preparation, therapeutic evaluation and pharmacokinetic study in rats. *Int. J. Pharm.*, *330*, 1-2, 155–163, 2007.
38. Wang, X., Jiang, Y., Wang, Y.W., Huang, M.T., Ho, C.T., Huang, Q., Enhancing anti-inflammation activity of curcumin through O/W nanoemulsions. *Food Chem.*, *108*, 2, 419–424, 2008.
39. Chen, J. and Hu, L., Nanoscale delivery system for nutraceuticals: Preparation, application, characterization, safety, and future trends. *Food Eng. Rev.*, *12*, 1, 14–31, 2020.
40. Shen, P., Zhang, R., McClements, D.J., Park, Y., Nanoemulsion-based delivery systems for testing nutraceutical efficacy using Caenorhabditis elegans: Demonstration of curcumin bioaccumulation and body-fat reduction. *Food Res. Int.*, *120*, 157–166, 2019.
41. Sun, Y., Xia, Z., Zheng, J., Qiu, P., Zhang, L., McClements, D.J., Xiao, H., Nanoemulsion-based delivery systems for nutraceuticals: Influence of carrier oil type on bioavailability of pterostilbene. *J. Funct. Foods*, *13*, 61–70, 2015.
42. Davidov-Pardo, G. and McClements, D.J., Nutraceutical delivery systems: Resveratrol encapsulation in grape seed oil nanoemulsions formed by spontaneous emulsification. *Food Chem.*, *167*, 205–212, 2015.
43. Rao, J., Decker, E.A., Xiao, H., McClements, D.J., Nutraceutical nanoemulsions: influence of carrier oil composition (digestible versus indigestible oil) on β-carotene bioavailability. *J. Sci. Food Agric.*, *93*, 13, 3175–3183, 2013.
44. Hatanaka, J., Chikamori, H., Sato, H., Uchida, S., Debari, K., Onoue, S., Yamada, S., Physicochemical and pharmacological characterization of α-tocopherol-loaded nano-emulsion system. *Int. J. Pharm.*, *396*, 1-2, 188–193, 2010.
45. Li, C., Zhang, Y., Su, T., Feng, L., Long, Y., Chen, Z., Silica-coated flexible liposomes as a nanohybrid delivery system for enhanced oral bioavailability of curcumin. *Int. J. Nanomed.*, *7*, 5995, 2012.
46. Liu, W., Liu, J., Liu, W., Li, T., Liu, C., Improved physical and *in vitro* digestion stability of a polyelectrolyte delivery system based on layer-by-layer self-assembly alginate–chitosan-coated nanoliposomes. *J. Agric. Food Chem.*, *61*, 17, 4133–4144, 2013.
47. Mineart, K.P., Kelley, E.G., Nagao, M., Prabhu, V.M., Processing–structure relationships of poly (ethylene glycol)-modified liposomes. *Soft Matter*, *13*, 31, 5228–5232, 2017.
48. Gibis, M., Ruedt, C., Weiss, J., *In vitro* release of grape-seed polyphenols encapsulated from uncoated and chitosan-coated liposomes. *Food Res. Int.*, *88*, 105–113, 2016.

49. Foteini, P. *et al.*, Physicochemical study of the protein–liposome interactions: Influence of liposome composition and concentration on protein binding. *J. Liposome Res.*, 29, 4, 313–321, 2019.
50. Mozafari, R.M., *Nanoliposomes: From fundamentals to recent developments*, Trafford, Iran, 2005.
51. Shoji, Y. and Nakashima, H., Nutraceutics and delivery systems. *J. Drug Targeting*, *12*, 6, 385–391, 2004.
52. Lin, C.H., Chen, C.H., Lin, Z.C., Fang, J.Y., Recent advances in oral delivery of drugs and bioactive natural products using solid lipid nanoparticles as the carriers. *J. Food Drug Anal.*, *25*, 2, 219–234, 2017.
53. Das, S. and Chaudhury, A., Recent advances in lipid nanoparticle formulations with solid matrix for oral drug delivery. *AAPS Pharmscitech*, *12*, 1, 62–76, 2011.
54. da Silva Santos, V., Ribeiro, A.P.B., Santana, M.H.A., Solid lipid nanoparticles as carriers for lipophilic compounds for applications in foods. *Food Res. Int.*, *122*, 610–626, 2019.
55. Fathi, M., Mozafari, M.R., Mohebbi, M., Nanoencapsulation of food ingredients using lipid based delivery systems. *Trends Food Sci. Technol.*, *23*, 1, 13–27, 2012.
56. Ravanfar, R., Tamaddon, A.M., Niakousari, M., Moein, M.R., Preservation of anthocyanins in solid lipid nanoparticles: Optimization of a microemulsion dilution method using the Placket–Burman and Box–Behnken designs. *Food Chem.*, *199*, 573–580, 2016.
57. Puglia, C., Offerta, A., Tirendi, G.G., Tarico, M.S., Curreri, S., Bonina, F., Perrotta, R.E., Design of solid lipid nanoparticles for caffeine topical administration. *Drug Deliv.*, *23*, 1, 36–40, 2016.
58. Fathi, M., Varshosaz, J., Mohebbi, M., Shahidi, F., Hesperetin-loaded solid lipid nanoparticles and nanostructure lipid carriers for food fortification: preparation, characterization, and modeling. *Food Bioprocess Technol.*, *6*, 6, 1464–1475, 2013.
59. Neves, A.R., Martins, S., Segundo, M.A., Reis, S., Nanoscale delivery of resveratrol towards enhancement of supplements and nutraceuticals. *Nutrients*, *8*, 3, 131, 2016.
60. Vijayakumar, M.R., Kumari, L., Patel, K.K., Vuddanda, P.R., Vajanthri, K.Y., Mahto, S.K., Singh, S., Intravenous administration of trans-resveratrol-loaded TPGS-coated solid lipid nanoparticles for prolonged systemic circulation, passive brain targeting and improved *in vitro* cytotoxicity against C6 glioma cell lines. *RSC Adv.*, *6*, 55, 50336–50348, 2016.
61. Liu, G.Y., Wang, J.M., Xia, Q., Application of nanostructured lipid carrier in food for the improved bioavailability. *Eur. Food Res. Technol.*, *234*, 3, 391–398, 2012.
62. Krausz, A.E., Adler, B.L., Cabral, V., Navati, M., Doerner, J., Charafeddine, R.A., Friedman, A.J., Curcumin-encapsulated nanoparticles as innovative

antimicrobial and wound healing agent. *Nanomed.: Nanotechnol. Biol. Med.*, *11*, 1, 195–206, 2015.

63. Renard, D., Robert, P., Lavenant, L., Melcion, D., Popineau, Y., Gueguen, J., Schmitt, C., Biopolymeric colloidal carriers for encapsulation or controlled release applications. *Int. J. Pharm.*, *242*, 1-2, 163–166, 2002.
64. Sinha, V.R. and Kumria, R., Polysaccharides in colon-specific drug delivery. *Int. J. Pharm.*, *224*, 1-2, 19–38, 2001.
65. Shin, G.H., Kim, J.T., Park, H.J., Recent developments in nanoformulations of lipophilic functional foods. *Trends Food Sci. Technol.*, *46*, 1, 144–157, 2015.
66. Mehanny, M., Hathout, R.M., Geneidi, A.S., Mansour, S., Exploring the use of nanocarrier systems to deliver the magical molecule; curcumin and its derivatives. *J. Controlled Release*, *225*, 1–30, 2016.
67. Emeje, M.O., Obidike, I.C., Akpabio, E.I., Ofoefule, S.I., Nanotechnology in drug delivery, in: *Recent advances in novel drug carrier systems*, pp. 69–106, 2012.
68. Bernela, M., Ahuja, M., Thakur, R., Enhancement of anti-inflammatory activity of glycyrrhizic acid by encapsulation in chitosan-katira gum nanoparticles. *Eur. J. Pharm. Biopharm. : Official Journal of Arbeitsgemeinschaft fur PharmazeutischeVerfahrenstechnike.V*, *105*, 141–147, 2016, https://doi.org/10.1016/j.ejpb.2016.06.003.
69. Rani, R., Dilbaghi, N., Dhingra, D., Kumar, S., Optimization and evaluation of bioactive drug-loaded polymeric nanoparticles for drug delivery. *Int. J. Biol. Macromol.*, *78*, 173–179, 2015, https://doi.org/10.1016/j.ijbiomac.2015.03.070.
70. Hong, D.Y., Lee, J.S., Lee, H.G., Chitosan/poly-γ-glutamic acid nanoparticles improve the solubility of lutein. *Int. J. Biol. Macromol.*, *85*, 9–15, 2016, https://doi.org/10.1016/j.ijbiomac.2015.12.044.
71. Chaiyasan, W. A. N. A. C. H. A. T., Srinivas, S.P., Tiyaboonchai, W. A. R. E. E., Development and characterization of topical ophthalmic formulations containing lutein-loaded mucoadhesive nanoparticles. *Int. J. Pharm. Pharm. Sci.*, *8*, 3, 261–266, 2016.
72. Guan, X., Gao, M., Xu, H., Zhang, C., Liu, H., Lv, L., Tian, Y., Quercetin-loaded poly (lactic-co-glycolic acid)-d-α-tocopheryl polyethylene glycol 1000 succinate nanoparticles for the targeted treatment of liver cancer. *Drug Delivery*, *23*, 9, 3307–3318, 2016.
73. Altındal, D. Ç. and Gümüşderelioğlu, M., Melatonin releasing PLGA micro/nanoparticles and their effect on osteosarcoma cells. *J. Microencapsulation*, *33*, 1, 53–63, 2016.
74. Blažević, F., Milekić, T., Romić, M.D., Juretić, M., Pepić, I., Filipović-Grčić, J., Hafner, A., Nanoparticle-mediated interplay of chitosan and melatonin for improved wound epithelialisation. *Carbohydr. Polym.*, *146*, 445–454, 2016.
75. Torchilin, V.P., Targeted polymeric micelles for delivery of poorly soluble drugs. *Cell. Mol. Life Sci. CMLS*, *61*, 19, 2549–2559, 2004.

76. Zhu, Y., Peng, W., Zhang, J., Wang, M., Firempong, C.K., Feng, C., Yu, J., Enhanced oral bioavailability of capsaicin in mixed polymeric micelles: Preparation, *in vitro* and *in vivo* evaluation. *J. Funct. Foods*, *8*, 358–366, 2014.
77. Assadpour, E. and Mahdi Jafari, S., A systematic review on nanoencapsulation of food bioactive ingredients and nutraceuticals by various nanocarriers. *Crit. Rev. Food Sci. Nutr.*, *59*, 19, 3129–3151, 2019, https://doi.org/10.1080/10408398.2018.1484687.
78. Elzoghby, A.O., Samy, W.M., Elgindy, N.A., Albumin-based nanoparticles as potential controlled release drug delivery systems. *J. Controlled Release*, *157*, 2, 168–182, 2012.
79. Singh, H., Nanotechnology applications in functional foods; opportunities and challenges. *Prev. Nutr. Food Sci.*, *21*, 1, 1, 2016.
80. Ali, A., Ahmad, U., Akhtar, J., Khan, M.M., Engineered nano scale formulation strategies to augment efficiency of nutraceuticals. *J. Funct. Foods*, 62, 103554, 2019.
81. Rangan, A., Manjula, M.V., Satyanarayana, K.G., Trends and methods for nanobased delivery for nutraceuticals, in: *Emulsions*, pp. 573–609, Academic Press, 2016.
82. Azzi, J., Jraij, A., Auezova, L., Fourmentin, S., Greige-Gerges, H., Novel findings for quercetin encapsulation and preservation with cyclodextrins, liposomes, and drug-in-cyclodextrin-in-liposomes. *Food Hydrocolloids*, 81, 328–340, 2018.
83. Semenova, M.G., Antipova, A.S., Zelikina, D.V., Martirosova, E.I., Plashchina, I.G., Palmina, N.P., Ozerova, N.S., Biopolymer nanovehicles for essential polyunsaturated fatty acids: Structure–functionality relationships. *Food Res. Int.*, 88, 70–78, 2016.
84. Dey, T.K., Banerjee, P., Chatterjee, R., Dhar, P., Designing of ω-3 PUFA enriched biocompatible nanoemulsion with sesame protein isolate as a natural surfactant: Focus on enhanced shelf-life stability and biocompatibility. *Colloids Surf. A: Physicochem. Eng. Asp.*, 538, 36–44, 2018.
85. Nunes, S., Madureira, A.R., Campos, D., Sarmento, B., Gomes, A.M., Pintado, M., Reis, F., Solid lipid nanoparticles as oral delivery systems of phenolic compounds: Overcoming pharmacokinetic limitations for nutraceutical applications. *Crit. Rev. Food Sci. Nutr.*, 57, 9, 1863–1873, 2017.
86. Domínguez Rubio, A.P., Martínez, J.H., Martínez Casillas, D.C., ColuccioLeskow, F., Piuri, M., Pérez, O.E., Lactobacillus casei BL23 produces microvesicles carrying proteins that have been associated with its probiotic effect. *Front. Microbiol.*, 8, 1783, 2017.
87. Ruiz-Rico, M., Pérez-Esteve, É., Lerma-García, M.J., Marcos, M.D., Martínez-Máñez, R., Barat, J.M., Protection of folic acid through encapsulation in mesoporous silica particles included in fruit juices. *Food Chem.*, 218, 471–478, 2017.

88. Salvia-Trujillo, L., Qian, C., Martín-Belloso, O., McClements, D.J., Influence of particle size on lipid digestion and β-carotene bioaccessibility in emulsions and nanoemulsions. *Food Chem.*, 141, 2, 1472–1480, 2013.
89. Sharma, S., Sudan, P., Arora, V., Goswami, M., Dorac, C.P., Nanotechnological advances for nutraceutical delivery, in: *Nanotechnology*, pp. 149–182, Jenny Stanford Publishing, 2021.
90. Livney, Y.D., Nanostructured delivery systems in food: Latest developments and potential future directions. *Curr. Opin. Food Sci.*, 3, 125–135, 2015.
91. Araiza-Calahorra, A., Akhtar, M., Sarkar, A., Recent advances in emulsion-based delivery approaches for curcumin: From encapsulation to bioaccessibility. *Trends Food Sci. Technol.*, 71, 155–169, 2018.
92. Gonçalves, R.F., Martins, J.T., Duarte, C.M., Vicente, A.A., Pinheiro, A.C., Advances in nutraceutical delivery systems: From formulation design for bioavailability enhancement to efficacy and safety evaluation. *Trends Food Sci. Technol.*, 78, 270–291, 2018.
93. Cushen, M., Kerry, J., Morris, M., Cruz-Romero, M., Cummins, E., Nanotechnologies in the food industry–Recent developments, risks and regulation. *Trends Food Sci. Technol.*, 24, 1, 30–46, 2012.
94. Benetti, F., Micheletti, C., Manodori, L., Regulatory perspectives on nanotechnology in nutraceuticals, *in: Nutraceuticals, Nanotechnology in the Agri-Food Industry, Volume 4*, A.M. Grumezescu (Ed.), Academic Press, Elsevier, London Wall, London, United Kingdom, 2016.
95. Szakal, C., Roberts, S.M., Westerhoff, P., Bartholomaeus, A., Buck, N., Illuminato, I., Rogers, M., Measurement of nanomaterials in foods: Integrative consideration of challenges and future prospects. *ACS Nano*, 8, 4, 3128–3135, 2014.
96. Peters, R., ten Dam, G., Bouwmeester, H., Helsper, H., Allmaier, G., vdKammer, F., Weigel, S., Identification and characterization of organic nanoparticles in food. *TrAC Trends Anal. Chem.*, 30, 1, 100–112, 2011.
97. Bouwmeester, H., Brandhoff, P., Marvin, H.J., Weigel, S., Peters, R.J., State of the safety assessment and current use of nanomaterials in food and food production. *Trends Food Sci. Technol.*, 40, 2, 200–210, 2014.
98. Linsinger, T., Roebben, G., Gilliland, D., Calzolai, L., Rossi, F., Gibson, N., Klein, C., *Requirements on measurements for the implementation of the European Commission definition of the term "nanomaterial"*, Publications Office of the European Union, Belgium, 2012.
99. Magnuson, B., Munro, I., Abbot, P., Baldwin, N., Lopez-Garcia, R., Ly, K., Socolovsky, S., Review of the regulation and safety assessment of food substances in various countries and jurisdictions. *Food Addit. Contam.: Part A*, 30, 7, 1147–1220, 2013.
100. Fúnez, A. Á., Duaso, A.I.H., Gómez, P.M., Nanotechnology in food industry II: Risk assessment and legislation. *Rev. Complut. Cienc. Vet.*, 10, 2, 18, 2016.

6

Challenges in Development of Prebiotic and Probiotics

Pradnya Jadhav, Sakshi Kor and Shadab Ahmed*

Institute of Bioinformatics and Biotechnology (merged with Department of Biotechnology), Savitribai Phule Pune University, Pune, India

Abstract

In recent times, the host microbiota and the microenvironment that lies there within has seen a huge leap in terms of understanding its importance, mechanism, and consequent health benefits. The research articles on gut microbiome has greatly been accumulated in recent years allowing us means to modulate gut microbiota and thereby providing us an opportunity to reap in benefits. In this chapter, we will discuss the scientific observation and inferences based on insights provided by various articles describing mechanism on how health benefits are connected to gut microbiome. The use of probiotics, prebiotics, and both of them together as synbiotic has made them a useful tool in gut microflora management. The chapter also touches on new insights and future trends like genetic manipulations, newer novel oligomers, etc., as tools for developing new generation prebiotics and probiotics and their collective use as synbiotics.

Keywords: Probiotics, prebiotics, synbiotics, gut microbiome, microflora

6.1 Introduction

Over the previous years, the production of functional food has become a major part of the food biotechnology industry. In other words, it is the need of the world to incorporate functional foods in the diet of people due to the reasons like increasing world population, enhanced healthcare services, and increased life expectancy, which ultimately leads to development

**Corresponding author*: sahmed@unipune.ac.in; shadabghazi@gmail.com

Rajesh K. Kesharwani, Tingirikari Jagan Mohan Rao and Raj K. Keservani (eds.) Prebiotics and Probiotics in Disease Regulation and Management, (161–184) © 2022 Scrivener Publishing LLC

of health-conscious customers [1]. The use of the term "functional foods" dates back to Japan which defined it as "to the processed food containing ingredients that aid specific bodily functions in addition to being nutritious" [2]. Many amendments were made later on in the definition by many governing bodies. The most widely accepted definition of the functional food was given by China State Food and Drug Administration (SFDA) in the year 2005. According to SFDA "Functional food is a food having special health functions or it is able to supply vitamins or minerals. It is suitable for consumption by specific group of people and has the function of regulating human body functions, and it will not cause any harm whether acute or subacute or chronic" [3]. The functional food category is further divided into classes like probiotics, prebiotics, and synbiotics.

6.1.1 Probiotics, Prebiotics, and Synbiotics

6.1.1.1 Probiotics

Probiotics are classified as living organisms, which include organisms like bacteria and yeasts, that have the ability to provide health benefits to the host and can be administered in adequate amounts [4]. Since the discovery of probiotics, it has often been used to treat a variety of diseases in humans. The diseases include diseases associated with brain, skin and gut microbiota [5]. The two major strains of bacteria which are considered as probiotic strains include *Lactobacillus* and *Bifidobacterium* [6]. Lactobacillus belongs to the lactic acid bacteria (LAB) family, which are most commonly used as probiotics in the food industry. LABs can be administered through ingestion and are able to survive the acidic environment of the gut. After colonization, they are able to reduce the pH of the gut, which prevents growth of pathogenic bacteria in gut [7]. The way in which probiotics works is the beneficial microorganisms colonize the areas like gastrointestinal (GI) tract and skin while offering the host with health benefits. The health benefits include regulation of hosts' immunity, protection against pathogens and sometimes energy acquisition and beneficial metabolite production [8]. Probiotics are traditionally considered as beneficial microorganisms in foods or in health supplements. The research in the field of probiotics suggested a new categorization in which the nutritive probiotics were differentiated from the therapeutic and pharmacological probiotics and the two new categories were suggested as neutribiotics and pharmabiotics [9]. Neutribiotics are probiotic microbes associated with a food, a food product or a dietary supplement with nutritive claim [10]. Pharmabiotics include pharmaceutic probiotics, which have a specific health claim against a disease.

In general terms, pharmabiotics have a specific physiological effect on a body function or have a pharmacological effect against a particular disease [11]. Kefir ointment gel prominently used to treat microbial contamination in burn wounds [12] and cosmetics for microbial contamination on the skin [13] are some of the examples of the pharmabiotics. This new categorization suggested that the categories neutribiotics and pharmabiotics under two different regulating bodies depending based upon if the product is food or a drug. The method employed by research industries all over the world to increase the efficiency of probiotics includes development of genetically engineered novel strains which express the functional gene for a particular metabolite or a gene that can improve survival [14].

6.1.1.2 Prebiotics

The most widely accepted definition of prebiotics was given by Gibson and Roberfroid in 1995 which defines prebiotic as "a nondigestible food ingredient that beneficially affects the host by selectively stimulating the growth and/or activity of one or a limited number of bacteria in the colon, and thus improving host health" [15]. The definition remain unaltered for many years until panellists in the Iinternational Scientific Association for Probiotics and Prebiotics (ISAPP) modified it to "a substrate that is selectively utilized by host microorganisms conferring health benefit" [16]. To understand the concept of prebiotics we have to consider a term known as "dysbiosis," which is a physiological condition resulting in reduction of the carbohydrate fermenting, short chain fatty acid producing bacteria and there might be presence of a gas producing pathogenic bacteria like clostridium [17]. Prebiotic compounds help in restoring these useful bacteria in a gut. In simple words, prebiotic compounds alter the beneficial gut microbiota's content and/or functioning providing the host with health advantages. Typically, the prebiotic compounds are oligosaccharides. Oligosaccharides are carbohydrates with low molecular weight having a low degree of polymerization and two to twenty monosaccharide units. There have been multiple reports in which a prebiotic is used as an additive in a food. A group of scientists studied the effect of addition of prebiotic compounds inulin and β-glucans in the cheese making process as fat replacers for the production of low-fat cheese [18]. The inclusion of inulin to yoghurt as a functional component was described by Moghadam, Keivaninahr, Fouladi, Mokarram, and Nazemi [19]. Apart from enriching the gut microbiome prebiotics are known to perform other functions as well. Short-chain fatty acid (SCFA) production can also be aided by prebiotics [20]. Prebiotics can help to improve gut health and function, lower gut pH, and lower nitrogenous metabolite levels [21].

6.1.1.3 *Synbiotics*

While explaining prebiotics, Gibson & Roberfroid also stated that probiotics and prebiotics can be combined together to form a new type of approach, which they called synbiotics. The term "synbiotics" is defined as follows: "mixtures of probiotics and prebiotics that beneficially affects the host by improving the survival and implantation of live microbial dietary supplements" [22]. A synbiotic approach should consist of a probiotic component that is a live organism in sufficient amount capable of providing advantages to the host's health and a prebiotic component, that is a compound or an additive capable of enrichment of the gut microbiome. As a result, the host's well-being and health are improved, as is the probiotic's survival and implantation in the GI tract [23]. From the introduction of synbiotics concept its definition has not changed in a way but it has been further subdivided in two approaches according to Kolida and Gibson [24]. The two approaches are termed as complementary approach and synergistic approach. In the complementary approach, selection of probiotic component and prebiotic component is mutually independent. Probiotic is chosen by considering its beneficial health effect on the host while prebiotic component is chosen by considering its effect on the population of the microbiome. As prebiotic enhances the growth and activity of microbiome, it can indirectly enhance it for the probiotic microorganism.

In synergistic approach, the selection of prebiotic is dependent on the probiotic chosen. In this case also, the probiotic is chosen by considering its beneficial health effect on the host. The selection of the prebiotic is done in a way such that it could specifically enhance the growth and activity of the probiotic microorganism chosen. Affinity of the prebiotic toward the probiotic is specifically considered in this approach and prebiotics having higher affinity for the probiotics are chosen specifically. As a part of its activity, the prebiotic could enhance the growth and activity of the other microbiome present but the effect is indirect [24]. Due to use of the prebiotics, it has been observed that the probiotic microorganisms become more tolerant to stress caused due to factors like temperature, oxygenation, and pH in the intestine.

6.1.2 History of Probiotics and Prebiotics

Probiotic is a word derived from Latin language, which means "for life." Ancient populations were using fermented products, such as cheese, yogurt, beer, and wine many years before the original concept of probiotics came into existence. It has been also reported that ancient population were aware of the therapeutic and nutritional value of the fermented foods [25]. Some reports claim that the first report for the use of products to voluntarily modify gut microbiome dates back to ancient China 500 years ago. The Chinese people used faeces for the treatment of infection and food poisoning [6]. Some reports claim that the use of fermented products to treat the disorders related to gut, dates to the time earlier than 2000 BC where Egyptians consumed fermented dairy products like "Laban Rayad" and "Laban Khed" [26]. Ancient Romans and Greek people also knew many recipes of fermented milk. A very popular delicacy "Jahurt" was consumed by people living in Balkan. Some reports claim that Indians were aware of the fermented food products 800 to 300 years BC and Turks were aware of the same in 8th Century. Certain reports describe the consumption of fermented milk drink knows as "ajran" in central Russia around 12th century. Around the 14th century, Hungary developed another fermented product "tarho" for consumption [27].

If we consider the modern probiotic history, since the last 50 years, the utilization of certain bacteria strains to achieve specific clinical effect has been of interest. In 1965, Lilly and Stillwell first defined probiotics, which describes probiotic as "a substance secreted by one bacterium to promote the growth of other bacteria" [28]. After the first definition, amendments were made two times in the definition. In 1989, Huis in't Veld *et al.* put forward the notion of the living bacterial complement [29]. One of the drawbacks of the notion was it was still considering probiotics only for nutritional purposes. The latest and widely accepted definition of probiotics classifies probiotics as a living microorganism that should be consumed in sufficient quantities to have a beneficial influence on one's health and is not restricted to nutritional effect (4).

In the first, probiotic products had only single species of microorganism belonging to *Saccharomyces* sp. or *Lactobacillus* sp. for treating and prevention of symptoms caused due to *Clostridium difficile* [30]. Later on, probiotics with a greater diversity and quantity of microbes (varying from 10^8 to more than 10^{10}) were created.

In case of prebiotics, the very first mention of factors enhancing the bacterial growth can be dated back to 1950s where a researcher described the presence of "bifidus factor" in human milk for the enrichment of *Lactobacillus bifidus* in infants [31]. In the 1980s and early 1990s, reports on the bifidogenic qualities of inulin and oligofructose which is derived from inulin, fructooligosaccharides (FOS) synthesised from sucrose, as well as galactose- and xylose-containing oligosaccharides surfaced [32].

In the year 1995, Gibson and Roberfroid gave the first working definition of the term "prebiotics." Scientific community quickly adapted to the new term and since then extensive research is going on to identify and study the effect of various prebiotic compounds on the gut microbiome.

6.2 Current Use of Probiotics and Prebiotics for Health Benefits

6.2.1 Prebiotic and Probiotic Health Benefits

6.2.1.1 Prebiotics Uses in Health Benefits

According to the definition of prebiotics, it must satisfy the following criteria for it to be beneficial for host.

a) Normalize the gastric pH via mammalian enzymes and gastrointestinal adsorption;
b) Specific microflora from the intestine should be able to ferment it;
c) Should increase the growth and/or activity of intestinal bacteria, which is linked to host's health and well-being [33].

There are various advantages for both animals and humans. We can categorize them according to the function

1) **Defense against pathogens**
   Short chain low-digestible carbohydrates (LDCs) like fructans (inulin, fructo-oligosaccharides), galacto-oligosaccharides and resistant starches have therapeutic and defense application. By modifying the host defence system and regulating the interplay between pathogenic and beneficial microbes, LDCs can prevent bacterial and viral infection [34]. The prebiotics administration will propagate beneficial bacteria, thus resulting in acidic pH and thus preventing the growth of other pathogenic microbes. Also, colonization of beneficial microbes will utilize the available nutrients with no nutrients for invading microbes [36]. The epithelium of the gut is protected by thick mucosal layer, which is referred to as the first line of defense for any rupture, injury, or against any pathogenic bacteria. This mucosal layer is made up of

mucin and other digestive enzymes, antimicrobial peptides, and immunoglobulins [35].

a) Acetate (a SCFAs) enhances the gut defense mechanism through epithelial cells, protecting the host from infection. Acetate like any other SCFA regulate the inflammation response by binding to G-protein coupled receptors 41 and 43 present on immune cells within the gut-associated lymphoid tissues (GALT) [38].
b) Butyrate which is produced by species like *Fecalibacteriumprausnitzii, Eubacterium rectale* and *Rose buria* spp. induce the expression of antimicrobial peptide like LL37, which prevents microbial infection [37].
c) Oligosaccharides and glycoproteins present in large diversity can prevent the adhesion of microbes by acting like their receptor analogous. Like milk and lactulose can prevent the adherence of *Campylobacter jejuni*, EPEC, *Helicobacter pylori*, etc. [39].

2) **Simulation of immune system**
In order to simulate the immune system, anti-inflammatory cytokines must be increased and proinflammatory cytokines must be decreased. Prebiotics have both direct and indirect impacts on the host's immune system. We can say that prebiotics indirectly increase the advantageous and protective bacterial population like bifidobacteria and lactobacillus and thus decreasing the chances of harmful bacteria [40]. For example, monomer of MOS has the ability to inhibit the infection of Salmonella, since it binds to mannose through type 1 fimbriae [41]. Oligosaccharides can be absorbed directly into the intestinal cells and alter gene expression.
Bifidobacterium longum and fructooligosaccharides (FOS)/inulin as prebiotic can be used for patients with active ulcerative colitis and thus reducing the inflammation in GIT [43]. Butyrate reduces the synthesis of proinflammatory IL-2 and IFN-γ, whereas acetate and propionate boost the production of anti-inflammatory cytokine, like IL-10 [44].
3) **Improvement in nutrient (mineral) absorption**
Uptake of minerals in small intestine is via active transport mechanisms. The SCFAs is produced by fermentation of

prebiotics, thus reducing the pH in the lumen. The decreased pH leads to active and increased uptake of calcium, thus applying a larger driving force for passive uptake of calcium [42]. Consumption of mixture of FOS and inulin or GOS by teenagers will result increase in absorption and mineralization of calcium, thus decreasing the chances of osteoporosis [45].

4) **Effect on satiety**

Satiety is defined as a state of noneating, characterized by absence of hunger due to indigestion. Studies show that SCFA can regulate the appetite through various ways like

a) SCFAs produced by fermentation in the GIT interact with fatty acid receptors like FFAR2 and FFAR3 and thus regulate liposysis [46].
b) SCFA and colonic cells leads to production of anorexigenic hormones (stimulate eating) like PYY and GLP-1 [47].
c) SCFA reaches liver through hepatic portal vein and here propanoiate triggers gluconeogenesis which is a satiety signal [48].

5) **Improved bowel function**

Functional bowel disorders (FBDs) are a group of chronic gastrointestinal disorders marked by symptoms such as abdominal discomfort, bloating, distension, and bowel anomalies [49] Consumption of dietary fibers can help in improvement of bowel functioning. Fermentable dietary fibers help the microbiota proliferate in the colon by providing them with vital nutrients. Because individual bacteria and groups of bacteria have varying ability to consume carbohydrates and must compete with other bacteria for them, there is a growing understanding that fiber combinations are more likely than single fibers to encourage the growth of a wider range of bacteria [50]. Also fermented SCFAs of prebiotics can regulate the gut hormones and improve the effect of bowels and softening the stools and regularizing the defecation frequency [51]. Dietary modulators of gut microbiota in pediatric obesity can restore symbiosis of healthy bacteria and reduce adiposity (adipose tissue–related inflammation in obesity) [52].

6.2.1.2 Probiotics Uses in Health Benefits

Probiotics can be considered as "good" bacteria, which can reside in our body and provide us with various health benefits. Microorganisms live in a complex functional ecosystem, in which they play multiply roles like converting dietary fibers into metabolites which can be in either good or bad way. Different sources of probiotics can be fermented dairy products like yoghurt cheese, fermented milk, fortified milk, pickles, chocolates, granola bars, juices, microalgae, probiotic supplements, etc.

1) **Helps in balancing the beneficial bacteria in GIT**
   The probiotics have very important property of antipathogenic activity. It is studied that probiotic inhibits the activity of pathogen by producing short-chain fatty acids (SCFAs) like acetate, propionate, butyrate and lactic acid. The probiotics help in maintaining the pH in the colonic lumen thus, preventing growth of invasive bacteria [53]. Studies also suggest that probiotics produce large number of antipathogenic compounds for their self-defense like bacteriocins, ethanol, organic acids, acetaldehydes, hydrogen peroxide, etc. [54].

   a) Compounds like bacteriocins and peptides increase the membrane permeability of the pathogenic cell, resulting in unstable membrane potential and thus death [55].
   b) Similarly, hydrogen peroxide causes oxidation of sulfhydryl groups, thus peroxidation of lipid membranes, thus rupturing the membrane and killing the pathogen [56].
   c) Probiotics can also stimulate the host defense system to prevent pathogenic invasion [57].
   d) Probiotics are healthy and beneficial microbes which can compete with pathogenic bacteria for binding sites and nutrients [57].

2) **Antidiabetic activity**
   Gram negative Bacteroidetes and gram-positive Firmicutes are predominantly residing in gut microenvironment. These bacterial phyla play important role in antidiabetic activity. In type II diabetic patients there is decreased number of firmicutes species, which leads to increased Bacteroidetes/firmicutes ratio and increasing concentration of plasma glucose levels [59].

3) **Maintaining the urogenital health**
Today the number of cases for urinary tract infection (UTI) have increased. There is a great number of microflora associated with the vaginal region. which includes *Lactobacillus* spp. Thus, this imbalance of microbial composition can lead to UTI and bacterial vaginosis which can be balanced using Lactobacillus probiotics [58].
4) **Can reduce allergies**
Increasing allergic diseases caused due to immunity disorder, needs solution. Probiotics play potential role in preventing allergies. Some probiotics like *Lactobacillus plantarum L67* are associated with preventing allergies associated with IL-12 and interferon-γ [63].
5) **Boost immunity**
Lactobacillus has the ability to enhance the immune system of the host. The probiotics like *Lactobacillus rhamnosus GG* helps in proliferation of murine T and B lymphocytes. The *Bifidobacterium breve YIT4064* can protect the host against influenza and rotaviral infections. The probiotics produce important immunological factors like IL-6, TNF-α, and nitric oxide (NO) [64].
6) **Reduce digestive disorders**
There can be inflammation in the intestinal tract, which can cause abnormal bowel function and thus indigestion. Such chronic inflammations are known as inflammatory bowel disorder (IBD), which includes Crohn's disease and ulcerative colitis. These disorders are associated with rupture and inflammation of mucosal lining. The SCFAs have main role in maintaining the colonic homeostasis. Thus, to overcome, we require SCFAs like acetate, butyrate, and propionate, and these levels can be restored using bacteria like *Lactobacillus*, *Bifidobacterium*, *Enterobacter*, and *E. coli* as probiotics [62].
7) **Loose weight and belly fats, reducing obesity**
Fats are lipids produced by lipogenesis. Probiotics like *Lactobacillus gasseri* BNR17 prevent the growth of adipose tissue [60]. Other probiotics which too show antiobesity property are *Lactobacillus acidophilus*, *Lactobacillus casei*, and *Bifidobacterium longum* [61].

6.2.2 Prebiotics and Probiotics Used in Combinatorial Approach for Health Benefits

After the introduction of concept of synbiotics by Gibson & Roberfroid, multiple efforts have been made to use the combinatorial approach of using probiotics and prebiotics together to treat a particular disorder. One of such examples is use of synbiotic approach in treating steatosis of liver. Steatosis occurs when bacterial metabolic products such as ethanol, lipopolysaccharides (LPS) and short-chain fatty acids (SCFA) penetrate the liver and accelerate the detoxifying process. This leads to storage of triacylglycerols resulting in steatosis. A randomized trial tried to check the effect of synbiotics approach to treat this condition by using five probiotics (*Lactobacillus plantarum, Lactobacillus delbrueckii* sphp. *bulgaricus, Lactobacillus acidophilus, Lactobacillus rhamnosus, Bifidobacterium bifidum*) in addition to employing inulin as a prebiotic. The study was conducted in adults with nonalcoholic steatosis. The results indicated reduction in the accumulation of intrahepatic triacylglycerol [65]. A lot of research has been done to check the effect of synbiotic approach on inflammatory bowel disease (IBD). IBD is a disorder comprising of four pathological conditions: ulcerative colitis (UC), Crohn's disease (CD), pouchitis, and microscopic colitis. The conditions primarily affect gastrointestinal tract [66]. In the presence of inulin as a prebiotic, the anti-inflammatory impact of the probiotic strains *Lactobacillus acidophilus, L. plantarum, Bifidobacterium lactis, B. breve* was investigated. The study was performed on Swiss mice with induced UC by using Dextran Sodium Sulphate. The effect of the treatment was measured in the form of NO levels in the peritoneal macrophage cultures. The study suggested that the severity of the UC reduced after inulin was given orally and probiotic strains, which was evident from the reduction in the NO concentration measured in peritoneal macrophage cultures [67]. A case study which used rats with chronic inflammation, effect of *L. plantarum* LS/07 CCM7766 on the condition was investigated alone and in conjugation with inulin. *L. plantarum* LS/07 CCM7766, alone and in conjugation with inulin, eliminated the inflammation in the jejunal mucosa by restricting the production of proinflammatory cytokines and enhancing the synthesis of IL-10 cytokine, although TGF-1 levels did not alter significantly [68].

Another short 4-week study looked into whether a twice-daily dose of 6 g Synergy 1VR and *Bifidobacterium longum* was useful in people with active UC [43].

Effect of synbiotic approach has also been tested on diseases like dementia and Alzheimer's disease by taking into consideration lacunar stroke as a potential cause. It is hypothesized that reducing the risk of lacunar stroke can decrease the risk of Alzheimer's disease [69]. In a case study which used the *L. acidophilus* LAFTI L10 (L10), *B. lactis* LAFTI B94 (B94), and *L. casei L26* LAFTI (L26) along with prebiotics inulin and fructooligosaccharides increased the probiotics organisms' survival and retention time *in vivo* [70].

In conclusion, many reports provide proof about the use of synbiotic approach in treating various disorders and diseases. The major limiting factor in the approach is finding the perfect match of probiotic microorganism and its prebiotic component, enhancing its growth and activity. A lot of research still needs to be done to better understand the concept of synbiotics in benefit of human health.

6.2.3 Limitations of Probiotics

Even though probiotics are "generally regarded as safe (GRAS)," adverse effects, such as septicemia and fungemia, have only been recorded in a small number of high-risk conditions [71]. Several studies have linked probiotic use to negative consequences, such as immunoreactivity, and gene transfer that leads to pathogenic antibiotic resistance [72, 73]. The people who are elders, immunocompromised and critical, belong to the vulnerable groups making probiotic usage in the context of pathology particularly dangerous.

Limitations of Probiotics are as follows:

a) Either resistance is transferred from the probiotic to human bacterial pathogens, directly or indirectly through the commensal flora or it could happen vice versa [74].
b) Within bacterial species, there is a lot of strain-to-strain diversity in features related to probiotic efficacy [75].
c) The research approach in the probiotic field uses a trial and error method but the approach should be mechanism-based [76].
d) The interactions like probiotics–host mucosal and probiotics–microbiome are absent *in vitro* models. In addition, in some cases the *in vivo* models may not be compatible with human probiotics, so the choice of model is important [76]. As for safety, especially long-term, the reports present are inadequate.

Prebiotics are certainly not appropriate for everyone. Many challenges are faced by the industry for the production of prebiotics and probiotics like the use of economic sources, novel techniques, low cost of production, and improvement in viability while storage [77].

6.3 Development of New Generation of Probiotics/Prebiotics

6.3.1 Development of New Generation of Probiotics

Probiotics production has risen significantly in recent years as public awareness of their unique characteristics like decrease in cholesterol, detoxification, maintenance of permeability and intestinal pH, stimulation of immune system, microbiome normalization [78–80]. The first generation of probiotics emerged in the last several decades because of efforts to create probiotic products. Due to reduction in probiotic population while storage, food processing, gastrointestinal conditions led to the development of a second-generation where the bacteria used were coated with polymers (natural or synthetic) before being lyophilized [81, 82]. Unfortunately, this strategy failed to address the sensitivity and vulnerability of the digestive system [83]. To solve the second-generation problems encapsulation method was used as the third generation. The microorganisms used were encapsulated in nanomaterials to ensure survivability and controlled release in the gastrointestinal tract [81, 83]. Still, the problems were not solved of targeted delivery so many researches are being conducted to overcome the challenges and to develop new generations of probiotics. A new product called paraprobiotics is made up of nonviable microorganism (inactivated) that provides health benefits to the consumers like regulation of the immune system, anti-inflammatory response, antiproliferative, and antioxidant properties. As nonviable microorganisms are used so the safety is ensured and risks are reduced and an even increase in shelf life is also observed [84]. Another significant benefit is that when used in combination with antibiotics or antifungal drugs, there is no loss of bioactivity [85]. The foods that do not offer an appropriate environment for probiotics efficient functions, in such foods paraprobiotics can be added. The addition of paraprobiotics in food does not change their organoleptic properties. The interaction with the food matrix is also not direct [86]. They can be added to food before thermal processing without completely compromising the health beneficial feature [87]. Physical or chemical treatments can be used to inactivate probiotic cells.

Generally, *Akkermansia muciniphila* is abundantly found in the intestinal tract. They are being considered as the next generation of probiotics. It belongs to the phylum Verrucomicrobia. It can be easily identified by the 16srRNA gene sequence. This symbiotic bacterium has many prebiotic properties- protection of growth health, regulation of the immune system, metabolic modulation. Different diseases like autoimmune disease and metabolic syndromes are related to an imbalance in *Akkermansia muciniphila* number [88].

Christensenella can be used as a probiotic due to health benefits provided by it like related to metabolic disorders and obesity [89]. *Christensenella* can form a co-occurring network with different bacteria. The presence of these bacteria in large numbers leads to a reduction in BMI [90]. For its use as next-generation probiotics, various studies are being conducted. Streptomyces can treat and prevent inflammatory disorders and due to this, it benefits it can be used as a candidate for next-generation probiotics [91].

6.3.2 New Prebiotics With Improved Effect on GIT Microbiota for Health Benefits

GIT microbiome has an important role in digesting various nutritional compounds for maintaining human health. Several types of research on probiotics are found to be done for efficiently maintaining the microbiome of the gastrointestinal tract to improve and maintain health conditions. The intestinal microbiome should be in the optimum range in the hosts. As gastric enzymes cannot act on prebiotic foods, so they remain undisturbed. Some notable prebiotics and advantages associated with them are shown in Table 6.1.

6.3.3 Improvement in Viability of Probiotics

Functional foods are becoming increasingly popular around the world because of their nutritional and health benefits. *Bifidobacterium* and *Lactobacillus,* these probiotic bacteria are commonly found in dairy products. Glycerol and oligofructose were added in different concentrations in frozen yogurt, and the viability of probiotics and yogurt culture was checked. The yogurt cultures used were of *Lactobacillus bulgaricus* and *Streptococcus thermophiles* and probiotics used were *Bifidobacterium lactis* and *Lactobacillus acidophilus.* The result showed positive effects on maintaining the probiotic's viability. Oligofructose and glycerol at concentrations of 6% and 4% respectively are proven to be more effective [100]. Another study was conducted for improvement in the viability of

Table 6.1 A few notable prebiotics and the documented benefits associated with them.

Prebiotics/dietary fibers	Changes in microbiome observed	Reference
Galacto-oligosaccharides	Increase in *Lactobacilli, bifidobacteria, butyrate*	[92]
Agave inulin	Increase in *Bifidobacterium* and decrease in *Lachnobacterium, Ruminococcus, Desulfovibrio,*	[93]
Soluble corn fiber	Increase in *Parabacteroides, Dialiste, Bifidobacterium*	[94]
Inulin + oligofructose	Increase in *Bifidobacterium longum, Bifidobacterium adolescentis* and *Bifidobacterium pseudocatenulatum*	[95]
Xylooligosaccharide	Increase in *Bifidobacterium,* increased propionate, butyrate while reducing the concentrations of *p*-cresol and acetate	[96]
Polydextrose	Decrease in *lactobacilli/ enterococci* and *C. histolyticum*	[97]
Fructo-oligosaccharides	Increase in *Lactobacillus* spp and decrease in *Clostridium* spp.	[98]
Arabinoxylo-oligosaccharides and inulin	Increase in *Bifidobacterium, Prevotella, Bacteroides,* acetate, butyrate, propionate	[99]

probiotics in frozen yogurt. In this study, the probiotics and the yogurt culture mixture were made by using the same species from the earlier report but the supplementations were different, here they used inulin and glycerol in different concentrations. They also observed positive results and the optimum concentration of inulin and glycerol was found to be 6% and 4%, respectively [101].

Traditional methods of probiotic delivery to farmed aquatic animals are ineffective because the probiotics' viability is lost before they reach their target site. Chitosan-coated alginate microparticles were used to encapsulate the probiotic bacteria to ensure controlled release, maintenance of viability, and targeted delivery [102].

6.3.4 Current Trends and Scope for Development

Nonetheless, there is growing interest in manipulating the genome of probiotic strains using the CRISPR/Cas system to create the next generation of strong probiotics with unique functionalities and the ability to supply new biomolecules, in addition to predicting probiotic qualities [103]. A new generation of probiotics could be introduced to the food and pharmaceutical industries using the probiotic biofilm approach [104]. Studies on seaweeds, such as red seaweed (*Gelidium sesquipedale*), laminarin, etc. have demonstrated that they can improve gut microbiota while also being cost-effective [105]. New strategies like pharmabiotics (butyrate-producing bacteria), psychobiotics, and phagebiotics are being introduced, and extensive researches are being conducted on them [105–108].

References

1. Dillard, C.J. and German, J.B., Phytochemicals: Nutraceuticals and human health. *J. Sci. Food Agric.*, *80*, 12, 1744–1756, 2000.
2. Swinbanks, D. and O'Brien, J., Japan explores the boundary between food and medicine. *Nature*, *364*, 6434, 180–180, 1993.
3. Sarao, L.K. and Arora, M., Probiotics, prebiotics, and microencapsulation: A review. *Crit. Rev. Food Sci. Nutr.*, *57*, 2, 344–371, 2017.
4. Hill, C., Guarner, F., Reid, G., Gibson, G.R., Merenstein, D.J., Pot, B., Sanders, M.E., The International Scientific Association for Probiotics and Prebiotics consensus statement on the scope and appropriate use of the term probiotic. *Nat. Rev. Gastroenterol. Hepatol.*, *11*, 8, 506–514, 2014.
5. Bowe, W.P. and Logan, A.C., Acne vulgaris, probiotics and the gut-brain-skin axis-back to the future? *Gut Pathog.*, *3*, 1, 1–11, 2011.
6. Wieërs, G., Belkhir, L., Enaud, R., Leclercq, S., Philippart de Foy, J.M., Dequenne, I., Cani, P.D., How probiotics affect the microbiota. *Front. Cell. Infect. Microbiol.*, 9, 454, 2020.
7. Peng, M., Tabashsum, Z., Anderson, M., Truong, A., Houser, A.K., Padilla, J., Biswas, D., Effectiveness of probiotics, prebiotics, and prebiotic-like components in common functional foods. *Compr. Rev. Food Sci. Food Saf.*, *19*, 4, 1908–1933, 2020.
8. Thursby, E. and Juge, N., Introduction to the human gut microbiota. *Biochem. J.*, *474*, 11, 1823–1836, 2017.

9. Arora, M. and Baldi, A., Regulatory categories of probiotics across the globe: A review representing existing and recommended categorization. *Indian J. Med. Microbiol.*, *33*, S2–S10, 2015.
10. Das, L., Bhaumik, E., Raychaudhuri, U., Chakraborty, R., Role of nutraceuticals in human health. *J. Food Sci. Technol.*, *49*, 2, 173–183, 2012.
11. Sreeja, V. and Prajapati, J.B., Probiotic formulations: Application and status as pharmaceuticals—A review. *Probiotics Antimicrob. Proteins*, *5*, 2, 81–91, 2013.
12. Cetik Yildiz, S., Demir, C., Cengiz, M., Ayhanci, A., Protective properties of kefir on burn wounds of mice that were infected with *S. aureus, P. auroginasa and E. coli. Cell. Mo. Biol.* (Noisy-le-Grand, France), 65, 7, 60–65, 2019.
13. Peng, M., Tabashsum, Z., Patel, P., Bernhardt, C., Biswas, D., Linoleic acids overproducing Lactobacillus casei limits growth, survival, and virulence of Salmonella Typhimurium and enterohaemorrhagic Escherichia coli. *Front. Microbiol.*, *9*, 2663, 2018.
14. Gibson, G.R. and Roberfroid, M.B., Dietary modulation of the human colonic microbiota: Introducing the concept of prebiotics. *J. Nutr.*, *125*, 6, 1401–1412, 1995.
15. Gibson, G.R., Hutkins, R., Sanders, M.E., Prescott, S.L., Reimer, R.A., Salminen, S.J., Reid, G., Expert consensus document: The International Scientific Association for Probiotics and Prebiotics (ISAPP) consensus statement on the definition and scope of prebiotics. *Nat. Rev. Gastroenterol. Hepatol.*, *14*, 8, 491–502, 2017.
16. Valcheva, R. and Dieleman, L.A., Prebiotics: Definition and protective mechanisms. *Best Pract. Res. Clin. Gastroenterol.*, *30*, 1, 27–37, 2016.
17. Aydinol, P. and Ozcan, T., Production of reduced-fat Labneh cheese with inulin and β-glucan fibre-based fat replacer. *Int. J. Dairy Technol.*, *71*, 2, 362–371, 2018.
18. Esmaeilnejad Moghadam, B., Keivaninahr, F., Fouladi, M., Rezaei Mokarram, R., Nazemi, A., Inulin addition to yoghurt: Prebiotic activity, health effects and sensory properties. *Int. J. Dairy Technol.*, *72*, 2, 183–198, 2019.
19. Peng, M., Tabashsum, Z., Anderson, M., Truong, A., Houser, A.K., Padilla, J., Biswas, D., Effectiveness of probiotics, prebiotics, and prebiotic-like components in common functional foods. *Compr. Rev. Food Sci. Food Saf.*, *19*, 4, 1908–1933, 2020.
20. Carvalho de Morais, E., Prebiotic addition in dairy products: Processing and health benefits, in: *Probiotics, Prebiotics, and Synbiotics: Bioactive Foods in Health Promotion*, Watson, R.R. and Preedy, V.R. (Eds.), Academic Press, Campinas, Brazil, 2015.
21. Bijle, M.N., Ekambaram, M., Lo, E.C., Yiu, C.K.Y., Synbiotics in caries prevention: A scoping review. *PLoS One*, *15*, 8, e0237547, 2020.
22. Anadon, A. *et al.*, Prebiotics and probiotics: An assessment of their safety and health benefits, in: Probiotics, *Prebiotics, and Synbiotics: Bioactive Foods in Health Promotion*, Watson, R.R. and Preedy, V.R. (Eds.), Academic Press, Madrid, Spain, 2015.

23. Bijle, M.N., Ekambaram, M., Lo, E.C., Yiu, C.K.Y., Synbiotics in caries prevention: A scoping review. *PLoS One*, *15*, 8, e0237547, 2020.
24. Kolida, S. and Gibson, G.R., Synbiotics in health and disease. *Annu. Rev. Food Sci. Technol.*, 2, 373–393, 2011.
25. Roberfroid, M., Gibson, G.R., Hoyles, L., McCartney, A.L., Rastall, R., Rowland, I., Meheust, A., Prebiotic concept and health. *Br. J. Nutr.*, *104*, Suppl 2, S1–63, 2010.
26. Abou-Donia, S.A., Origin, history and manufacturing process of Egyptian dairy products: An overview. *Alexandria J. Food Sci. Technol.*, *5*, 1, 51–62, 2008.
27. Hosono, A. and Nakazawa, Y. (Eds.), *Functions of fermented milk: Challenges for the health sciences*, Elsevier Applied Science, London, 1992.
28. Lilly, D.M. and Stillwell, R.H., Probiotics: Growth-promoting factors produced by microorganisms. *Science*, *147*, 3659, 747–748, 1965.
29. Havenaar, R. and Marteau, P., Establishing a scientific basis for probiotic R&D. *Trends Biotechnol.*, *12*, 1, 6–8, 1994.
30. Goldenberg, J.Z., Yap, C., Lytvyn, L., Lo, C.K.F., Beardsley, J., Mertz, D., Johnston, B.C., Probiotics for the prevention of Clostridium difficile-associated diarrhea in adults and children. *Cochrane Database Syst. Rev.*, 12, 2017.
31. Enam, F. and Mansell, T.J., Prebiotics: Tools to manipulate the gut microbiome and metabolome. *J. Ind. Microbiol. Biotechnol.*, *46*, 9-10, 1445–1459, 2019.
32. Hutkins, R.W., Krumbeck, J.A., Bindels, L.B., Cani, P.D., Fahey Jr., G., Goh, Y.J., Sanders, M.E., Prebiotics: Why definitions matter. *Curr. Opin. Biotechnol.*, *37*, 1–7, 2016.
33. Shokryazdan, P., Jahromi, M.F., Navidshad, B., Liang, J.B., Effects of prebiotics on immune system and cytokine expression. *Med. Microbiol. Immunol.*, *206*, 1, 1–9, 2017.
34. Di Bartolomeo, F., Startek, J.B., Van den Ende, W., Prebiotics to fight diseases: Reality or fiction? *Phytother. Res.*, *27*, 10, 1457–1473, 2013.
35. Liévin-Le Moal, V. and Servin, A.L., The front line of enteric host defense against unwelcome intrusion of harmful microorganisms: Mucins, antimicrobial peptides, and microbiota. *Clin. Microbiol. Rev.*, *19*, 2, 315–337, 2006.
36. Sanders, M.E., Merenstein, D.J., Reid, G., Gibson, G.R., Rastall, R.A., Probiotics and prebiotics in intestinal health and disease: From biology to the clinic. *Nat. Rev. Gastroenterol. Hepatol.*, *16*, 10, 605–616, 2019.
37. Ashida, H., Ogawa, M., Kim, M., Mimuro, H., Sasakawa, C., Bacteria and host interactions in the gut epithelial barrier. *Nat. Chem. Biol.*, *8*, 1, 36–45, 2012.
38. Maslowski, K.M., Vieira, A.T., Ng, A., Kranich, J., Sierro, F., Yu, D., Mackay, C.R., Regulation of inflammatory responses by gut microbiota and chemoattractant receptor GPR43. *Nature*, *461*, 7268, 1282–1286, 2009.
39. Miller, J.B. and McVeagh, P., Human milk oligosaccharides: 130 reasons to breast-feed. *Br. J. Nutr.*, *82*, 5, 333–335, 1999.

40. Shokryazdan, P., Jahromi, M.F., Navidshad, B., Liang, J.B., Effects of prebiotics on immune system and cytokine expression. *Med. Microbiol. Immunol.*, *206*, 1, 1–9, 2017.
41. Oyofo, B.A., DeLoach, J.R., Corrier, D.E., Norman, J.O., Ziprin, R.L., Mollenhauer, H.H., Prevention of Salmonella typhimurium colonization of broilers with D-mannose. *Poult. Sci.*, *68*, 10, 1357–1360, 1989.
42. Goss, S.L., Lemons, K.A., Kerstetter, J.E., Bogner, R.H., Determination of calcium salt solubility with changes in pH and PCO2, simulating varying gastrointestinal environments. *J. Pharm. Pharmacol.*, *59*, 11, 1485–1492, 2007.
43. Furrie, E., Macfarlane, S., Kennedy, A., Cummings, J.H., Walsh, S.V., O'neil, D.A., Macfarlane, G.T., Synbiotic therapy (Bifidobacterium longum/Synergy 1) initiates resolution of inflammation in patients with active ulcerative colitis: A randomised controlled pilot trial. *Gut*, *54*, 2, 242–249, 2005.
44. Cavaglieri, C.R., Nishiyama, A., Fernandes, L.C., Curi, R., Miles, E.A., Calder, P.C., Differential effects of short-chain fatty acids on proliferation and production of pro-and anti-inflammatory cytokines by cultured lymphocytes. *Life Sci.*, *73*, 13, 1683–1690, 2003.
45. Whisner, C.M., Martin, B.R., Schoterman, M.H., Nakatsu, C.H., McCabe, L.D., McCabe, G.P., Weaver, C.M., Galacto-oligosaccharides increase calcium absorption and gut bifidobacteria in young girls: A double-blind crossover trial. *Br. J. Nutr.*, *110*, 7, 1292–1303, 2013.
46. Stoddart, L.A., Smith, N.J., Milligan, G., International Union of Pharmacology. LXXI. Free fatty acid receptors FFA1,-2, and-3: Pharmacology and pathophysiological functions. *Pharmacol. Rev.*, *60*, 4, 405–417, 2008.
47. Chambers, E.S., Morrison, D.J., Frost, G., Control of appetite and energy intake by SCFA: What are the potential underlying mechanisms? *Proc. Nutr. Soc.*, *74*, 3, 328–336, 2015.
48. Mithieux, G., Metabolic effects of portal vein sensing. *Diabetes Obes. Metab.*, *16*, S1, 56–60, 2014.
49. Wilson, B., Rossi, M., Dimidi, E., Whelan, K., Prebiotics in irritable bowel syndrome and other functional bowel disorders in adults: A systematic review and meta-analysis of randomized controlled trials. *Am. J. Clin. Nutr.*, *109*, 4, 1098–1111, 2019.
50. Rasmussen, H. and Hamaker, B.R., Prebiotics and inflammatory bowel disease. *Gastroenterol. Clin.*, 46, 4, 783–795, 2017.
51. Buddington, R.K., Kapadia, C., Neumer, F., Theis, S., Oligofructose provides laxation for irregularity associated with low fiber intake. *Nutrients*, *9*, 12, 1372, 2017.
52. Nicolucci, A.C. and Reimer, R.A., Prebiotics as a modulator of gut microbiota in paediatric obesity. *Pediatr. Obes.*, *12*, 4, 265–273, 2017.
53. Kareem, K.Y., Ling, F.H., Chwen, L.T., Foong, O.M., Asmara, S.A., Inhibitory activity of postbiotic produced by strains of Lactobacillus plantarum using reconstituted media supplemented with inulin. *Gut Pathog.*, *6*, 1, 1–7, 2014.
54. Islam, S.U., Clinical uses of probiotics. *Medicine*, *95*, 5, 1536–5964, 2016.

55. Simova, E.D., Beshkova, D.B., Dimitrov, Z.P., Characterization and antimicrobial spectrum of bacteriocins produced by lactic acid bacteria isolated from traditional Bulgarian dairy products. *J. Appl. Microbiol.*, *106*, 2, 692–701, 2009.
56. Ammor, S., Tauveron, G., Dufour, E., Chevallier, I., Antibacterial activity of lactic acid bacteria against spoilage and pathogenic bacteria isolated from the same meat small-scale facility: 1—Screening and characterization of the antibacterial compounds. *Food Control*, *17*, 6, 454–461, 2006.
57. Figueroa-González, I., Cruz-Guerrero, A., Quijano, G., The benefits of probiotics on human health. *J. Microb. Biochem. Technol. S*, *1*, 1948–5948, 2011.
58. Waigankar, S.S. and Patel, V., Role of probiotics in urogenital healthcare. *J. Mid-Life Health*, *2*, 1, 5, 2011.
59. Barrett, H.L., Callaway, L.K., Nitert, M.D., Probiotics: A potential role in the prevention of gestational diabetes? *Acta Diabetol.*, *49*, 1, 1–13, 2012.
60. Kang, J.H., Yun, S.I., Park, M.H., Park, J.H., Jeong, S.Y., Park, H.O., Anti-obesity effect of Lactobacillus gasseri BNR17 in high-sucrose diet-induced obese mice. *PLoS One*, *8*, 1, e54617, 2013.
61. Karimi, G., Sabran, M.R., Jamaluddin, R., Parvaneh, K., Mohtarrudin, N., Ahmad, Z., Khodavandi, A., The anti-obesity effects of Lactobacillus casei strain Shirota versus Orlistat on high fat diet-induced obese rats. *Food Nutr. Res.*, *59*, 1, 29273, 2015.
62. Gowri, R.S., Meenambigai, P., Prabhavathi, P., Rajeswari, P.R., Yesudoss, L.A., Probiotics and its effects on human health-A review. *Int. J. Curr. Microbiol. Appl. Sci.*, *5*, 4, 384–392, 2016.
63. Song, S., Lee, S.J., Park, D.J., Oh, S., Lim, K.T., The anti-allergic activity of Lactobacillus plantarum L67 and its application to yogurt. *J. Dairy Sci.*, *99*, 12, 9372–9382, 2016.
64. Sanap, D.S., Garje, M.A., Godge, G.R., Probiotics, their health benefits and applications for development of human health: A review. *J. Drug Deliv. Ther.*, *9*, 4-s, 631–640, 2019.
65. Wong, V.W.S., Wong, G.L.H., Chim, A.M.L., Chu, W.C.W., Yeung, D.K.W., Li, K.C.T., Chan, H.L.Y., Treatment of nonalcoholic steatohepatitis with probiotics. A proof-of-concept study. *Ann. Hepatol.*, *12*, 2, 256–262, 2013.
66. Plaza-Díaz, J., Ruiz-Ojeda, F.J., Vilchez-Padial, L.M., Gil, A., Evidence of the anti-inflammatory effects of probiotics and synbiotics in intestinal chronic diseases. *Nutrients*, *9*, 6, 555, 2017.
67. Abdelouhab, K., Rafa, H., Toumi, R., Bouaziz, S., Medjeber, O., Touil-Boukoffa, C., Mucosal intestinal alteration in experimental colitis correlates with nitric oxide production by peritoneal macrophages: Effect of probiotics and prebiotics. *Immunopharmacol. Immunotoxicol.*, *34*, 4, 590–597, 2012.
68. Štofilová, J., Szabadosová, V., Hrčková, G., Salaj, R., Bertková, I., Hijová, E., Bomba, A., Co-administration of a probiotic strain Lactobacillus plantarum LS/07 CCM7766 with prebiotic inulin alleviates the intestinal inflammation in rats exposed to N, N-dimethylhydrazine. *Int. Immunopharmacol.*, *24*, 2, 361–368, 2015.

69. Lye, H.S., Lee, Y.T., Ooi, S.Y., Teh, L.K., Lim, L.N., Wei, L.K., Modifying progression of aging and reducing the risk of neurodegenerative diseases by probiotics and synbiotics. *Front. Biosci.*, *10*, 344–51, 2018.
70. Su, P., Henriksson, A., Mitchell, H., Prebiotics enhance survival and prolong the retention period of specific probiotic inocula in an *in vivo* murine model. *J. Appl. Microbiol.*, *103*, 6, 2392–2400, 2007.
71. Vandenplas, Y., Salvatore, S., Viera, M., Devreker, T., Hauser, B., Probiotics in infectious diarrhoea in children: Are they indicated? *Eur. J. Pediatr.*, *166*, 12, 1211–1218, 2007.
72. Boyle, R.J., Robins-Browne, R.M., Tang, M.L., Probiotic use in clinical practice: what are the risks? *Am. J. Clin. Nutr.*, *83*, 6, 1256–1264, 2006.
73. Ayichew, T., Belete, A., Alebachew, T., Tsehaye, H., Berhanu, H., Minwuyelet, A., Bacterial probiotics their importances and limitations: A review. *J. Nutr. Health Sci.*, *4*, 2, 202, 2017.
74. Montassier, E., Valdés-Mas, R., Batard, E. *et al.*, Probiotics impact the antibiotic resistance gene reservoir along the human GI tract in a person-specific and antibiotic-dependent manner. *Nat. Microbiol.*, 6, 1043–1054, 2021, https://doi.org/10.1038/s41564-021-00920-0.
75. Crittenden, R., Bird, A.R., Gopal, P., Henriksson, A., Lee, Y.K., Playne, M.J., Probiotic research in Australia, New Zealand and the Asia-Pacific region. *Curr. Pharm. Des.*, *11*, 1, 37–53, 2005.
76. Suez, J., Zmora, N., Segal, E., Elinav, E., The pros, cons, and many unknowns of probiotics. *Nat. Med.*, *25*, 5, 716–729, 2019.
77. Figueroa-González, I., Quijano, G., Ramírez, G., Cruz-Guerrero, A., Probiotics and prebiotics–perspectives and challenges. *J. Sci. Food Agric.*, *91*, 8, 1341–1348, 2011, https://doi.org/10.1002/jsfa.4367.
78. Aoudia, N., Rieu, A., Briandet, R., Deschamps, J., Chluba, J., Jego, G., Guzzo, J., Biofilms of Lactobacillus plantarum and Lactobacillus fermentum: Effect on stress responses, antagonistic effects on pathogen growth and immunomodulatory properties. *Food Microbiol.*, *53*, 51–59, 2016.
79. Hu, M.X., Li, J.N., Guo, Q., Zhu, Y.Q., Niu, H.M., Probiotics biofilm-integrated electrospun nanofiber membranes: A new starter culture for fermented milk production. *J. Agric. Food Chem.*, *67*, 11, 3198–3208, 2019.
80. Watson, R.R. and Preedy, V.R. (Eds.), *Probiotics, prebiotics, and synbiotics: Bioactive foods in health promotion*, Academic Press, 2015.
81. de Vos, P., Faas, M.M., Spasojevic, M., Sikkema, J., Encapsulation for preservation of functionality and targeted delivery of bioactive food components. *Int. Dairy J.*, *20*, 4, 292–302, 2010.
82. Salas-Jara, M.J., Ilabaca, A., Vega, M., García, A., Biofilm forming Lactobacillus: New challenges for the development of probiotics. *Microorganisms*, 4, 3, 2016.
83. Burgain, J., Gaiani, C., Linder, M., Scher, J., Encapsulation of probiotic living cells: From laboratory scale to industrial applications. *J. Food Eng.*, *104*, 4, 467–483, 2011.

84. Aguilar-Toalá, J.E., Garcia-Varela, R., Garcia, H.S., Mata-Haro, V., González-Córdova, A.F., Vallejo-Cordoba, B., Hernández-Mendoza, A., Postbiotics: An evolving term within the functional foods field. *Trends Food Sci. Technol.*, *75*, 105–114, 2018.
85. Warda, A.K., Rea, K., Fitzgerald, P., Hueston, C., Gonzalez-Tortuero, E., Dinan, T.G., Hill, C., Heat-killed lactobacilli alter both microbiota composition and behaviour. *Behav. Brain Res.*, *362*, 213–223, 2019.
86. Guimarães, J.T., Balthazar, C.F., Silva, R., Rocha, R.S., Graça, J.S., Esmerino, E.A., Cruz, A.G., Impact of probiotics and prebiotics on food texture. *Curr. Opin. Food Sci.*, *33*, 38–44, 2020.
87. de Almada, C.N., Almada, C.N., Martinez, R.C., Sant'Ana, A.S., Paraprobiotics: evidences on their ability to modify biological responses, inactivation methods and perspectives on their application in foods. *Trends Food Sci. Technol.*, *58*, 96–114, 2016.
88. Zhai, Q., Feng, S., Arjan, N., Chen, W., A next generation probiotic, Akkermansiamuciniphila. *Crit. Rev. Food Sci. Nutr.*, *59*, 19, 3227–3236, 2019.
89. Bertazzoni, E., Donelli, G., Midtvedt, T., Nicoli, J., Sanz, Y., Probiotics and clinical effects: Is the number what counts? *J. Chemother. (Florence, Italy)*, *25*, 4, 193–212, 2013, https://doi.org/10.1179/1973947813Y.0000000078.
90. Goodrich, J.K., Davenport, E.R., Beaumont, M., Jackson, M.A., Knight, R., Ober, C., Ley, R.E., Genetic determinants of the gut microbiome in UK twins. *Cell Host Microbe*, *19*, 5, 731–743, 2016.
91. Bolourian, A. and Mojtahedi, Z., Immunosuppressants produced by Streptomyces: Evolution, hygiene hypothesis, tumourrapalog resistance and probiotics. *Environ. Microbiol. Rep.*, *10*, 2, 123–126, 2018.
92. Walton, G.E., van den Heuvel, E.G., Kosters, M.H., Rastall, R.A., Tuohy, K.M., Gibson, G.R., A randomised crossover study investigating the effects of galacto-oligosaccharides on the faecal microbiota in men and women over 50 years of age. *Br. J. Nutr.*, *107*, 10, 1466–1475, 2012.
93. Holscher, H.D., Bauer, L.L., Gourineni, V., Pelkman, C.L., Fahey Jr., G.C., Swanson, K.S., Agave inulin supplementation affects the fecal microbiota of healthy adults participating in a randomized, double-blind, placebo-controlled, crossover trial. *J. Nutr.*, *145*, 9, 2025–2032, 2015.
94. Whisner, C.M., Martin, B.R., Nakatsu, C.H., Story, J.A., MacDonald-Clarke, C.J., McCabe, L.D., Weaver, C.M., Soluble corn fiber increases calcium absorption associated with shifts in the gut microbiome: A randomized dose-response trial in free-living pubertal females. *J. Nutr.*, *146*, 7, 1298–1306, 2016.
95. Salazar, N., Dewulf, E.M., Neyrinck, A.M., Bindels, L.B., Cani, P.D., Mahillon, J., Delzenne, N.M., Inulin-type fructans modulate intestinal Bifidobacterium species populations and decrease fecal short-chain fatty acids in obese women. *Clin. Nutr.*, *34*, 3, 501–507, 2015.
96. Lecerf, J.M., Dépeint, F., Clerc, E., Dugenet, Y., Niamba, C.N., Rhazi, L., Pouillart, P.R., Xylo-oligosaccharide (XOS) in combination with inulin

modulates both the intestinal environment and immune status in healthy subjects, while XOS alone only shows prebiotic properties. *Br. J. Nutr., 108,* 10, 1847–1858, 2012.
97. Costabile, A., Fava, F., Röytiö, H., Forssten, S.D., Olli, K., Klievink, J., Walton, G.E., Impact of polydextrose on the faecal microbiota: A double-blind, cross-over, placebo-controlled feeding study in healthy human subjects. *Br. J. Nutr., 108,* 3, 471–481, 2012.
98. Matsumoto, K., Ichimura, M., Tsuneyama, K., Moritoki, Y., Tsunashima, H., Omagari, K., Kikuchi, K., Fructo-oligosaccharides and intestinal barrier function in a methionine–choline-deficient mouse model of nonalcoholic steatohepatitis. *PLoS One, 12,* 6, e0175406, 2017.
99. Van den Abbeele, P., Taminiau, B., Pinheiro, I., Duysburgh, C., Jacobs, H., Pijls, L., Marzorati, M., Arabinoxylo-oligosaccharides and inulin impact inter-individual variation on microbial metabolism and composition, which immunomodulates human cells. *J. Agric. Food Chem., 66,* 5, 1121–1130, 2018.
100. Muzammil, H.S. and Rasco, B., Probiotics viability in frozen yoghurt supplemented with oligofructose and glycerol. *Int. J. Hortic. Agric. Food Sci., 2,* 70–74, 2018.
101. Muzammil, H., Rasca, B., Junaid, M., Viability of Probiotics in Frozen Yogurt Supplemented with Inulin and Glycerol. *Int. J. Nutr. Food Sci., 7,* 4, 116, 2018.
102. MasoomiDezfooli, S., Gutierrez-Maddox, N., Alfaro, A.C., Seyfoddin, A., Development of a microencapsulated probiotic delivery system for New Zealand black-footed abalone (Haliotis iris). *Pharm. Dev. Technol., 26,* 4, 390–402, 2021.
103. Tenea, G.N. and Ortega, C., Genome Characterization of Lactiplantibacillus plantarum Strain UTNGt2 Originated from Theobroma grandiflorum (White Cacao) of Ecuadorian Amazon: Antimicrobial Peptides from Safety to Potential Applications. *Antibiotics, 10,* 4, 383, 2021.
104. Rezaei, Z., Salari, A., Khanzadi, S., Probiotic Biofilm: A Novel Approach to Produce a New Generation of Probiotics and Probiotic Foods, 2021.
105. Goyal, N., Yadav, V., Rastogi, M., A New era probiotics, prebiotics & synbiotics. *Food Agric. Spectr. J., 1,* 01, 6–13, 2020.
106. Paton, A.W., Morona, R., Paton, J.C., Bioengineered microbes in disease therapy. *Trends Mol. Med., 18,* 7, 417–425, 2012.
107. Shanahan, F., Dinan, T.G., Ross, P., Hill, C., Probiotics in transition. *Clin. Gastroenterol. Hepatol., 10,* 11, 1220–1224, 2012.
108. Eeckhaut, V., Ducatelle, R., Sas, B., Vermeire, S., Van Immerseel, F., Progress towards butyrate-producing pharmabiotics: Butyricicoccuspullicaecorum capsule and efficacy in TNBS models in comparison with therapeutics. *Gut, 63,* 2, 367–367, 2014.

7

Immunostimulatory Role of Prebiotics and Probiotics

Tanuja Mohanty[†], Bhanu Pratap Gurjar[†], Sudheer BabuYangala and Usha Nagarajan[*]

Department of Biochemistry, School of Interdisciplinary and Applied Sciences, Central University of Haryana, Mahendergarh, India

Abstract

The symbiotic association has been one of the most significant relationships of nature. Many microbes are symbiotically associated with humans specifically in the gut region. Both microbe and organism coevolve to endure any alteration in the environment. Deficits of normal microbiome enhance the probability of occurrence of dreadful diseases in the organism. Moreover, microbial dysbiosis and pathogenesis have attracted much attentions of researchers to develop new strategies, such as application of prebiotics and probiotics. Both of these are essential nutrient components that play a significant role in managing overall health conditions, as well as aid in maintaining a proper functional immune system in the host. In this current chapter, we discuss the numerous features of prebiotics and probiotics along with their history of development and their role in combating some common but dangerous diseases. We have also given emphasis on their impact and their immune-modulatory mechanism, as well as their contribution in ameliorating immune-related diseases. This chapter aims to draw the attention of investigators involved in various fields of the health sector for the development of vaccines, pharmaceutical components, and drugs.

Keywords: Prebiotics, probiotics, immune system, immunostimulant, gut microbiome, galacto-oligosaccharide, fructo-oligosaccharide, *Lactobacillus*

[*]*Corresponding author*: usha@cuh.ac.in
[†]Authors contributed equally

Rajesh K. Kesharwani, Tingirikari Jagan Mohan Rao and Raj K. Keservani (eds.) Prebiotics and Probiotics in Disease Regulation and Management, (185–218) © 2022 Scrivener Publishing LLC

7.1 Introduction

In the last few decades, scientific advances have unraveled the significance of several minute organisms based on their living, coexisting behaviors with other organisms, including humans [1]. However, the behavior of humans have also coevolved with the emergence of new technologies. As the times passed, gradually technological growth influenced both the individual and the ecosystem in a positive, as well as in negative manner [2]. Changing lifestyle of people in the modern age, as well as unhealthy eating behavior, has provided opportunity for diseases development mostly related to defects in the diet. As food being the primary focus of all the organisms for survival, different organism has developed various strategies to obtain their resources. This coevolution has also expanded to tiny organisms, which are collectively now known as microorganisms. These organisms show diversified functions and are implicated to resolve food and health-related issues [2]. They have shown a massive impact on other organism through probiotic or prebiotic actions. These actions are interdependent and interlinked with each other. They regulate the health of host organism by synthesizing nutrient products, which maintain the homeostasis of the commensal microbiome in the gut of the host. They also degrade toxic substances synthesized by the disease causative strains and suppress diseases development by acting against the pathogens [3]. Recent research updates show that these prebiotics and probiotics are widely utilized in the pharmaceutical industry as they have become very essential for designing therapeutic approaches. Demand for these products has soared up as they are both ecofriendly, as well as cost effective. However, extended research is required in this field to completely understand their working principle [4]. Exploring these microbes would aid in designing suitable prebiotics and probiotics. In this chapter, we have discussed already existing views about the probiotics involved in several immune-related diseases, and we have attempted to highlight their underlying immunomodulatory mechanisms. Here, we have also discussed on the significance of gut microbiome maintaining a healthy immune system.

7.2 Prebiotics

FAO/WHO has defined the "prebiotics" as the group of nutrients that selectively escalates the growth of beneficial bacteria in the host gut (especially in the colonic region) [5]. However, the definition has undergone massive alteration in last few years as now a few carbohydrates are considered in the category [3]. They maintain the intestinal homeostasis via many metabolic activities, such as decontamination, nutrient production, drug metabolism, antipathogenicity, and immune regulation [3]. The history of the prebiotics began with the discovery of one of the components of milk N-acetyl glucosamine, which promoted the growth of *Bifidobacterium* strain in 1954 by Gyorgy [6]. Later, in 1957, researchers recognized that lactulose is acting as one of the Bifidus factor [7]. Gradually, further studies on this area concluded many nondigestible oligosaccharides acting as Bifidus factor. In 1995, ultimately, these bacterial-growth promoting substances were named as prebiotics by a group of scientists. Consumption of these substances favored selective growth of microbes in the colonic region and are of prime importance to maintain the host's health [8]. And in 2007, mounting evidences indicated about its wide application other than just limiting its effect to gut region only. They also modulated the immune system to prevent pathogen entry and were even involved in managing the metabolic functions. These substances were able to perform the task of eliminating pathogen by releasing SCFA, which upregulated the mucin production and reduced the translocation activity using SCFA receptors found on immune cells [9]. Along with exerting action through SCFAs, the diverse sugar unit present in the nondigestible carbohydrates also possesses some prebiotic properties. Each sugar molecule may influence the animals differently, but energy derived by the fermentation of these prebiotics is widened by the action of probiotics to regularize their metabolic processing [10]. However, there are few criteria which must be fulfilled before considering a suitable prebiotic candidate, such as easy hydrolyzation, resistance to low pH, permitting selective growth of advantageous microbiota, as well as exerting beneficial effects on the health of the host. Beneficial gut microbiota, such as *Bifidobacteria* and *Lactobacilli* species, have been quite promising in meeting these criteria. They are the substrates for selective growth of beneficial bacteria along with eliminating the pathogenic ones [11]. Along with these, few chemical components, such as fructo-oligosaccharides (FOS), galacto-oligosaccharides (GOS), and trans-galacto-oligosaccharides (TOS) have been determined to be prebiotic in action. They are involved in impacting the host in multiple ways. They are acted by the gut microbiome, which produces SCFAs regulating immune cells, such as T helper 2 cells, dendritic cells (in bone marrow). These fatty acid stimulate GPCR for AMP production and also regulate the epigenetic activity by suppressing HDAC activity [12]. Another fermented product from prebiotic includes peptidoglycan, which is also shown to modulate innate immune system for pathogen exclusion [3].

These compounds escape the lumina side of the mucosa into blood and are recognized by a type of pattern recognition receptor, nuclear oligomerization domain-1 (NOD-1). This receptor activates neutrophils, thereby priming innate immune system against pathogen [13]. The prebiotics also stimulate the growth of selective microbes as in the case of Fructans which particularly promote lactic acid–producing bacteria, whereas *Bifidobacteria* and *Lactobacilli* mainly thrive in the presence of GOS [14]. The immunostimulatory effects of prebiotics are significant for older people as any alterations in immune responsiveness leads to increase in susceptibilities for age-related disabilities. Besides, some noncarbohydrates prebiotics, such as flavanols, extracted from cocoa has shown to encourage the growth of lactic-acid producing bacteria [14]. Another study reported the involvement of prebiotic kestose (FOS) in strengthening the epithelial barrier upon infection. Further, it is also highlighted that administration of prebiotics to animal upregulated glucagon-like peptide level to combat inflammation and disorders related to obesity. They are growing evidences about mimicking the pathogen binding site by prebiotics for the purpose of pathogen exclusion [12]. In the current century, prebiotics have gained attention in utilization to treat various diseases like muscle wasting, colorectal cancers, respiratory tract infections and also in aging intestines. In addition, it has been rigorously used as a criterion for strain selection to evaluate beneficial aspects of probiotics [15]. Some of the Prebiotics and their mechanism has been discussed and summarized in the Table 7.1.

7.2.1 Galacto-Oligosaccharides (GOS)

This nondigestible carbohydrate is derived from the lactose with the help of enzyme b-galactosidases by the process of enzymatic transglycosylation. It consists of mixture of oligosaccharides, such as lactose, glucose, and galactose. Several *in vitro* experiments have shown its resistant to salivary ad pancreatic amylase, making it a suitable candidate for prebiotic. GOS is fermented by many strains of *Lactobacillus, Bifidobacterium, Bacteroides,* and *Clostridium* [16]. A notable variation in the cytokines level in the distal colon of the individuals fed with GOS is also observed. There was little reduction in IL-12 and IL-6 but TNF-α was upregulated [17]. Moreover, the glycosidic linkages in the oligosaccharide demonstrated a protective action against colorectal cancer. They were also observed to suppress the microbial enzymatic activity (β-glucuronidase) to reduce carcinogenesis [18]. Through the production of SCFA, GOS strengthen the epithelial barrier by enhancing the expression of junction protein claudin-1 and zonula occluden-1 (ZO-1)p as well as reduced MUC-2 expression [19].

Table 7.1 Well-known prebiotics and their related probiotic enhancement roles.

S. no.	Prebiotics	Probiotics	Mechanism	Reference
1.	Pectin	*Eubacteriumeligans* *Roseburia*	Affected the microbial diversity by changing pH	[105]
2.	Apple Pectin	*Faecalibacterium prausnitzii* *Anaerostipes hadrus*	Exerts anti-inflammatory effects on host cells	[105]
3.	Lactic acid or SCFA (Short Chain Fatty Acids)	*Lactobacillus* *Bifidobacterium, Clostridium leptum, Roseburia*	Modulate the cytokine production or (peripheral blood mononuclear cell (PBMC). Expression of cluaudin-1 and mucin -2	[105, 106]
4.	Dietary Fructans in various fruits vegetables, food products.	*Lactobacillus* *Bifidobacterium*	Reduces abdominal discomfort Downregulate Inflammatory Cytokines (IL)-6, IL-8, IL-17a, IFNγ	[107–110]

(*Continued*)

Table 7.1 Well-known prebiotics and their related probiotic enhancement roles. (*Continued*)

S. no.	Prebiotics	Probiotics	Mechanism	Reference
5.	Galacto-oligosaccharides (GOS)	*Lactobacillus, Bifidobacterium, Bacteroides, and Clostridium.*	reduction in IL-12 and IL-6 but TNF-α was upregulated suppress the microbial enzymatic activity β-glucuronidase production of SCFA expression of junction protein Claudin-1 and zonula occluden-1 (ZO-1) reduce MUC-2	[16, 17]
6.	Raffinose	*lactate producing bacteria*	increase in IgG, TNF-α and IL-6 Increase villus height Increase in goblet cells Downregulated amylase and Lipase activity	[24, 26]
7.	Human Milk Oligosaccharides	*Bifidobacterium (B. breve* and *B. infantis)*	upregulate cytokines like IFN-g and IL-10 downregulated IL-4 elevation Toll-Like Receptors (TLR-2 and TLR-4)	[27, 28, 30]

(*Continued*)

Table 7.1 Well-known prebiotics and their related probiotic enhancement roles. (*Continued*)

S. no.	Prebiotics	Probiotics	Mechanism	Reference
8.	Flavanols	*Bifidobacterium Lactobacillus*	dampened NO production hindered the production of Prostanoids and leukotrienes Downregulated TNF-α, IL-1β, IL-4, and IL-6	[33, 34]
9.	Poly Unsaturated Fatty Acids	*Roseburia*	suppress the production of cytokine prostaglandin E2, TNF-α, IL-6, IL-1β, E selectin and C-reactive protein.	[36]

7.2.2 Fructo-Oligosaccharides and Polysaccharides

These are another class of nondigestible carbohydrates which are derived from plant-based products. There are many varieties of prebiotic kestose (FOS), such as inulin, oligo-fructose, and short chain FOS. Though escape the hydrolysis by human digestive enzymes but are acted by few commensal microbiomes and undergo thorough fermentation in the colonic region of human gut, thus not excreted in the fecal matter. Upon hydrolyzation, they produce SCFA in the interior of the cells. These fatty acids lower the pH favoring the growth of beneficial bacteria such as *Bifidobacteria* and *Lactobacillus.* Moreover, during the fermentation, few important minerals such as zinc, magnesium and calcium are made available for absorption. In another studies, it was found that consumption of 100 g of FOS down-regulated triglycerides level in the mice model; however, no effect was seen on hepatic triglycerides. However, propionate, an SCFA negatively regulated hepatic triglycerides. In some instances, they have been able to inhibit constipation [20]. In other clinical studies, increase of Butyrate level upon inulin rich diet consumption in Crohn disease patients was reported [21]. Besides, inulin extracted from burdock roots has shown to possess immunomodulatory properties, such as stimulation of splenocytes and peritoneal macrophages, delaying the progression of tumor, activation of NO-stimulated innate immune system, as well as in vivo acid phosphatase production. However, these activities are dose-dependent [22], whereas fructans have shown to possess anti-viral properties by triggering the release of cytokines IL-1β, IL-6, IL-10, IFN-γ, and TNF-α, which block viral replication. They also account for upregulating the antibodies against influenza A virus. However, fructans are acid-sensitive and are partially digestible. Gases (like hydrogen) and SCFAs are responsible for modulating various signaling processes by regulating redox potential. They also contribute in phenol assimilation and inulin encourages glucose absorption. Many authors have mentioned the involvement of FOS-derived metabolites and phenolic compound in activating AMPK signaling pathway [21]. This signaling pathway has been targeted by many researchers for designing treatment against dreadful diseases, such as cancer, type 2 diabetes as they are central regulator of many overall metabolic processes of human body [23].

7.2.3 Raffinose

Growing evidences on the prebiotic role of Raffinose have made it to the list of prebiotics. They are made of trisaccharide galactose, glucose, and fructose. Since, this prebiotic is isolated from soya bean waste, thus they are ecofriendly as well. Like other prebiotics, it also aided in the production of SCFAs (primarily acetate but not butyrate), stimulated the growth of lactate producing bacteria, lowering of pH, reduction in ammonia content, increase CO_2 production [24]. Moreover, there are studies indicating the positive role of raffinose in iron absorption [25]. Considering its impact on immune system, raffinose causes increase in IgG, TNF-α, and IL-6, thereby uplifting humoral immune response. The groups fed with the prebiotic exhibited soaring up in the villus height along with the increase in goblet cells. However, the activity of certain enzymes, like amylase and lipase, was downregulated [26].

7.2.4 Human Milk Oligosaccharides

Not limiting to the focus on the nutrients provided to infants, recent studies have explained the prebiotic action of human milk oligosaccharides (HMO). They act as a decoy and mimic the pathogen binding site for inhibiting pathogen entry. Studies reveal that they favor selective growth of microbes as in case of *Bifidobacterium* where *B. breve* and *B. infantis* growth was supported [27]. They have been found to inhibit the progression of diseases, such as diarrhea, respiratory tract infection (RTI), sepsis. They upregulate cytokines like IFN-g and IL-10, whereas downregulated IL-4 induction [28]. Further, components of milk oligosaccharide increase the level of bone marrow derived dendritic cells primarily CD40+ and CD86+. Acidic HMOs from milk also caused some immunological changes, such as increase in IFNγ and IL-10 and decrease in IL-13. Fucosylated and sialylated HMOs generally exert their effect on mast cells and with the induction of T_{reg} cells, they lessen food-related allergic responses [29]. Interestingly, 3′-sialyllactose HMO has been observed to induce immune cells IFN-γ, TNF-α, IL-12, and TGF-β1 [30], whereas few HMOs turned down the release of IL-8 from cell lines infected with *E. coli* [31]. Some are involved in the maturation of dendritic cells (DCs). They are also responsible for the elevation of different types of toll-like receptors (TLR-2 and TLR-4), which stimulate the release of anti-inflammatory cytokines [30] and 2′-FL HMO has been reported to dampen inflammation via TLR-4. Other than TLRs, C-type lectins, selectins, are also reported in various literature to be interacting with HMOs. They also maintain the integrity of the mucosal barrier by interacting with the glycans present on the intestinal epithelial cells. Some changes in a type of lectin, galectins, which are profusely involved in regulating many immune cells. HMOs mainly play a crucial role in managing neonatal immune system and promoting a good microbial diversity [31]. Though the intestinal immune system is immature, it undergoes a dynamic shift under the influence of HMOs which aid in maturation. Glycocalyx layer is the most important part of intestinal epithelium as it inhibits pathogen adherence. Many experimental data have shown the effect of HMOs in enhancing intestinal barrier by stimulating glycocalyx. Moreover, these reinforcing effects are dependent on the structure of HMO as both 2′-FL and 3-FL showed variable results [32].

7.2.5 Flavanols

Flavanols are types of polyphenols, which are highly abundant in fruits, vegetables, nuts and other plant-based products [33]. These noncarbohydrates prebiotics are acted upon by commensal gut microbiome and converted into different forms to exert beneficial effects. Few microbes, such as *Bifidobacterium and Lactobacillus*, caused biotransformation of flavanols to some bioactive components, which dampened NO production induced by LPS [34]. Quercetin or kaempferol are some of the flavanols, which hindered the production of prostanoids and leukotrienes, which are inflammatory in nature by blocking the activity of the enzyme Cyclooxygenase

(COX-2). Moreover, many are involved in the hampering the release of inflammation provoking cytokines such as TNF-α, IL-1β, IL-4, and IL-6. Taxifolin glycoside has been suggested to downregulate immune response influenced by dendritic cell. They reinforce activity of many immune cells like natural killer cells, cytotoxic T lymphocyte, and also promote phagocytosis by macrophages. Many flavanols, such as apigenin, flavones, reso-kaempferol, synchronize the immune response by modulating the few signaling pathways like JAK/STAT pathway [33].

7.2.6 Polyunsaturated Fatty Acids

The prebiotic effects are not just limited to SCFAs, rather it is also noticed in the case of poly unsaturated fatty acids (PUFA) as well. The enzymes produced by gut microbiome specially belonging to *Lactobacillus* strain aid in the production of many bioactive intermediates such as oxo fatty acids, hydro fatty acids, conjugated fatty acids. PUFAs like a-linolenic acid and linolenic act as a precursor for these intermediates [35]. Many studies indicate the interaction between n-3PUFA and fatty acid receptor GPR120 suppress the production of cytokine prostaglandin E2, TNF-α, IL-6, IL-1β, E selectin and C-reactive protein. N-3 PUFA has been suggested to attenuate polarization of CD4+T cell and promote B-cell development. These fatty acids encourage the growth of butyrate producing bacteria like *Roseburia* and reduce the abundance of *Coprococcus* and *Facecalibacterium* [36].

7.3 Probiotics

Probiotics are host-friendly microbiota which possess numerous beneficial properties, such as inhibition of bowel disorders, maintaining a proper functional immune system, thereby improving the overall health of an individual [37]. In 2002, FDA/WHO considered those microbes as probiotics which upon consummation provided health benefits to the host [38]. Many literatures mention the discovery of probiotic in 2000 BC; however, the use of yeast in beverages began long before it [39]. Élie Metchnikoff first proposed the idea of controlling gastrointestinal defects using selected microbiota which later became a very hot topic for research. Since ancient times, traditional fermented food has become the part of various communities which has played a crucial role in maintain microbial diversity. During Babylonian, Egyptian, and Indus valley civilization i.e., 6000 years ago, lactic acid bacteria has been introduced for milk fermentation. These bacteria confer long shelf life and good flavor and texture to

Table 7.2 Various strains of gut microbiota possessing disease causing as well as disease preventing functions.

S. no.	Name of the disease	Disease causing/enhancing agent	Disease preventive/reducing agent	Reference
1.	Multiple sclerosis (MS)	*Streptococcus*	*Prevotella*	[46]
2.	Respiratory tract infection (RTI)	*Streptococcus pneumoniae, Haemophilus influenzae, Moraxella catarrhalis Staphylococcus aureus*	*Lactobacillus pentosus Lactobacillus reuteri, Bifidobacterium lactis Bb12, Lactobacillus casei Bifidobacterium Longum*	[53, 57, 59]
3.	Cardiovascular disease (CVD)	*Helicobacter pylori, Chlamydia pneumonia, Mycoplasma pneumonia Porphyromonas gingivalis*	*Streptococcus thermophilus, Lactobacillus acidophilus, Lactobacillus rhamnosus Enterococcus faecium Pediococcusacidilactici*	[62, 96]

(*Continued*)

Table 7.2 Various strains of gut microbiota possessing disease causing as well as disease preventing functions (*Continued*)

S. no.	Name of the disease	Disease causing/enhancing agent	Disease preventive/reducing agent	Reference
4.	Rheumatoid arthritis (RA)	*Prevotella copri, Porphyromonas gingivalis*	*Bacteroides fragilis, Bifidobacterium* species, and *Eubacterium rectale–Clostridium coccoides* *Faecalibacterium* *Lactobacillus casei* *Lactobacillus acidophilus*	[89, 97, 98]
5.	Inflammatory bowel disease (IBD)	*Gamma proteobacteria* *E. coli* *Enterobacteriaceae, Pasteurellaceae, Veillonellaceae, and Fusobacteriaceae*	*L. casei, L. plantarum, L. acidophilus, L. delbrueckii* subsp.*bulgaricus, B. longum, B. breve, B. infantis* and *Streptococcus salivarius subsp. Thermophiles.* *Clostridia, Ruminococcaceae, F. prausnitzii* *Leuconostoc* *Saccharomyces boulardii*	[81, 82, 99]

(*Continued*)

Table 7.2 Various strains of gut microbiota possessing disease causing as well as disease preventing functions (*Continued*)

S. no.	Name of the disease	Disease causing/enhancing agent	Disease preventive/reducing agent	Reference
6.	Vulvovaginal candidiasis	*Candida glabrata* *Candida albicans*	*L. acidophilus*, *L. rhamnosus GR-1* *L. fermentum RC-14* *L. casei*	[100–102]
7.	T1D (type 1 diabetes) in children	Altered *Bacteroidetes*/ *Firmicutes* ratio *Bacteroides fragilis* *Streptococcus mitis*	*Bifidobacterium* *Lactobacillus plantarum* *Clostridium* *Faecalibacterium prausnitzii*	[68, 103]
8.	Colorectal cancer (CRC)	*H. pylori* *Fusobacterium nucleatum*	*L. rhamnosus*, *L. kefiri*, *L. acidophilus*, *B. breve*	[75, 77]
9.	Muscle wasting	*Mycobacterium ulcerans* *E. coli*	*Lactobacillus plantarum*	[104, 60]

milk due to which this process has been continuing for many generations. Currently, probiotics, which fulfill the Food and Drug Administration—Generally Recognized as Safe (FDA GRAS) status, are being selected for various applications. However, a deep understanding is required about the underlying mechanism behind their immunomodulatory roles for making it suitable for therapeutic approaches [40]. In recent days, researchers are mainly focusing on the use of probiotics in various disease treatments acute infectious like diarrhea, inflammatory bowel disease and many more (summarized in Table 7.2) [41]. However, FAO and WHO has jointly come out with the strict guidelines for evaluation of efficacy of probiotics before implementing in food or health-related purposes [42].

7.4 Role of Prebiotics and Probiotics in Immunorelated Diseases

7.4.1 Multiple Sclerosis (MS)

Lesions in the central nervous system cause emergence of diseases named multiple sclerosis, which leads to both physical and neurological defects. Death of oligodendrocyte followed by inflammation driven by macrophage and T-lymphocyte cause development of the disease. This leads to the formation of plaques filled with the inflammatory cells, axons lacking in myelin both in gray and white matter of CNS, ultimately, leading to neuronal impairment [43]. Like other autoimmune disorders, MS is a chronic immune disorder arising out of multiple factors, such as genetic, environmental and immunological factors, and so on. This disease is not only caused by a single gene rather cluster of genes are involved in the progression of MS. It is reported that HLA class II are associated with risk increment [44]. Demyelination, insulin resistance, axonal degeneration, and oxidative stress are few of the consequences of the disease [45]. T-helper cells as well as the intercommunication between APC and T-lymphocytes aid in the initiation of the disease. The cytokines IL-17, IL-21, IL-22, and IL-26 are some of the pro-inflammatory cytokines released by Th-17 (CD4+ T-cells) [43]. The cytokines IL-6, tumor necrosis factor alpha (TNF-α), and interferon (IFN)-γ disrupt the blood-brain barrier. The cytokines produced by B-lymphocytes, such as lymphotoxin (or transforming growth factor beta [TGF-β]) and TNF-α are inflammatory in action. However, this lymphocyte has both positive and negative influence as B-cell driven cytokine IL-10 has anti-inflammatory action. Along with CD4+ T cells, CD8+ cells too help in the progression of the disease as they stimulate oligodendrocyte's death and elevate vascular permeability [43]. Thus, designing immunomodulatory strategies can have therapeutic effect. Such actions can be linked with the involvement of gut microbiome as reports have suggested a vivid distinction in abundance of commensal microbiome among diseased and healthy individuals [45]. Since Th-17 are key players in the progression of the disease, it is also associated with the shift in the mucosa-related microbiota in the small intestine. When compared to healthy subjects, relapsing-remitting MS patients exhibited increment in *Firmicutes/Bacteroidetes* ratio, increment in *Streptococcus* (mainly *Streptococcus mitis* and *Streptococcus oralis*) proportion, as well as decrease in abundance of *Prevotella*(anti-inflammatory)in the fecal matter. Such alterations are observed due to the fact that many microbiota, such as segmented filamentous bacteria are associated with enhanced Th17 differentiation. Hence, certain immunomodulatory drugs, such as IFN-b, glatiramer acetate (GA), or fingolimod targeting MS are suggested. Inference from these clinical data show the increase in the abundance of anti-inflammatory and butyrate producing microbe, such as *Faecalibacterium, Coprococcus.* However, a notable increment in the *Prevotella* strain was observed in IFN-treated patients [46, 47]. Findings have concluded that consumption of probiotics can negatively regulate the population of *Akkermansia* and *Blautia,* whereas up stimulate the abundance of beneficial microbes, such as Lactobacillus, Streptococcus, and Bifidobacterium. Some researchers associate the decrease level of short chain fatty acids (SCFAs) with increase of progression of MS. As seen in the case of propionic acid, which restored the mitochondrial impairment, as well as normalized Treg/TH17 cell ratio. Also, colonization in mice with *Bacteroides fragilis* (produce polysaccharide A) and Th-17 inducer segmented filamentous bacteria has shown to ameliorate MS progression. Aryl hydrocarbon receptor ligands released by commensal microbiome are also observed to downregulate inflammation and neurodegeneration [45, 48]. Other function of probiotics includes production of hormones GLP-1 and PYY, which help in improvising the insulin resistance in the brain. It is concluded that microbial metabolites travel to brain and interact with astrocytes to lower the inflammation. However, a vivid illustration of dietary impacts of probiotics can help in devising strain specific treatments [45].

7.4.2 Respiratory Tract Infections

Respiratory tract infection (RTI) has been categorized as upper RTI and Lower RTI. Upper RTI comprises of nose, pharynx, larynx, sinus, larger airways. This region is attacked by many pathogens, which leads to many infections, such as common cold, pharyngitis, tonsillitis, etc. [49]. About 87.5% of RTI occur in the upper respiratory tract of human [49]. Whereas the rest of the RTI belongs to lower respiratory infection, which mostly includes acute bronchitis and pneumonia [50]. Along with another chronic respiratory infection, i.e., lung cancer has been the cause for most of the cancer-related death and is very prominent in males when compared to females. Although particular probiotic could not be indicated as a solution, however, one of the clinical studies have demonstrated the involvement of probiotic strains along with chemotherapy in improving the health conditions of the patients [51]. While understanding the immunological changes in RTI, a significant reduction in immune cells, such as T and B lymphocytes, natural killer cells was observed in severe acute respiratory syndrome. Among T-lymphocytes, CD4+ type reduction was prevalent in almost all patients [52]. Moreover, patients suffering from chronic obstructive pulmonary disease (COPD) have inflamed airway due to elevation in inflammatory cytokines such as IL-1β, IL-6, TNF-α, and IL-17 in the bronchoalveolar lavage (BAL) fluid [53]. Normally, Th1 and Th2 control allergic reaction by suppressing the related receptors during eczema. However, in the diseased condition, their activity is altered [54]. Allergic reactions are more commonly observed in small age group peoples due to environmental factors, but in addition to these, intestinal flora also contribute in initiation of these allergic diseases through mucosal immunity causing shifts in Th1/Th2 cells balance. However, probiotic application improve the Th1 response and reduce the production of the inflammatory cytokines [55].Sputum samples, bronchoalveolar fluid, and bronchial biopsies obtained from the asthmatic patients showed soaring up in the inflammatory cells, such as T-lymphocytes, neutrophils, and eosinophils [56]. Although upper respiratory tract is home to many commensal microbiomes and the most prominent genera include *Staphylococcus, Streptococcus, Corynebacterium, Prevotella, Veillonella, Propionibacterium*, and *Fusobacterium,* whereas *Moraxella* (mostly in Children). However, many reports claim about the involvement of pathogens *Streptococcus pneumoniae, Haemophilus influenzae, Moraxella catarrhalis,* and *Staphylococcus aureus* as a key players in progression of respiratory tract infection [57]. *Haemophilus influenzae* and *Streptococcus pneumoniae* have become the most common cause for the death of million infants aged under 5 years of old [58]. Further, *Moraxella catarrhalis* and *Streptococcus pneumonia* have been considered as the prime mediators of COPD [53]. Therefore, probiotic action downregulates the deleterious effects of this pathogenic microbes. Several

LAB (*Lactobacillus, Streptococcus, Bifidobacterium,* and *Enterococcus* sp.) strains have been efficient in regulating immune responses. They interact with gut lymphoid-associated tissue (GALT) to heighten the respiratory immunity. Findings have suggested the involvement of *Lactobacillus pentosus* in the augmentation of IFN-g and IL-12 in the airways aiming to protect the host respiratory tract. Several probiotics strains, such as *Lactobacillus reuteri, Bifidobacterium lactis Bb12, LGG,* and *Lactobacillus casei* have been noted to regulate the T-cell responses by synchronizing Treg cells. These strains also downregulated airway inflammation and hyperresponsiveness in animal models. Beneficial bacteria exert their probiotic effect by inhibiting the activity of pathogenic strains as in case of *Salmonella typhimurium* infection, which is inhibited by the Foxp3+ T cells inducer *Bifidobacterium infantis* [59]. *Lactobacillus gasseri* inhibited Th17 proinflammatory cytokines in asthmatic individuals, whereas *B. breve* M-16V *downregulated L-4, IL-5, and IL-10* [51]. *Also, during Bifidobacterium longum* which when orally administered to mice soared up Alveolar macrophage-reactive oxygen species (ROS) in order to protect against *K. pneumoniae* infection. Many commensal microorganisms have been reported to upregulate cytokine production mainly IL-22 and IL-17 A in mouse suffering pneumonia. The metabolites from these bacteria also regulate the immunity in the pulmonary region. Antimicrobial peptide production has been used by few as one of the strategies [57]. Other than just focusing on the route of oral administration, the probiotic administration via intranasal path, such as in case of *LGG* has been quite efficient in providing the protection against H1N1 influenza virus infection [59]. In case of lung cancer, supplementation of *Lactobacillus acidophilus* exerted beneficial effect by increasing the rate of survival along with the decrease in the tumor size. They elevated the CD4+ lymphocytes and downregulated the macrophage infiltration. Also, upon analyzing the data from western blotting, a marked reduction in oncogenic gene and elevation in tumor suppression gene was concluded. In addition to this, several strains of *Lactobacillus (L. lactis KC24, L. lactis NK34, L. casei CRL 431)* have been demonstrated to possess anti-cancer properties. Further few Bifidobacterial strains, such as *B. bifidum, B. longum, B. lactis,* and *B. breve* have also successful in suspended tumor progression. Moreover, researchers have also found few strains, such as *Enterococcus faecium K-50* and *Saccharomyces cerevisiae* when administered along with the vaccine [51]. All these studies support the usage of probiotics and prebiotics in curing RTI. However, further knowledge on the appropriate probiotic strain and its dosage amount must be acquired to minimize its side effects.

7.4.3 Cardiovascular Disease (CVD)

In recent years CVDs have been a severe cause of death, mostly in the western countries. An unhealthy diet has been recognized as a major factor for cardiovascular disease morbidity. However, the relation of morbidities and dietary components was yet to be explored to acknowledge the significance of gut microbiota and their metabolites in combating the disease [60]. There are several clinical studies which have emphasized on the immunological changes leading to the development of the CVD-related diseases, such as atherosclerosis, cardiac arrest, stroke, cardiomyopathies, and defects in cardiac rhythm. Mounting evidence suggest the dysregulation in chemokines in the progression of the disorder. For example, researchers have shown the role of chemokine receptor CXC3 as one of the contributing factors towards atherosclerosis and myocardial infarction. Other immune cells such as mast cells, neutrophils T-helper (Th) 2 cells and several cytokines have also shown to aid in pathogenesis, whereas Leukotrienes has been observed to propel vascular inflammation. Hence, these immune cells can act as biomarkers for detecting many coronary diseases. As in the case of C-reactive protein (CRP) and N-terminal probrain natriuretic peptide (NT-proBNP), which has been linked with heart failure. The levels of this biomarkers determine the cardiorespiratory fitness in the patients. Further, CD8+ T cells has been concluded to have the major impact on the heightening the severity of the heart failure. Many studies have demonstrated that the alterations of the mediators from the mast cells to be one of the efficient therapeutic approaches for ameliorating the disease [61]. Moreover, little is known about the roles of probiotic and prebiotic supplements that can act as an important dietary component in the prevention and treatment of CVD. Microbiota living in symbiosis with the host and in turn influences the health of the host by modulating the metabolism, protecting against pathogens, and by maintaining immunological homeostasis. Studies are connecting the gut microbiota with several cardiometabolic diseases, including obesity and coronary disease [60]. Emerging data have shown the role of probiotics in increasing LDL/HDL ratio, downregulation of blood pressure, blood glucose level, and BMI. Fermented milk having *Lactobacillus* has shown to bring reduction in the cholesterol level as hypercholesteremia patients are more prone to atherosclerosis, ultimately leading to chronic heart attack. Researchers have also designed multiple yogurt having variety of probiotics, such as *Streptococcus thermophilus, Lactobacillus acidophilus, Lactobacillus rhamnosus,* and *Enterococcus faecium* in different composition to comprehend the role of these strains on CVD. The yogurt consisting

S. thermophilus and *Enterococcus faecium* has been shown to decrease CVD risk by 20%. Another symbiotic yogurt containing *Lactobacillus acidophilus, Bifidobacterium longum* and 1% of oligo-fructose caused elevation in HDL-level. Another study revealed about the anti-inflammatory role of *Lactobacillus rhamnosus GG* (*LGG*), which brought shift in lysophosphatidylcholine level, a putative factor for angiogenesis and carcinogenesis. Other immunomodulatory roles of the probiotic, specially *Lactobacillus and Bifidobacterium* includes, deconjugation of bile salts and assimilation of cholesterol in Bacterial cell Membrane. Consumption of the strain *L. acidophilus ATCC 43121* in another placebo studies have revealed to cause decrement in serum cholesterol level by 25% in hypercholesterolemic rats, whereas *L. acidophilus 145* and *B. longum 913* caused upregulation in HDL-cholesterol level. Moreover, some commercially available product such as PROBIOS-23, Cardioviva have been extremely beneficial for patients. PROBIOS-23 containing *Lactobacillus rhamnosus, Bifidobacterium adolescentis* and *Pediococcusacidilactici* brought remarkable reduction in cholesterol, triglycerides and LDL-C levels whereas *Lactobacillus reuteri NCIMB 30242* in Cardioviva downregulated LDL-cholesterol levels by almost 11.6% [62]. The microbiome occupying the colonic region are primarily responsible for fermenting food into an important metabolite, such as short chain fatty acids and secondary bile acids. Hence, these products are quite necessary to maintain the gut homeostasis, as well as cardiovascular health. There was a notable distinction in the microbial composition in patients if compared to healthy individuals. Placebo studies have indicated increment in the abundance of *Prevotella, Hungatella,* and *Succinclasticum* in individuals suffering from chronic heart failure along with the decrement in *Lachnospiraceae* family, which includes *Faecalibacterium* and *Bifidobacterium.* Also, *Enterobacteriaceae* and *Streptococcus* spp. was abundant in atherosclerotic patients. These gut microbes use several metabolites to gain access to different organs of the body releasing various metabolites, such as SCFA, trimethylamine N-oxide (TMAO), lipopolysaccharides (LPS). The severity of the coronary diseases is reduced in the presence of butyrate, propionate and acetate-producing microbes, whereas the presence of TMAO-producing microbes, such as *Roseburia intestinalis* and *Faecalibacterium prausnitzii* exhibited deleterious effect on the health of the host as it dysregulates lipid metabolism. It is evident from the experimental studies on animal models that TMAO is responsible for elevating inflammatory cytokines tumor necrosis factor (TNFα) and interleukin-1β) aiding in the atherosclerotic plaque formation. Dysregulation of endothelial cells in the vessels and the presence of LDL in the macrophages stimulates inflammatory responses. This eventually leads to the development of foam cells, hence causing plaque formation. This condition is associated with dysfunction in lipid metabolism. Alteration of gut microbiome especially the change in the ratio of Firmicutes and Bacteroidetes is notable in the patients. However, emerging data suggest about various commensal bacteria exerting immunomodulatory changes for inhibiting CVD. One of them being, *Akkermansia muciniphila* considered to be an appropriate probiotic candidate for downregulating fat deposition and insulin resistance in the mouse model [63, 64]. Upon exploring its immunomodulatory effect, it was observed to regulate both systemic and organ-specific immune system. It causes alteration in mesenteric lymph nodes. It downregulates MHC-II expression on dendritic cells and also scales down the expression of CD-86, the costimulatory molecule expression on B cells. The microbe was found to escalate IL-10/TNF-alpha ratio. Hence, we can conclude that *A. muciniphila* upregulated the anti-inflammatory responses [65]. Among the prebiotics, a flavanol chrysin has been observed to ameliorate myocardial injuries and inflammation in rats suffering from diabetes, whereas bilobetin reduced insulin resistance in animal models fed with food enriched in fats. Some are also responsible for preventing cardiotoxicity due to oxidative stress-induced mitochondrial dysfunction [33]. Moreover, fish oil enriched in n-3 PUFA has shown to reduce the severity of many CVD. It downregulates the factors propelling atherosclerosis formation [36].

7.4.4 Type 1 Diabetes (T1D)

It is an autoimmune disorder caused due to the destruction of beta-pancreatic cells, causing impairment in glucose production. This causes the dependence on the exogenous insulin. So far, these insulin and pro-insulin peptides are targets for autoreactive T1D pathogenesis [66]. Therefore, understanding the anti-islet immune response would be essential in developing intervening strategies against TID. Many studies have been conducted on the animal model to understand the type of immune component involved in the disease. For example, few studies have verified that without T cells (CD8+ and CD4+ T cells) and MHC-I, TID could not be detected in the mice model. CD4+ T cells escalate cytokine production to generate an immune response against the beta-cells as the type of cytokine produced was different from that of healthy individuals. IFN-g was reported in the patients, whereas IL-10 was observed in nondiabetic individuals [67]. Additionally, the absence of *Bifidobacterium* species along with elevated levels of bacteria from genus Bacteroides in the fecal matter of patients show a positive correlation with the observation of autoantibodies targeting pancreatic islet b-cells in children with T1D). Thus, deficiencies of the bacterial species in the gut can be related to the onset and progression of local and systemic inflammatory disorders. However, supplementing the suitable composition of probiotic strains will give protection from autoimmune disorders [68]. In one of the pilot studies, a probiotic capsule was orally administered to children to evaluate the efficacy of the probiotics in glycemic control. A significant reduction in glycated hemoglobin A1c (HbA1c) was noticed in the subjects. The capsule consists of strains of *Lactobacillus, Bifidobacterium,* and *Streptococcus.* However, immunological activity of the capsule is yet to be speculated [69]. These bacteria are also responsible suppressing IL-1β, thereby attenuating T1D. Probiotics belonging to *Lactobacillus* genus ameliorates TID progression by reduced TNF-α and boosted the release of IL-10 and pre/pro insulin. Few probiotic strains control Free fatty acid receptor (FFAR2 and FFAR3) activity which further stimulates glucagon-like peptide-1 (GLP-1), which downregulates blood glucose level. Moreover, it is also reported that early exposure to probiotics can reduce the risk of autoimmunity and hindered TLR4 signaling process [70]. Few clinical researches on pediatric TID patients have revealed about the link between tryptophan metabolism and progression of the disease. Kynurenine, a byproduct of the metabolism, was found in very small amount in the serum of the patients if compared to that of nondiabetic individuals due to dysfunction in the enzyme indoleamine 2,3 dioxygenase 1 (IDO1). However, regular administration of Probiotic *Lactobacillus rhamnosus* GG for almost 3 months led to an increase in the tryptophan level in the serum. A remarkable reduction in the cytokines IFN-γ and IL-17F were also observed in patients when treated with this probiotic [71]. Besides, prebiotics also attenuated TID progression. One of the examples is high amylose maize starch (HAMS), which stimulates SCFA for exhibiting immunomodulatory effects and also promote insulin sensitivity [72]. Moreover, many placebo-controlled studies have recommended inulin for treating T1D patients [73].

7.4.5 Colorectal Cancer

Among all the type of cancers, colorectal cancer (CRC) occupies the third position in affecting millions of people worldwide. There are many contributing factors, such as poor eating habits, unhealthy lifestyle, increase consumption of preservative foods, etc., which aid in pathogenesis of CRC. While understanding the immune mechanism reports claim about the interaction between programmed cell death-1(PD-1) and programmed cell death-1 ligand (PDL-1) which downregulates the expression of IL-2 production propagating carcinogenesis. CD4+, Th17, CD8+ T and CD4+ regulatory T (Treg) have also been used as therapeutic means against tumor progression. However, many studies suggest constructing checkpoint blockers one of the efficient ways to mitigate the disease. Hence, these immunological pathways can be explored while designing the appropriate probiotic to combat CRC [74]. Recently, attention has been given to the role of gut microbiota, like *Fusobacterium nucleatum, Escherichia coli, Enterococcus faecalis, Streptococcus gallolyticus, Bacteroides fragilis* in colorectal carcinogenesis. Some studies also link the role of *Helicobacter pylori* with the progression of gastric carcinogenesis; however, the mechanism is not yet clear [75]. *Fusobacterium nucleatum* has been reported to soar up the tumor progression by selectively recruiting myeloid cells, whereas IL-17 is upregulated in the presence of *Bacteroides fragilis*. Another gut microbe named *Helicobacter hepaticus* secrete proinflammatory cytokines, such as IL-6, IL-8, TNF-α, IFN-γ. Moreover, the most commonly known pathogen *Helicobacter pylori* has been reported to stimulate colonic mucosal cells by increasing secretion of gastrin [76]. The microbes aiding in carcinogenesis, usually secrete genotoxins (like cytolethal distending toxin (CDT), *B. fragilis* toxin (BFT), Colibactin), which deliberately cause double-strand break and arrest cell cycle ultimately leading to the swelling of the cell. CDT usually stimulate the activation of proinflammatory factors like IL-6 [75]. Extensive research in this area revealed many Lactobacilli strains (*L. rhamnosus, L. kefiri, L. acidophilus)* to be more effective in combating carcinogenesis. They use Toll-like receptors specially TLR-2 for promoting apoptosis and downregulating inflammation by IL-10 stimulation. They also modulate few proteins involved in cell junctions like claudin, occluding, and JAM-1. One of the studies reported that administration of both *L. rhamnosus* and *B. breve* downregulated biomarkers of CRC [77], whereas *Lactobacillus rhamnosus* and *Bifidobacterium lactis* showed positive results when administered in colon-cancer induced rats. Efficacy of role of prebiotics like Fructo-oligosaccharides and galacto-oligosaccharides are highly explored for the attenuation of CRC. These components possess various functions including regulation of immune response, production of metabolites, as well as aid in alteration of gene expression in the bacteria inhabiting caecum and colonic region [76]. Other reported increase in the abundance of *Firmicutes*, *Paraprevotella*, and *Parabacteroides* genus which are anti-inflammatory in nature [78]. However, more advance research is required to understand the underlying mechanism to inhibit the CRC progression [76].

7.4.6 Inflammatory Bowel Diseases

It is gastrointestinal disease associated with inflammation and injuries in the epithelial layer of the intestine. A combination of genetic, environmental and inflammatory factors is responsible for progression of the disease. Crohn's disease (CD) and ulcerative colitis (UC) are the two forms of IBD. The presence of inflammatory cytokines is involved in the pathogenesis. Diminished amount of anti-inflammatory cytokines IL-10 has been correlated with the initiation of IBD. Many antigen-presenting cell (APC)-derived cytokines such as IL-6, IL-18, and TNF is concentrated in the intestinal mucosa of the patients. IL-6 dampened the T-cell apoptosis and further stimulated anti-inflammatory factors. Some clinical studies have mentioned about the beneficial role of inhibiting IL-1 activity in curing chronic colitis. Among TNF, only soluble form is reported to be majorly involved in intestinal inflammation, however, both soluble and membrane bound has been proposed for treatment of colitis. Thus, probiotics targeting this cytokines can be another way of treating IBD [79]. The interaction between immune cells Th1, Th2, Th17, and Treg cells are involved in increasing the proinflammatory components. The disturbance in the abundance of phyla *Bacteroidetes* and *Firmicutes* is notable in the patients of IBD due to which low amount of SCFA in fecal matter is reported. SCFAs use few transporters to exert its effect; however, the inflammation reduces the expression of these transporters. Hence, low quantity of butyrate is one of the important characteristics of IBD. Butyrate is stated to promote acetylation of Foxp3, which eventually stabilize peripherally induced Treg cells (p Tregs). However, in case of IBD, in spite of a high amount of Tregs in the inflammatory induced lesions, no control on inflammation can be witnessed. Rather, decrease in butyrate increase the proinflammatory ability of Treg cells [80]. In newly diagnosed children with CD, an increased abundance of *Enterobacteriaceae, Pasteurellaceae*, *Veillonellaceae*, and *Fusobacteriaceae* and decreased levels of *Bacteroidales* and *Clostridia* were observed in ileal and rectal biopsies [81]. Although *Lactobacillus* and *Bifidobacterium* are dominant ones, but there are number of strains which has been recommended as a probiotic for IBD, such as *Escherichia coli Nissle 1917, Streptococcus, Enterococcus, Saccharomyces boulardii* and *Leuconostoc,* whereas some prebiotics like poly-ols, oligosaccharides, and soluble fiber are also employed. Sometimes, the combination of both, i.e., synbiotics are also considered for therapeutic purposes [82]. The prebiotic galacto-oligosaccharides has been reported to augment the IL-15 level, which is usually involved in antibody synthesis and T-cell proliferation [83], whereas some studies aimed to evaluate the efficacy of fructo-oligosaccharide in inhibiting the UC reemission [84]. One of the clinical studies were performed to assess the role of few lactobacillus strain (*L. casei, L. acidophilus,* and *L. rhamnosus*) in reducing murine colitis. These probiotics promoted antioxidants and downregulated TLR4 signaling. They even accelerated the healing process of LPS-induced intestinal injury. However, among the three strains, *L. acidophilus* demonstrated highest probiotic effects [85].

7.4.7 Rheumatoid Arthritis (RA)

The disease emerges when the antibodies are made against self-antigen i.e., Fc portion of IgG, leading to autoimmunity and ultimately become a major cause of death due to multi-organ failure [86]. Moreover, patients suffering from Rheumatoid Arthritis(RA) are prone to cardiovascular disease such as atherosclerotic plaque formation, myocardial infarction, congestive heart failure [87]. MHC-II has a strong correlation in the pathogenesis; however, some environmental factors can also be taken into consideration [86]. Storage of fluid and migration of inflammatory cells to the joints are some of the characteristics of the disease. IL-11, IL-13, and IL-10 are some of the proinflammatory cytokines involved RA. Helper T17 (Th17) has been reported in the contribution to the pathogenesis. Besides immunological factors, certain environmental agents, such as low vegetable diet, high fat-containing foods, and smoking led to RA. Findings reveal that women are more susceptible to the disease. Moreover, gut microbiome dysbiosis and RA are correlated. *Prevotell. Copri,* another probiotic is observed to elevate the proinflammatory cytokines IL-1β, IL-6, and IL-23 level and also trigger TLR-2 receptors in the intestinal epithelium. It also prompted Th17 cells activation thereby leading to enormous secretion of IL-17 and causing inflammation. Clinical trials on patients revealed that probiotics consumption downregulated IL-6 level. Among the probiotics *L. casei* or *L. acidophilus* have been successful in decreasing the concentration of inflammatory cytokines and inhibiting arthritis. *L. acidophilus* downregulated the Th-17 mediated pathways [88]. Many butyrate producing microbes *Faecali bacterium* are found to be diminished in the patients. Some probiotics upregulate secretory IgA, which support the B-cell differentiation into plasma cells. These cells block pathogenic adherence. They also regulate the host metabolism via indirect ways, such as increase mucin (MUC 2 and MUC 3) production, heightening the mucus layer thickness, regulation cell junction proteins, and boost up AMP production [89]. There are increasing evidences about the antiarthritic effects of prebiotic. One of them being berberine, which has shown to downregulate some inflammatory cytokines like IFNγ, IL-17, and IL-2 as these are associated with bone erosion and joint destruction [90]. Through experimental verification, it has been concluded that the administration of the prebiotic Thalidomide suppress inflammation in joints [91].

7.4.8 Muscle Wasting

Muscle Wasting is a comorbidity observed in individuals suffering life-threatening diseases such as chronic CVD, renal diseases, COPD. It is associated with reduction in the muscle mass, making patients resistant towards treatments. Patients suffering from this condition undergo a huge weight loss accompanied by skeletal muscle atrophy. Their response to chemotherapy is very poor. It reported that dysfunction macrophages alter the homeostasis of the skeletal muscle. Many experiments suggest the involvement of neutrophils and T cells in the maintenance of these macrophages [92], whereas sarcopenia is the condition associated with the loss of muscle mass and increase of fragility with the progression of age [93]. Along with it, cachexia is another muscle wasting syndrome linked with involuntary deprivation of lean body mass due to alteration in the pattern of cytokine production [94]. From numerous data, it is concluded that shift in gut microbiome can be correlated with muscle wasting syndromes. Colonization of the gut with *E. coli* provoked inflammation, whereas colonization with *Lactobacillus plantarum* promoted muscle endurance and elevated muscle mass. A significant amount of *Enterobacteriaceae* was notable in the gut of the patient [60]. Data indicate about the several strains of *Lactobacilli* involved in strengthening muscle integrity. Probiotic administration also downregulated interleukin (IL)-6 in the serum, thereby attenuating the cachexia progression. Supplementation of prebiotics like inulin and fructooligosaccharides (FOS) improved muscle functionality [95].

7.5 Conclusion

Prebiotics are ingredients that stimulate the growth and or function of the gastrointestinal microbes, but these products modulate the immune function in direct or indirect ways. The direct pathway is usually employed by probiotics; however, for prebiotics, it is a topic of debate. However, recent studies suggest regarding some bacterial strains present in the microbiota which can also act on enterocytes and cause susceptible diseases and can modulate those enterocytes through our diet [111]. Different probiotics strains and their genera show different immune effects in different types of individuals, but the exact effect of many genera, species of both for prebiotic and probiotic immunomodulatory mechanisms is still not clear.

Inflammatory Bowel Disease is the best example of prebiotic and probiotic-mediated disorder, which is caused due to the interaction between the Intestinal Epithelium Mucous Immune System. However, insufficient data inhibit clinical trials for treatments of Ulcerative colitis or Crohn's disease by using these prebiotics and probiotics supplements. Both prebiotics and probiotics may help in restoring normal microbiota communities in the intestine or may stimulate specific mucosal immune functions, thereby contributing reducing the severity diseases. For example, mild inflammation in the intestinal mucosa may be amenable to prebiotic and probiotic treatment, and it has been suggested that probiotics could improve the inflammatory immune status in the elderly. Hence, it is quite clear from all the existing data that many prebiotics and probiotics can be employed against immunomodulatory diseases. However, the effect is dose- and strain-dependent. Although many literatures indicate about the usage of it; however, no clinical trial has been approved yet for the treatment.

Acknowledgment

This work is supported by Science and Engineering Research Board (SERB), Department of Science and Technology (DST), Government of India for the research grants (YSS/2014/000896 and CRG/2018/003725) to UN.

References

1. Rybakova, D., Fischer, D., Cernava, T., Vergès, M.C., Charles, T., Chen, X., Cocolin, L., Eversole, K., Corral, G. H., Kazou, M., Kinkel, L., Lange, L., Lima, N., Loy, A., Macklin, J.A., Maguin, E., Mauchline, T., McClure, R., Mitter, B., ... Schloter, M., Microbiome definition re-visited: Old concepts and new challenges. *Microbiome*, 8, 1, 103, 2020.
2. Roberfroid, M., Prebiotics: The Concept Revisited. *J. Nutr.*, 137, 3, 830S–837S, Mar. 2007.
3. Davani-Davari, D. Negahdaripour, M., Karimzadeh, I., Seifan, M., Mohkam, M., Masoumi, S. J., Berenjian, A., & Ghasemi, Y., Prebiotics: Definition, types, sources, mechanisms, and clinical applications. *Foods*, 8, 3, 92, 2019.
4. Parvez, S., Malik, K.A., Ah Kang, S., Kim, H.Y., "Probiotics and their fermented food products are beneficial for health. *J. Appl. Microbiol.*, 100, 6, 1171–1185, Jun.2006.
5. de Vrese, M. and Schrezenmeir, J., Probiotics, prebiotics, and synbiotics. *Adv. Biochem. Eng. Biotechnol.*, 111, 1–66, 2008.

6. Tymczyszyn, E.E., Santos, M., II, Costa, M.C., Illanes, A., History, synthesis, properties, applications and regulatory issues of prebiotic oligosaccharides. *Carbohydrates Appl. Med.*, 661, 2, 127–154, 2014.
7. Petuely, F., The Lactobacillus bifidus factor. *Dtsch. Med. Wochenschr.*, 82, 46, 1957–1960, Nov. 1957.
8. Gibson, G.R. and Roberfroid, M.B., Dietary modulation of the human colonic microbiota: Introducing the concept of prebiotics. *J. Nutr.*, 125, 6, 1401–1412, Jun.1995.
9. Lomax, A.R. and Calder, P.C., Prebiotics, immune function, infection and inflammation: A review of the evidence. *Br. J. Nutr.*, 101, 5, 633–658, 2009.
10. Rasmussen, H.E. and Hamaker, B.R., Prebiotics and Inflammatory Bowel Disease. *Gastroenterol. Clin. North Am.*, 46, 4, 783–795, 2017.
11. Scantlebury-Manning, T. and Gibson, G., Microbial-gut interactions in health and disease. Prebiotics. *Best Pract. Res. Clin. Gastroenterol.*, 18, 287–298, May 2004.
12. Pujari, R. and Banerjee, G., Impact of prebiotics on immune response: from the bench to the clinic. *Immunol. Cell Biol.*, 99, 3, 255–273, 2021.
13. Clarke, T.B., Davis, K.M., Lysenko, E.S., Zhou, A.Y., Yu, Y., Weiser, J.N., Recognition of peptidoglycan from the microbiota by Nod1 enhances systemic innate immunity. *Nat. Med.*, 16, 2, 228–231.
14. Davani-Davari, D., Negahdaripour, M., Karimzadeh, I., Seifan, M., Mohkam, M., Masoumi, S.J., Berenjian, A., Ghasemi, Y., Prebiotics: Definition, types, sources, mechanisms, and clinical applications.,". *Foods (Basel, Switzerland)*, 8, 3, 92, Mar. 2019.
15. Leghari, A. Shahid, S., Farid, M., Saeed, M., Hameed, H., Anwar, S., Nishat, Z., Shahid, M., Meraj, A., Beneficial aspects of probiotics, strain selection criteria and microencapsulation using natural biopolymers to enhance gastric survival: A review. *Life Sci. J.*, 18, 30–47, Jan. 2021.
16. Sako, T., Matsumoto, K., Tanaka, R., Recent progress on research and applications of non-digestible galacto-oligosaccharides. *Int. Dairy J.*, 9, 1, 69–80, 1999.
17. Monteagudo-Mera, A., Arthur, J.C., Jobin, C., Keku, T., Bruno-Barcena, J.M., Azcarate-Peril, M.A., High purity galacto-oligosaccharides enhance specific Bifidobacterium species and their metabolic activity in the mouse gut microbiome. *Benef. Microbes*, 7, 2, 247–264, 2016.
18. Qamar, T.R. Iqbal, S., Syed, F., Nasir, M., Rehman, H., Iqbal, M.A., Liu, R. H., Impact of novel prebiotic galacto-oligosaccharides on various biomarkers of colorectal cancer in wister rats. *Int. J. Mol. Sci.*, 18, 9, 1785, 2017.
19. Gao, R., Tian, S., Wang, J., Zhu, W., Galacto-oligosaccharides improve barrier function and relieve colonic inflammation via modulating mucosa-associated microbiota composition in lipopolysaccharides-challenged piglets. *J. Anim. Sci. Biotechnol.*, 12, 1, 92, Dec. 2021.

20. Sabater-Molina, M., Larqué, E., Torrella, F., Zamora, S., Dietary fructooligosaccharides and potential benefits on health. *J. Physiol. Biochem. 2009 653*, 65, 3, 315–328, Sep. 2009.
21. Peshev, D. and Van den Ende, W., Fructans: Prebiotics and immunomodulators. *J. Funct. Foods*, 8, 1, 348–357, May 2014.
22. Zhang, X.J., Liu, S.F., Lu., Y., Wang, J.Y., Chen, K.S., Immunomodulatory activity of a fructooligosaccharide isolated from burdock roots. *RSC Adv.*, 9, 20, 11092–11100, Apr. 2019.
23. Carling, D., AMPK signalling in health and disease. *Curr. Opin. Cell Biol.*, 31–37, Apr. 2017.
24. Amorim, C., Silvério, S.C., Cardoso, B.B., Alves, J., II, Pereira, M.A., Rodrigues, L.R., *In vitro* fermentation of raffinose to unravel its potential as prebiotic ingredient. *LWT*, 126, 109322, May 2020.
25. Pacifici, S., Song, J., Zhang, C.K., Tako, E., Evaluating the effect of plant origin prebiotics (Raffinose and Stachyose) on iron status, intestinal functionality and intestinal bacterial populations *in vivo. FASEB J.*, 30, 692.17–692.17, 2016.
26. Zeng, Z., Zhang, Y., He, J., Yu, J., Mao, X., Zheng, P., Luo, Y., Luo, J., Huang, Z., Yu, B., Chen, D., Effects of soybean raffinose on growth performance, digestibility, humoral immunity and intestinal morphology of growing pigs. *Anim. Nutr.*, 7, 2, 393–399, Jun. 2021.
27. Barile, D. and Rastall, R.A., Human milk and related oligosaccharides as prebiotics. *Curr. Opin. Biotechnol.*, 24, 2, 214–219, Apr. 2013.
28. Triantis, V., Bode, L., van Neerven, J.R.J., Immunological effects of human milk oligosaccharides. *Front. Pediatr.*, 6, 190, 2018.
29. Zuurveld, M. van Witzenburg, N.P., Garssen, J., Folkerts, G., Stahl, B., Van't Land, B., Willemsen, L., Immunomodulation by human milk oligosaccharides: The potential role in prevention of allergic diseases. *Front. Immunol.*, 11, 801, May 2020.
30. Cheng, L., Kiewiet, M.B.G., Groeneveld, A., Nauta, A., de Vos, P., Human milk oligosaccharides and its acid hydrolysate LNT2 show immunomodulatory effects via TLRs in a dose and structure-dependent way. *J. Funct. Foods*, 59, 174–184, Aug. 2019.
31. Ayechu-Muruzabal, V. van Stigt, A. H., Mank, M., Willemsen, L., Stahl, B., Garssen, J., Van't Land, B., Diversity of human milk oligosaccharides and effects on early life immune development. *Front. Pediatr.*, 6, 239, 2018.
32. Kong, C.Elderman, M., Cheng, L., de Haan, B. J., Nauta, A., de Vos, P., Modulation of intestinal epithelial glycocalyx development by human milk oligosaccharides and non-digestible carbohydrates. *Mol. Nutr. Food Res.*, 63, 17, 1900303, Sep. 2019.
33. González-Gallego, J., García-Mediavilla, M.V., Sánchez-Campos, S., Tuñón, M.J., Anti-inflammatory, Immunomodulatory, and Prebiotic Properties of Dietary Flavonoids. *Polyphenols Prev. Treat. Hum. Dis.*, 22, 3, 327–345, Jan. 2018.

34. Kawabata, K., Sugiyama, Y., Sakano, T., Ohigashi, H., Flavonols enhanced production of anti-inflammatory substance(s) by Bifidobacterium adolescentis: Prebiotic actions of galangin, quercetin, and fisetin. *undefined*, 39, 4, 422–429, 2013.
35. Rinninella, E. and Costantini, L., Polyunsaturated fatty acids as prebiotics: Innovation or confirmation?. *Foods*, 11, 2, 146, Jan. 2022.
36. Parolini, C., Effects of fish n-3 PUFAs on intestinal microbiota and immune system. *Mar. Drugs*, 17, 6, 374, Jun. 2019.
37. Shi, L.H., Balakrishnan, K., Thiagarajah, K., Ismail, N., II, Yin, O.S., Beneficial properties of probiotics. *Trop. Life Sci. Res.*, 27, 2, 73, 2016.
38. Hill, C. Guarner, F., Reid, G., Gibson, G.R., Merenstein, D.J., Pot, B., Morelli, L., Canani, R.B., Flint, H.J., Salminen, S., Calder, P.C., Sanders, M.E., The International Scientific Association for Probiotics and Prebiotics consensus statement on the scope and appropriate use of the term probiotic. *Nat. Rev. Gastroenterol. Hepatol. 2014 118*, 11, 8, 506–514, Jun. 2014.
39. Ozen, M. and Dinleyici, E.C., The history of probiotics: The untold story. *Benef. Microbes*, 6, 2, 159–165, 2015.
40. Ghosh, T., Beniwal, A., Semwal, A., Navani, N.K., Mechanistic insights into probiotic properties of lactic acid bacteria associated with ethnic fermented dairy products. *Front. Microbiol.*, 10, 502, 2019.
41. Remus, D.M., Kleerebezem, M., Bron, P.A., An intimate tête-à-tête — How probiotic lactobacilli communicate with the host. *Eur. J. Pharmacol.*, 668, S33–S42, 2011.
42. Pandey, K.R., Naik, S.R., Vakil, B.V., Probiotics, prebiotics and synbiotics- A review. *J. Food Sci. Technol.*, 52, 12, 7577–7587, Dec. 2015.
43. Ghasemi, N., Razavi, S., Nikzad, E., Multiple Sclerosis: Pathogenesis, symptoms, diagnoses and cell-based Therapy. *Cell J.*, 19, 1, 1–10, Apr. 2017.
44. Hemmer, B., Kerschensteiner, M., Korn, T., Role of the innate and adaptive immune responses in the course of multiple sclerosis. *Lancet Neurol.*, 14, 4, 406–419, Apr. 2015.
45. Jiang, J., Chu, C., Wu, C., Wang, C., Zhang, C., Li, T., Zhai, Q., Yu, L., Tian, F., Chen, W., Efficacy of probiotics in multiple sclerosis: A systematic review of preclinical trials and meta-analysis of randomized controlled trials. *Food Funct.*, 12, 6, 2354–2377, Mar.2021.
46. Cosorich, I., Dalla-Costa, G., Sorini, C., Ferrarese, R., Messina, M. J., Dolpady, J., Radice, E., Mariani, A., Testoni, P. A., Canducci, F., Comi, G., Martinelli, V., Falcone, M., High frequency of intestinal TH17 cells correlates with microbiota alterations and disease activity in multiple sclerosis. *Sci. Adv.*, 3, 7, e1700492, 2017.
47. Cantarel, B.L. Waubant, E., Chehoud, C., Kuczynski, J., DeSantis, T.Z., Warrington, J., Venkatesan, A., Fraser, C.M., Mowry, E. M., Gut Microbiota in Multiple Sclerosis. *J. Investig. Med.*, 63, 5, 729–734, Jun. 2015.
48. Tankou, S.K., Regev, K., Healy, B. C., Cox, L. M., Tjon, E., Kivisakk, P., Vanande, I. P., Cook, S., Gandhi, R., Glanz, B., Stankiewicz, J., Weiner, H. L.

Investigation of probiotics in multiple sclerosis. *Mult. Scler.*, 24, 1, 58–63, Jan. 2018.
49. Jain, N., Lodha, R., Kabra, S.K., Upper respiratory tract infections. *Indian J. Pediatr.*, 68, 12, 1135–1138, 2001.
50. Mahowald, M., Shahan, B., Forbes, D., Respiratory Conditions: Lower Respiratory Tract Infections. *FP Essent.*, 486, 19–25, Nov. 2019.
51. Sharma, A., Viswanath, B., Park, Y.S., Role of probiotics in the management of lung cancer and related diseases: An update. *J. Funct. Foods*, 40, 625–633, Jan. 2018.
52. Cui, W., Fan, Y., Wu, W., Zhang, F., Wang, J.Y., Ni, A.P., Expression of lymphocytes and lymphocyte subsets in patients with severe acute respiratory syndrome. *Clin. Infect. Dis.*, 37, 6, 857–859, Sep. 2003.
53. Bhat, T.A., Panzica, L., Kalathil, S.G., Thanavala, Y., Immune Dysfunction in Patients with Chronic Obstructive Pulmonary Disease. *Ann. Am. Thorac. Soc*, 12, 2, S169–S175, Nov. 2015.
54. Renz, H., Brandtzaeg, P., Hornef, M., The impact of perinatal immune development on mucosal homeostasis and chronic inflammation. *Nat. Rev. Immunol.*, 12, 1, 9–23, 2012.
55. Michail, S., The role of Probiotics in allergic diseases. *Allergy, Asthma Clin. Immunol.*, 5, 13–17, 2009.
56. Mathur, S.K. and Nyenhuis, S.M., Changes in immune function in asthma in the elderly. *Aging Health*, 5, 4, 551–559, Jul. 2009.
57. Clark, S.E., Commensal bacteria in the upper respiratory tract regulate susceptibility to infection. *Curr. Opin. Immunol.*, 66, 42–49, Oct. 2020.
58. Lambert, L. and Culley, F.J., Innate Immunity to Respiratory Infection in Early Life. *Front. Immunol.*, 8, 1570, Nov. 2017.
59. Mortaz, E., Adcock, I.M., Folkerts, G., Barnes, P.J., Paul Vos, A., Garssen, J., Probiotics in the management of lung diseases. *Mediators Inflamm.*, 751068 2013.
60. Ziemons, J., Smidt, M.L., Damink, S.O., Rensen, S.S., Gut microbiota and metabolic aspects of cancer cachexia. *Best Pract. Res. Clin. Endocrinol. Metab.*, 35, 3, 101508, 2021.
61. Lazzerini, P.E., Hamilton, R.M., Boutjdir, M., Editorial: Cardioimmunology: inflammation and immunity in cardiovascular disease. *Front. Cardiovasc. Med.*, 6, 181, Dec. 2019.
62. Thushara, R.M., Gangadaran, S., Solati, Z., Moghadasian, M.H., Cardiovascular benefits of probiotics: A review of experimental and clinical studies. *Food Funct.*, 7, 2, 632–642, Feb. 2016.
63. Oniszczuk, A., Oniszczuk, T., Gancarz, M., Szymańska, J., Role of gut microbiota, probiotics and prebiotics in the cardiovascular diseases. *Molecules*, 26, 4, 1–15, Feb. 2021.
64. Zhao, X., Oduro, P.K., Tong, W., Wang, Y., Gao, X., Wang, Q., Therapeutic potential of natural products against atherosclerosis: Targeting on gut microbiota. *Pharmacol. Res.*, 163, 105362, 2021.

65. Katiraei, S., de Vries, M.R., Costain, A.H., Thiem, K., Hoving, L.R., van Diepen, J.A., Smits, H.H., Bouter, K.E., Rensen, P., Quax, P., Nieuwdorp, M., Netea, M.G., de Vos, W.M., Cani, P.D., Belzer, C., van Dijk, K.W., Berbée, J., van Harmelen, V., Akkermansia muciniphila Exerts Lipid-Lowering and Immunomodulatory Effects without Affecting Neointima Formation in Hyperlipidemic APOE*3-Leiden.CETP Mice. *Mol. Nutr. Food Res.*, 64, 15, e1900732, Aug. 2020.
66. Strollo, R., Vinci, C., Napoli, N., Pozzilli, P., Ludvigsson, J., Nissim, A., Antibodies to post-translationally modified insulin as a novel biomarker for prediction of type 1 diabetes in children. *Diabetologia*, 60, 8, 1467–1474, 2017.
67. Wållberg, M. and Cooke, A., Immune mechanisms in type 1 diabetes. *Trends Immunol.*, 34, 12, 583–591, 2013.
68. Uusitalo, U. Liu, X., Yang, J., Aronsson, C. A., Hummel, S., Butterworth, M., Lernmark, Å., Rewers, M., Hagopian, W., She, J. X., Simell, O., Toppari, J., Ziegler, A. G., Akolkar, B., Krischer, J., Norris, J. M., Virtanen, S. M., TEDDY Study Group, Association of Early Exposure of Probiotics and Islet Autoimmunity in the TEDDY Study. *JAMA Pediatr.*, 170, 1, 20–28, 2016, doi: 10.1001/jamapediatrics.2015.2757.
69. Kumar, S., Kumar, R., Rohilla, L., Jacob, N., Yadav, J., Sachdeva, N., A high potency multi-strain probiotic improves glycemic control in children with new-onset type 1 diabetes mellitus: A randomized, double-blind, and placebo-controlled pilot study. *Pediatr. Diabetes*, 22, 7, 1014–1022, Nov. 2021.
70. Mishra, S.P. Wang, S., Nagpal, R., Miller, B., Singh, R., Taraphder, S., & Yadav, H., Probiotics and Prebiotics for the Amelioration of Type 1 Diabetes: Present and Future Perspectives. *Microorganisms*, 7, 3, 67, Mar. 2019.
71. Mondanelli, G., Orecchini, E., Volpi, C., Panfili, E., Belladonna, M. L., Pallotta, M.T., Moretti, S., Galarini, R., Esposito, S., & Orabona, C., Effect of Probiotic Administration on Serum Tryptophan Metabolites in Pediatric Type 1 Diabetes Patients. *Int. J. Tryptophan Res.*, 13, 1178646920956646, 2020.
72. Ismail, H.M., BCh, M., Spall, M., Evans-Molina, C., DiMeglio, L.A., Evaluating the effect of Prebiotics on the gut microbiome profile and β-cell function in youth with newly-diagnosed Type 1 diabetes: Protocol of a randomized controlled trial. *medRxiv*, 2020.10.05.20207142, Apr. 2021.
73. Ho, J., Nicolucci, A. C., Virtanen, H., Schick, A., Meddings, J., Reimer, R. A., & Huang, C. Effect of Prebiotic on microbiota, intestinal permeability, and glycemic control in children with Type 1 diabetes. *J. Clin. Endocrinol. Metab.*, 104, 10, 4427–4440, Oct. 2019.
74. Payandeh, Z. *et al.*, PD-1/PD-L1-dependent immune response in colorectal cancer. *J. Cell. Physiol.*, 235, 7–8, 5461–5475, Jul. 2020.
75. Gagnière, J., Khalili, S., Somi, M.H., Mard-Soltani, M., Baghbanzadeh, A., Hajiasgharzadeh, K., Samadi, N., Baradaran, B., Gut microbiota imbalance and colorectal cancer. *World J. Gastroenterol.*, 22, 2, 501–518, Jan. 2016.

76. Kazmierczak-Siedlecka, K., Daca, A., Fic, M., van de Wetering, T., Folwarski, M., Makarewicz, W., Therapeutic methods of gut microbiota modification in colorectal cancer management - fecal microbiota transplantation, prebiotics, probiotics, and synbiotics. *Gut Microbes*, 11, 6, 1518–1530, Nov. 2020.
77. Drago, L., Probiotics and Colon Cancer. *Microorg.*, 7, 3, 66, Feb. 2019.
78. Mahdavi, M., Laforest-Lapointe, I., Massé, E., Preventing Colorectal Cancer through Prebiotics. *Microorg.*, 9, 6, 1325, Jun. 2021.
79. Neurath, M.F., Cytokines in inflammatory bowel disease. *Nat. Rev. Immunol.*, 14, 5, 329–342, Apr. 2014.
80. Gonçalves, P., Araújo, J.R., Di Santo, J.P., A cross-talk between microbiota-derived short-chain fatty acids and the host mucosal immune system regulates intestinal homeostasis and inflammatory bowel disease. *Inflamm. Bowel Dis.*, 24, 3, 558–572, Feb. 2018.
81. Kostic, A.D., Xavier, R.J., Gevers, D., The microbiome in inflammatory bowel disease: Current status and the future ahead. *Gastroenterology*, 146, 6, 1489–1499, 2014.
82. Zhang, X.F., Guan, X. X., Tang, Y. J., Sun, J. F., Wang, X. K., Wang, W. D., & Fan, J. M., Clinical effects and gut microbiota changes of using probiotics, prebiotics or synbiotics in inflammatory bowel disease: A systematic review and meta-analysis. *Eur. J. Nutr. 2021 605*, 60, 5, 2855–2875, Feb. 2021.
83. Gopalakrishnan, A., Clinthorne, J. F., Rondini, E. A., McCaskey, S. J., Gurzell, E. A., Langohr, I. M., Gardner, E. M., & Fenton, J. I., Supplementation with galacto-oligosaccharides increases the percentage of NK cells and reduces colitis severity in Smad3-deficient mice. *J. Nutr.*, 142, 7, 1336–1342, Jul. 2012.
84. Caviglia, G.P., De Blasio, F., Vernero, M., Armandi, A., Rosso, C., Saracco, G. M., Bugianesi, E., Astegiano, M., Ribaldone, D. G., Efficacy of a Preparation Based on Calcium Butyrate, Bifidobacterium bifidum, Bifidobacterium lactis, and Fructooligosaccharides in the Prevention of Relapse in Ulcerative Colitis: A prospective observational Study. *J. Clin. Med.*, 10, 21, 4961, Oct. 2021.
85. Chorawala, M.R., Chauhan, S., Patel, R., Shah, G., Cell wall contents of probiotics (Lactobacillus species) protect against lipopolysaccharide (LPS)-induced murine colitis by limiting immuno-inflammation and oxidative stress. *Probiotics Antimicrob. Proteins 2021 134*, 13, 4, 1005–1017, Feb. 2021.
86. Weyand, C.M. and Goronzy, J.J., The immunology of rheumatoid arthritis. *Nat. Immunol. 2020 221*, 22, 1, 10–18, Nov. 2020.
87. Hansildaar, R., Vedder, D., Baniaamam, M., Tausche, A.K., Gerritsen, M., Nurmohamed, M.T., Cardiovascular risk in inflammatory arthritis: rheumatoid arthritis and gout. *Lancet Rheumatol.*, 3, 1, e58–e70, Jan. 2021.
88. Paul, A.K. *et al.*, Probiotics and Amelioration of Rheumatoid Arthritis: Significant Roles of Lactobacillus casei and Lactobacillus acidophilus. *Microorganisms*, 9, 5, 1070, May 2021.
89. Ferro, M., Charneca, S., Dourado, E., Guerreiro, C.S., Fonseca, J.E., Probiotic supplementation for rheumatoid arthritis: A promising adjuvant therapy in the gut microbiome Era. *Front. Pharmacol.*, 12, 711788, Jul. 2021.

90. Shen, P., Jiao, Y., Miao, L., Chen, J.H., Momtazi-Borojeni, A.A., Immunomodulatory effects of berberine on the inflamed joint reveal new therapeutic targets for rheumatoid arthritis management. *J. Cell. Mol. Med.*, 24, 21, 12234–12245, Nov. 2020.
91. Gutiérrez-Rodríguez, O., Thalidomide a promising new treatment for rheumatoid arthritis. *Arthritis Rheumatol.*, 27, 10, 1118–1121, Oct. 1984.
92. VanderVeen, B.N., Murphy, E.A., Carson, J.A., The Impact of Immune Cells on the Skeletal Muscle Microenvironment During Cancer Cachexia. *Front. Physiol.*, 11, 1037, 2020.
93. Lee, M.-C., Tu, Y.T., Lee, C.C., Tsai, S.C., Hsu, H.Y., Tsai, T.Y., Liu, T.H., Young, S.L., Lin, J.S., Huang, C.C., Lactobacillus plantarum TWK10 improves muscle mass and functional performance in frail older adults: A randomized, double-blind clinical trial. *Microorganisms*, 9, 7, 1466, Jul. 2021.
94. Furrer, R. and Handschin, C., Muscle wasting diseases: Novel targets and treatments. *Annu. Rev. Pharmacol. Toxicol.*, 59, 315–339, Jan. 2019.
95. van Krimpen, S.J., Jansen, F.A.C., Ottenheim, V.L., Belzer, C., van der Ende, M., van Norren, K., The effects of pro-, pre-, and synbiotics on muscle wasting, a systematic review-gut permeability as potential treatment target. *Nutrients*, 13, 4, 1115, Mar. 2021.
96. Khademi, F., Vaez, H., Momtazi-Borojeni, A.A., Majnooni, A., Banach, M., Sahebkar, A., Bacterial infections are associated with cardiovascular disease in Iran: A meta-analysis. *Arch. Med. Sci.*, 15, 4, 902–911, 2019.
97. Vaahtovuo, J., Munukka, E., Korkeamäki, M., Luukkainen, R., Toivanen, P., Fecal microbiota in early rheumatoid arthritis. *J. Rheumatol.*, 35, 8, 1500–1505, 2008.
98. Vaghef-Mehrabany, E., Alipour, B., Homayouni-Rad, A., Sharif, S.-K., Asghari-Jafarabadi, M., Zavvari, S., Probiotic supplementation improves inflammatory status in patients with rheumatoid arthritis. *Nutrition*, 30, 4, 430–435, 2014.
99. Ghosh, S., Van Heel, D., Playford, R.J., Probiotics in inflammatory bowel disease: Is it all gut flora modulation?. *Gut*, 53, 5, 620–622, May 2004.
100. Fidel, P.L., Vazquez, J.A., Sobel, J.D., Candida glabrata: Review of epidemiology, pathogenesis, and clinical disease with comparison to C. albicans. *Clin. Microbiol. Rev.*, 12, 1, 80–96, 1999.
101. Falagas, M.E., Betsi, G., II, Athanasiou, S., Probiotics for prevention of recurrent vulvovaginal candidiasis: A review. *J. Antimicrob. Chemother.*, 58, 2, 266–272, Aug. 2006.
102. Han, Y. and ling Ren, Q., "Does probiotics work for bacterial vaginosis and vulvovaginal candidiasis,". *Curr. Opin. Pharmacol.*, 61, 83–90, Dec. 2021.
103. De Goffau, M.C., Fuentes, S., van den Bogert, B., Honkanen, H., de Vos, W. M., Welling, G. W., Hyöty, H., & Harmsen, H. J., "Aberrant gut microbiota composition at the onset of type 1 diabetes in young children,". *Diabetologia*, 57, 1569–1577, 8, Aug 2014.

104. Houngbédji, G.M., Bouchard, P., Frenette, J., Mycobacterium ulcerans infections cause progressive muscle atrophy and dysfunction, and mycolactone impairs satellite cell proliferation. *Am. J. Physiol. Regul. Integr. Comp. Physiol.*, 300, 3, R724–R732, Mar. 2011.
105. Chung, W.S.F., Walker, A.W., Louis, P., Parkhill, J., Vermeiren, J., Bosscher, D., Duncan, S. H., Flint, H. J., Modulation of the human gut microbiota by dietary fibres occurs at the species level. *BMC Biol.*, 14, 1, 3, 2016.
106. Markowiak-Kopeć, P. and Slizewska, K., The effect of probiotics on the production of short-chain fatty acids by human intestinal microbiome. *Nutr.*, 12, 4, 1107, Apr. 2020.
107. Delzenne, N.M., Neyrinck, A.M., Bäckhed, F., Cani, P.D., Targeting gut microbiota in obesity: Effects of prebiotics and probiotics. *Nat. Rev. Endocrinol.*, 7, 11, 639–646, 2011.
108. Franco-Robles, E. and López, M.G., Implication of fructans in health: Immunomodulatory and antioxidant mechanisms. *Sci. World J.*, 2015, 289267, 2015.
109. Paineau, D., Carcano, D., Leyer, G., Darquy, S., Alyanakian, M. A., Simoneau, G., Bergmann, J. F., Brassart, D., Bornet, F., & Ouwehand, A.C., Effects of seven potential probiotic strains on specific immune responses in healthy adults: A double-blind, randomized, controlled trial. *FEMS Immunol. Med. Microbiol.*, 53, 1, 107–113, 2008.
110. Finne-Soveri, H. and Ouwehand, A.C., Fermented cereal with specific bifidobacteria normalizes bowel movements in elderly nursing home residents. A randomized, controlled trial. *J. Nutr. Health Aging*, 11, 4, 305, 2007.
111. Klaenhammer, T.R., Kleerebezem, M., Kopp, M.V., Rescigno, M., The impact of probiotics and prebiotics on the immune system. *Nat. Rev. Immunol.*, 12, 10, 728–734, 2012.

8

Bioinformatics and Advanced Research in Gut Microflora

Arabinda Ghosh[1]*, Muddukrishnaiah Kotakonda[2], VedantVikrom Borah[3] and Nobendu Mukerjee[4,5]

[1]*Department of Botany, Microbiology Division, Gauhati University, Guwahati, Assam, India*
[2]*Department of Technology, Anna University, Chennai, India*
[3]*Department of Bio-Sciences, School of Life Sciences, Assam, Don Bosco University, Sonapur, Assam, India*
[4]*Department of Microbiology; Ramakrishna Mission Vivekananda Centenary College, West Bengal, Kolkata, India*
[5]*Department of Health Sciences, Novel Global Community Educational Foundation, Australia*

Abstract

Probiotics have attracted increasing interest in the scientific, healthcare, and public sectors in recent years. Publicity around microbiome research has also changed the popular perspective of microbes, moving away from disease-causing entities that should be avoided and toward a more reasonable approach that incorporates an awareness of microorganisms' beneficial roles in human health. Human microbiome composition has been associated with considerable gains in human health. Changes in the intestinal microbial population relative to control groups are now associated with a number of intestinal and extraintestinal illnesses. Modification of the human microbiome in order to restore equilibrium to microbial populations is a potential strategy for improving human health in the context of a variety of illnesses. The human microbiome is vital for metabolic functions, such as vitamin synthesis, short-chain fatty acid synthesis, and other key chemical digestion, gut homeostasis maintenance, and host immune response regulation. Molecular cross-talk is a process by which intestinal bacteria and human cells communicate via surface-associated proteins or extracellular components. Additionally, structural components of bacteria have their own receptors in the innate immune system;

**Corresponding author*: dra.ghosh@gauhati.ac.in: ORCID: 0000-0002-3891-5949

Rajesh K. Kesharwani, Tingirikari Jagan Mohan Rao and Raj K. Keservani (eds.) Prebiotics and Probiotics in Disease Regulation and Management, (219–238) © 2022 Scrivener Publishing LLC

for example, Toll-like receptor 5 recognizes a constant percentage of surface-associated flagellin, whereas Toll-like receptor-4 recognizes the cell wall component lipopolysaccharide. This chapter will highlight the importance of probiotic and their advancement with special reference to bioinformatics and classical methods.

Keywords: Prebiotics, gut microbiota, bioinformatics, sequencing, metagomics, computational biology, intestinal microbes, beneficial microbes, microflora

8.1 Introduction

The human gut microbiota's makeup has been linked to both health and disease, but to understand specific microbial species, it is required first to identify them. Despite scientists' best efforts at cultivation and sequencing, the bacteria that live in the human gut microbiota remain a mystery to them. We discovered 1,952 previously unknown bacterial species using 92,143 metagenome-assembled genomes from 11,850 human gut microbiomes and compared them to previously published data on bacterial diversity. According to the findings, adopting these uncultured genomes boosted the phylogenetic diversity of the aggregate human gut microbiota by 281%, resulting in a significant extension of the known species repertoire. Compared to understudied African and South American samples, the newly recognized species are more abundant in well-studied populations than reference isolate genomes, resulting in a more than 200% rise in the newly described species' category. A large number of newly identified biosynthetic gene clusters and a variety of odd functional capacities are among these hypothetical animals, which may help explain their enigmatic position in the evolution of life on Earth. A rise in the number of uncultured gut bacteria in researchers' collections could lead to new discoveries concerning intestinal bacteria' taxonomic and trigonal diversity. Even though the human gut microbiota is one of the most researched microbial ecosystems on the planet, we have been unable to collect and sequence the entire microbiota's species diversity due to technological and practical constraints. We were able to uncover 1,952 previously uncultured possible bacterial species thanks to the results of this study's metagenomic analysis, allowing us to conduct the first-ever investigation into previously uncultured microbial diversity. Over half of the potential species were not recognized at the genus level, indicating that there is still a great deal of bacterial variety that has yet to be discovered. The findings of this resource are used to build on and expand upon the findings of a recent study published in Nature [1, 2], which looked into the hitherto unknown diversity of human microbiomes throughout the body.

Our research findings have resulted in the creation of example genomes for 92,143 MAGs derived from human gut assemblies, in addition to the ability to classify 73% of the read data collected. Because culture and de novo analysis techniques are biased toward the most common organisms, less common species are more likely to be neglected regularly than more common species. Aside from that, geographical countries, such as Africa and South America, are underrepresented in scientific research. To gain a comprehensive understanding of the human gut microbial ecology, we must expand our research to encompass vast cohorts of people from all over the world. As a result, we concentrated our efforts on bacterial genomes since they have more extensive reference libraries and well-established protocols and criteria for this type of investigation [2].

8.2 Computational and Metagenomic Approaches

Fundamental questions in the field of metagenomics research are frequently raised, such as how we have learned so much about the microbiome and how we have arrived at this position after decades of speculation: What exactly is the microbiome's composition, and how do we go about determining it? It suggests that discovering interactions among microflora populations is a possible task. How did we establish a link between specific microflora members and their metabolic products, as well as such a diverse range of health problems and manifestations? The answer for uncultured microflora can be found in the technological advantage that gene and next-generation sequencing (NGS) has supplied and the rapid advancement of bioinformatics [3, 4], which has resulted in the rapid advancement of bioinformatics.

Having high sensitivity and specificity to detect microbial communities in disease pathogenesis is essential before examining the functional implications of these communities in disease pathogenesis. With the introduction of shotgun 16S ribosomal RNA (rRNA) sequencing [5, 6], NGS has considerably increased these capabilities [5, 6]. A gene known as the 16S rRNA gene is widely recognized as the de facto housekeeping gene in bacterial and archaeal populations. In studying the microbiome, the first compromise is that researchers tend to concentrate on the implications of the bacteriome (bacterial microbiome) while neglecting those of the mycobiome (fungal microbiome) and virome [7–10], both of which have been linked to pathological conditions but have remained largely unexplored. Although bacterial populations have a greater diversity (number of unique species) and abundance (number of members per species) than fungi and viruses, this concession is also based on the fact that bacteria are easier to detect and that we have a better understanding of the biological processes that they undergo.

Metagenomics [11, 12] is a term that originated in the field of genomics to characterize the study of metagenomes, which are the complete DNA content of environmental samples and the subject matter of this paper's examination. The metagenome, the total DNA content of all environmental components, is the subject of this research investigation, which is now underway. Metagenomics, which is the study of the metagenome, which is a collection of genes, is a relatively new issue in biology, has emerged very recently. It is now in the very early stages of development, as mentioned. This phrase refers to the identification and quantification of the genetic contributions of microbial subpopulations [13] in human microflora samples taken from faeces and histology biopsy specimens and the identification and quantification of their genetic contributions.

On the other hand, shotgun metagenomics [14], which combines all microbes and host DNA in a sample, complicates the results and is consequently more expensive, even though it produces more precise results. However, when the investigation is focused on bacteria and archaea discovered in large numbers of control samples and patient samples, as was the case in the current study, 16S rRNA metagenomics are less challenging to do in a laboratory setting. We must emphasize that both strategies make use of an approach that introduces significant variation between studies, particularly the use of next-generation sequencing (NGS) library creation for RNA or DNA [15], which is used in both procedures and introduces significant variability between studies. It is necessary to use multiplex polymerase chain reaction (PCR) primers in order to amplify hypervariable sections of the 16S rRNA gene [16] because of the high amount of uncertainty involved in the library building process. Multiplex polymerase chain reaction (PCR) primers are used to amplify hypervariable portions of the 16S rRNA gene, which is a gene that is found in bacteria.

Additionally, this phase is outlined in the 16S rRNA standard operating procedure, which is available on the internet. The use of several bioinformatics tools [17], in addition to standard bioinformatics tools, is required to preprocess these data to produce the best possible results correctly. In addition to basic trimming and assembly tools, there are also scaffolding and mapping tools available for you to choose from on the list of accessible options for you to consider. These pieces of information must be preprocessed appropriately, which means having the relevant tools available is crucial.

8.3 Antibiotic Resistance Genes Have Been Revealed in the Gut Microbiota of People Across the Globe

Antibiotic resistance genes in the gut microbiome of individuals ranging in age and geographic region were analyzed in silico. Antibiotic resistance has become a serious global public health problem during the last few decades due to the extensive and unregulated use of antibiotics in humans and animals. This is exacerbated further by a recent study that discovered the gut microbiota serves as a reservoir for antibiotic resistance. Researchers evaluated patients from eight countries, including the United States, for antibiotic resistance genes in their gut flora. The researchers were able to accomplish this by utilizing publicly available metagenomic data sets from 275 gut microbiomes. Using sequence similarity searches against 240 different drugs, we searched for genes that confer drug resistance on the genomic segments that form each of these metagenomes. During this study, researchers discovered 53 different antibiotic resistance genes in the human gut microbiota. The researchers identified four unique "resistotypes" of gut microbiomes, each with a similar profile of antibiotic resistance, as well as a slew of geographic and country-specific tendencies. Within each of these clusters, it was feasible to identify subgroups of medicines with similar resistance patterns. Multidrug resistance operons that are transportable have also been found in specific gut microbiomes, demonstrating their transportability. The researchers discovered an unusually high number of antibiotic resistance genes in the gut microbiomes of two babies. According to this study, the human gut microbiota can be considered a "big picture" of antibiotic resistance across multiple locations. With these facts in hand, new laws or the reinforcement of current legislation may be possible [18].

The identification and binding of microbial-associated chemical patterns to pattern recognition receptors activates several intracellular signaling pathways, altering the surface molecules of immune cells, as well as their effector, secretion profiles, including cytokines and interleukins. Finally, the type, number, and temporal pattern of interactions between microbial associated molecular patterns and pattern recognition receptors will influence the type of immune response, which can be categorized generically as proinflammatory or regulatory [19]. Extracellular and surface-associated proteins from the gut microbiota have been investigated as possible candidates for a portion of the immunomodulatory action of intestinal bacteria in recent years, considering their critical roles in the host-microbiota interaction. Numerous researches have focused on discovering the substances that promote the proliferation of Treg cells, a T-cell subset that is crucial for maintaining the gut mucosa's controlled and low-grade inflammatory condition. Until now, only a few proteins critical for maintaining gut homeostasis and produced by gut bacteria have been identified. Lactic acid bacteria [20] are transient members of the human gut microbiota in individuals who consume fermented foods. It has been proven that certain lactobacilli species produce immunomodulatory peptides encoded in larger extracellular proteins.

8.4 Microbiota in the Human Intestine

The human gastrointestinal tract (GIT) is home to a diverse and dynamic microbial community that is unique to each individual and is influenced by environmental and genetic variables. Each person carries roughly 1.5 kg of germs, which can account for up to 60% of faeces weight. This microbial population, which includes hundreds of species, changes along the GIT, with the stomach being sparsely populated and the colon being densely populated. This gut microbiota is crucial for human health not only because of its role in digesting, but also because of its critical role in the development of the gut and immune system [21]. The GIT microbiota has also been shown to play a role in the control of lipid absorption and storage, making this an interesting field of research in the fight against obesity. Furthermore, new research suggests that specific changes in gut microbiota composition are linked to a variety of disorders. This proof of the impact of gut bacteria on host health provides the basis for altering the gut microbiota with probiotics.

Probiotics are defined as "live bacteria that benefit the host when administered in appropriate doses." According to this definition, the term "probiotic" refers to strains that have been scientifically confirmed to have particular beneficial properties. As a result, each strain's qualities and attributes should be exhaustively detailed, and each strain's effect should be demonstrated on an individual basis [22]. While some of the beneficial effects ascribed to specific probiotic strains are backed up by strong scientific evidence from human intervention trials, others, while promising, remain purely hypothetical at the moment. Probiotics have been manufactured using a variety of microorganisms, the most prevalent of which being Lactobacillus and Bifidobacterium [23]. The majority of currently used strains were isolated from the intestinal microbiota of healthy persons, creating a strong relationship between probiotics and research on the gut microbiota. Furthermore, it is hypothesized that the majority of their effects on human health are mediated by changes in the composition and/or activity of the gut microbiota.

8.5 Probiotics Modes of Action

It was anticipated that probiotics had an effect on the gastrointestinal tract, and that effects on the incidence of diarrhoea and other gut illnesses were to be expected. Recent research in a number of countries, however, suggests that the consequences may be more widespread. The explanation for the divergent mechanisms could be related to the various types of probiotics. Probiotics are thought to boost an animal's general health by balancing the microbial balance in its gut [24]. In general, probiotic feed additives work primarily through competitive exclusion, bacterial antagonism, and immunological modulation.

8.6 Exclusion from Competition

The ability of normal microflora to protect against pathogen establishment is termed as competitive exclusion. Competitive exclusion states that cultures of selected, beneficial microbes added to feed compete with potentially hazardous bacteria for adhesion sites and organic substrates. The adherence to the digestive system wall could be for a variety of reasons, including preventing harmful microbe colonization or competing for nutrition [25] (Figure 8.1).

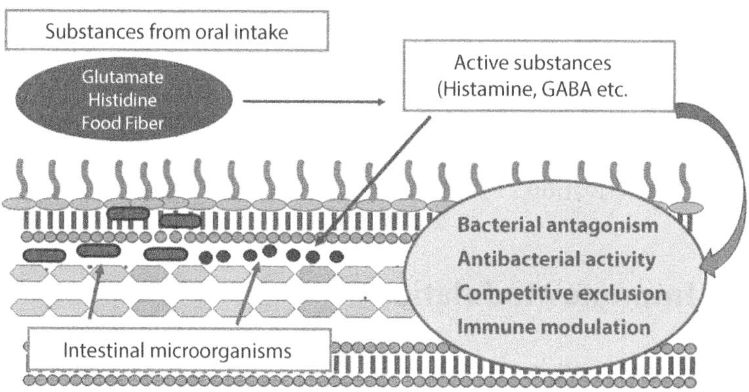

Figure 8.1 The conversion of luminal active compounds by intestinal bacteria may play a significant role in host–microbiota interactions.

8.7 Bacterial Antagonism

Probiotic bacteria may convert essential compounds to bioactive compounds with bactericidal or bacteriostatic characteristics.

8.8 Antibacterial Activity

Lactobacilli convert lactose to lactic acid, lowering the pH to a point where pathogenic bacteria cannot survive. Hydrogen peroxide is also created, which stops Gram-negative bacteria from growing. These compounds have a negative effect on pathogenic microorganisms, mostly due to a decrease in stomach pH. The poor secretion of hydrochloric acid in the stomach of weanling piglets may be somewhat countered by lowering the pH. Furthermore, living yeasts compete with lactic acid-producing bacteria to digest sugars obtained from starch breakdown, thereby stabilizing rumen pH and reducing the danger of acidosis. Changes in the amount and species of microbes in the rumen cause improvements in early digestion and intake.

8.9 Neutralization of Pathogenic Bacteria-Produced Enterotoxins

Probiotic bacteria generate organic acids, antioxidants, and bacteriocins, among other substances. These compounds have the potential to affect bacterial metabolism and toxin production, as well as reduce the number of live dangerous organisms [26]. When paired with additional antimicrobial environmental factors, such as low temperatures, organic acids, and detergent, bacteriocins generated by lactic acid bacteria have been demonstrated to penetrate the outer membrane of gram-negative bacteria, resulting in their inactivation.

8.10 Immune Modulation

The immune system is stimulated by probiotics. However, research and analysis into the ability of probiotics to alter the immune systems of animals and humans is still in its early stages. By boosting the gastrointestinal immune response, microbial populations can aid an animal's defence against invading diseases. This could help the immune system develop by stimulating antibody synthesis and increasing phagocytic activity. Because the immune system is activated after being exposed to probiotic bacteria, any hostile bacteria are detected due to heightened leukocyte monitoring, and so possible infections are destroyed [27].

8.11 Adhesion to the Digestive System Wall to Prevent Harmful Bacteria From Colonizing

In order to cause harm, dangerous bacteria must attach themselves to the gut wall. As a result, adding probiotics to the gastrointestinal tract is expected to result in an increase in normal microflora colonization as well as inhibition of harmful pathogen adhesion on the intestinal epithelium, blocking receptor sites and preventing the attachment of other bacteria, including harmful species. By doing so, the probiotic bacteria are able to keep pathogens out and so avoid infection. The colonization mechanism is thought to be linked to certain microflora species that can alter the development of glycol conjugates on epithelial cells, which can act as receptors for bacterial adherence.

8.12 Competing with Pathogenic Bacteria for Nutrients in the Gut

Probiotics and pathogenic microorganisms may compete for nutrients and absorption sites. In addition, pathogenic species may be suppressed as a result of competition for energy and nutrients between probiotic and other bacteria. It may appear odd that bacteria could not find enough food to flourish in the gut because it is such a rich source of nutrients. Probiotics have a lot of fermentative activity and help with digestion. Lactobacilli create lactic acid and proteolytic enzymes that aid in nutrition breakdown in the gastrointestinal tract.

8.13 Metagenomics in Microbiome and Probiotics Research

Our understanding of microbiota composition and development was largely focused on the use of classic culture-based approaches until the last decade. Culturing has yielded interesting results, but it has also resulted in a skewed understanding of the gut microbial makeup. Because only a small portion of the microbiota is culturable, most of the microorganisms found in the gut have escaped scientific attention until now, thanks to the recent development of molecular culture-independent approaches. Several culture-independent qualitative and quantitative approaches, largely based on PCR and DNA hybridization, have been developed and applied to microbiota assessment over the last 20 years [28]. More recently, the development of fast and low-cost DNA sequencing methods has allowed these modern techniques to be applied to the study of microbial communities directly in their environment to characterize the human gut microbiome without the need for species cultivation and isolation. These techniques, which are based on comprehensive DNA sequencing, have greatly expanded our understanding of microbiome makeup and function. The use of metagenomic techniques to investigate entire microbial communities has shown far more diversity than previously imagined and has aided in determining the community structure of some previously unknown ecosystems. The advancement of these methodologies has a significant impact on a variety of aspects of probiotics research. So far, over 3 million genes from the intestinal microbiome have been sequenced, revealing the existence of various

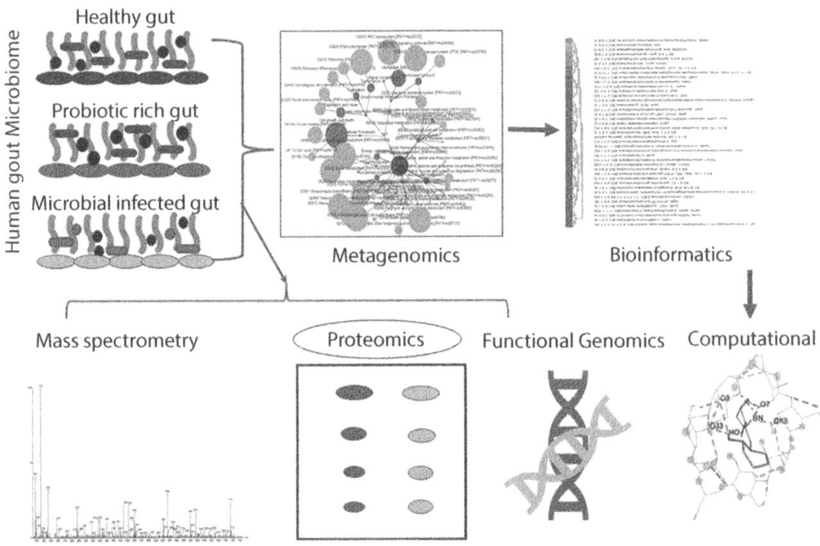

Figure 8.2 A new computational approach for the construction of prediction models predicting the behavior of probiotic bacteria based on laboratory data is proposed.

human enterotypes. Using metagenomics, the process of microbiota establishment in new-borns was detailed in detail, and the effect of nutrition was investigated. By comparing the microbiomes of healthy and unhealthy people, researchers have been able to identify abnormalities linked to a variety of human disorders, such as inflammatory disease and obesity. In the realm of probiotics, these anomalies are evident objectives for future product development aimed at correcting them. Similarly, the genomes of probiotics and intestinal commensal microorganisms have been sequenced in various investigations. This is allowing researchers to better understand the impact of microbiota and probiotics in human health. Genomic data on major elements of the intestinal microbiota, such as Bifidobacterium or Bacteroides, has revealed the genetic foundation for these microbes' adaption to the intestinal environment (Figure 8.2). Genome sequencing of individual probiotic strains has also revealed new information about probiotic features like as processes of adherence to the gut mucosa and interactions with the immune system, among other things.

8.14 Microbiome and Probiotics Research Challenges

Determining the structure and function of the healthy normal microbiota is one of the most difficult tasks in this subject. Recent research has revealed variances in the microbiota makeup of healthy people from various geographical areas, highlighting the difficulty of defining the normal microbiome at the species level. Metagenomic investigations, on the other hand, have revealed fresh information, indicating that the normal microbiota may be better described at the functional level than at the phylogenetic level. Thus, metagenomic investigations should go beyond the taxonomic composition inferred by the 16S rRNA gene in order to define the whole genetic repertoire of the community in order to understand the functional shift and restoration of the healthy condition generated by the probiotic. After defining a healthy human gut microbiota, the next stage will be to design intervention strategies aimed at reversing aberrant microbiota composition and activity. Probiotics are a potential choice for achieving this goal in this regard. As a result, a better understanding of various probiotic strains' microbiome-modulating capacities is required. So yet, there is a scarcity of metagenomic data from probiotic intervention research in humans. Nonetheless, a flood of such information is likely in the near future, and some research is already underway. By combining these findings with research on host gene responses to microbiota alterations and probiotic treatment, we will be able to better understand microbe-host microbe interactions and, as a result, how the gut microbiota affects our health and, more broadly, our physiology [29].

8.15 Potential Prebiotic Screening for Promoting Probiotic Health

Prebiotics are the dietary fiber that gut bacteria utilize as nutrition and break down into short-chain fatty acids (SCFA). In turn, these SCFA have a physiological effect on the human body. To be classified as prebiotics, a compound must satisfy three criteria: it must withstand host digestion, be fermentable by intestinal microbes, and selectively stimulate the growth and activity of gut bacteria linked to health and well-being [30, 31]. Prebiotics are "nondigestible compounds that, through its metabolization by microorganisms in the gut, modulate the composition and activity of the gut microbiota, conferring a beneficial physiological effect on the host" [30, 32]. Another point to remember is that, while not all prebiotics are carbohydrates, to differentiate fiber from carbohydrate-derived prebiotics: fibers are carbohydrates with a degree of polymerization (DP) of 3 or higher comprising of oligosaccharides and polysaccharides, and that endogenous enzyme cannot hydrolyze them in the small intestine [33]. Prebiotics are oligosaccharides such as fructans (inulin and fructo-oligosaccharide or FOS), galactooligosaccharides (GOS), resistant starch, and pectin oligosaccharide (POS) [31]. Cocoa-derived flavanols, on the other hand, have been reported to be noncarbohydrate prebiotics [34]. Various fermentable carbohydrates have shown a prebiotic effect, but the nondigestible oligosaccharides, fructans, and galactans are the dietary prebiotics with the most substantial evidence of health benefits in humans [35]. Inulin and its fructo- and galacto-oligosaccharides, as well as arabinoxylan oligosaccharides from wheat bran, have been researched as possible prebiotics since the prebiotic idea was introduced 20 years ago and the definition for dietary fiber was created 10 years ago [36, 37]. These prebiotics has been reported to stimulate the growth of *Bifidobacteria* and *Lactobacilli*, *Enterobacteria*, *Bacteroidetes*, and *Firmicutes* [38, 39]. In recent years, their link with human health has piqued people's curiosity.

8.15.1 Extraction and Characterization of Prebiotics

Prebiotics are found naturally in fruits and vegetables such as asparagus, onion, cereals, garlic, Jerusalem artichoke, chicory, sugar beet, wheat, barley, tomato, rye, soybean, peas, beans, banana, honey, and tiny amounts are present in human milk and animal colostrum's in the form of free sugars or glycoconjugates [40] and, more recently, in seaweeds and microalgae [41]. The following procedures are used to extract prebiotics or prebiotic candidate compounds:

(i) Extraction
Select plant samples are extracted in 95% or an 80% (v/v) ethanol solution or water to extract prebiotics [40]. Maceration is a method of extraction in which dried powdered material is immersed in a solution for a specified time (≤5 hours), with or without agitation. Hot water bath extraction at 90°C may be followed maceration is completed [42]. Extraction using ultrasound cleaning bath at 40 Hz performed for 40 min at 70°C [43], gives a substantial yield of prebiotics.

(ii) Precipitation
After extraction, the resultant slurry is filtered through the Buchner funnel (43–48 μm filter) [43] or concentrated in a rotary evaporator and centrifuged to remove large particles [42]. The filtrate, or the supernatant, is then precipitated in ethanol to isolate the polysaccharides. Dialysis in water at 4°C for 24 hours further helps in the isolation process. The precipitate is then oven-dried at 50°C till constant weight is obtained.

(iii) Resistance to acid and enzymatic digestion
Nondigestibility of oligosaccharides be it in form of resistance toward gastric acidity, hydrolysis by mammalian enzymes and gastrointestinal absorption determines whether oligosaccharides could be potential prebiotics [44]. After hydrochloric acid digestion and α-amylase treatment, the reducing sugar content is determined using FOS as a control. The difference in the reducing sugar content before and after treatment gives the estimate of nondigestible oligosaccharides [42].

8.15.2 Screening Prebiotics for Probiotic Growth Promotion

In vitro fermentation of prebiotics in carbon-free MRS medium supplemented with the extractable oligosaccharides provides valuable insights for screening of prebiotics. *Lactobacillus* strain is inoculated and incubated at 37°C for 48 hours; its growth rate and the acidification of the growth medium are determined. The growth rate is determined by plating the fermentation medium in an agar plate for counting the viable colonies [45, 46]. Such simulation could provide for important observation on the fermentability of the oligosaccharides in a mixture of extracted prebiotics. More so for the synthesis of symbiotic — a combination of prebiotics and selective probiotics [47].

8.15.3 Database System for Prebiotic Research

Online databases and Internet resources for science organize material and offer URLs and hyperlinks for any scholar to access relevant data with the least effort, time, and expense [48]. This feasibility, although not extensively developed, is available for information on prebiotics and probiotics alike. Some useful resources include—Global Prebiotic Association, https://prebioticassociation.org/, a database that raises awareness and educates on the field of prebiotics and its associated research. Derived from this resource, a team of researchers designed the freely available ODRAP database, https://rs-pharmcenter.com/rnf2019/db2/index.html?page=1 [48, 49]. The database houses important research activities carried out by researchers concerning prebiotics. It includes information on the evaluation of prebiotic activities *in vitro* and their associated methodologies. Continued efforts are made to enhance the organization and compilation of data related to prebiotics which is an arduous task considering the large volume of scientific information available [50]. Prebiotics and probiotics are the most used dietary ingredients in functional foods. Online databases allow people to familiarize themselves with information on prebiotics and their activity, sort by the genus and species of bacteria, the name of the prebiotic, and other factors [48].

8.16 Conclusion

Biological data can be used to assist scientists in analyzing and discovering patterns in computer-generated data. It is a computer science subject that combines programming, big data, and biology to help scientists analyse and uncover patterns in biological data. It is a branch in the field of information technology. The ability of this technology to organize enormous amounts of data is vital in conducting genome and DNA sequencing research, and this technology is critical in this regard. Nearly 2500 years after Hippocrates' discoveries about health and their direct connection with the gastrointestinal tract were discovered, the digestive tract, as well as the microbes that live there (bacteria, fungi, archea, and viruses), have revealed that they are a point of convergence for scientific investigation. Researchers are testing a new approach to microbial dysbiosis by using cognitive profiling of the gut-brain axis to gain new insights into the diseases and causes of neurological disorders. Most scientists generally agree that a person's digestive tract microbiome's genetic variety affects his or her overall health and that this diversity can provide preliminary insights into disease development and therapy success. Changes in the microbiome's biodiversity have been connected to contributions to the host's phenotype due to the microbiome's participation in immunological and physiological research. This is also linked to a neurological study that showed the existence of the gut-brain axis, which was previously thought to be a myth until its existence was discovered. The final bidirectional link will focus on our inquiry because it presents a new physics challenge for academics. We will examine the literature for computational analysis methodologies that satisfy the requirement for a better understanding of the microbiome-gut-brain interactions and the development and progression of neurological illnesses, using cross-disciplinary systems biology applications. In order to investigate these synergies, researchers used bioinformatics tools to aid in the construction and interpretation of microbial 16S ribosomal RNA data sets obtained by shotgun sequencing, as well as high-throughput sequencing of healthy and neurological disease samples housed in biobanks. Because of the advancement of these methodologies, researchers may now create hypotheses for their investigations in a more timely, cost-effective, and precise manner than was before possible. Combining metagenomics and metabolomics analysis to achieve their objectives will boost the project's chances of success.

In conclusion, our findings demonstrate that gut microbiota metagenome assemblies comprise a diverse variety of various species, such as archaea, eukaryotes, and viruses, all of which warrant further exploration. It is now possible to conduct precise and computationally efficient reference-based genome analyses on massive datasets of bacterial genomes, allowing for the construction of a comprehensive taxonomy of the composition of the microbial ecosystem. This is made possible by the availability of massive datasets of bacterial genes. Our goal is to develop high-quality reference genomes spanning from pure cultures to metagenomic assemblies (MAGs) as part of this work, which will serve as a model for understanding the human microbiota at the metagenomic level. Shortly, more than 2,000 more species will be made available for association and mechanistic investigations, helping researchers better understand the function of the microbiota in human health and disease.

References

1. Pasolli, E., Asnicar, F., Manara, S., Zolfo, M., Karcher, N., Armanini, F., Beghini, F., Manghi, P., Tett, A., Ghensi, P., Collado, M.C., Extensive unexplored human microbiome diversity revealed by over 150,000 genomes from metagenomes spanning age, geography, and lifestyle. *Cell*, 176, 3, 649–62, 2019 Jan 24.
2. Almeida, A., Mitchell, A.L., Boland, M., Forster, S.C., Gloor, G.B., Tarkowska, A., Lawley, T.D., Finn, R.D., A new genomic blueprint of the human gut microbiota. *Nature.*, 568, 7753, 499–504, 2019 Apr.
3. Schuster, S.C., Next-generation sequencing transforms today's biology. *Nat. Methods*, 5, 1, 16–8, 2008 Jan.
4. Metzker, M.L., Sequencing technologies—The next generation. *Nat. Rev. Genet.*, 11, 1, 31–46, 2010 Jan.
5. Jovel, J., Patterson, J., Wang, W., Hotte, N., O'Keefe, S., Mitchel, T., Perry, T., Kao, D., Mason, A.L., Madsen, K.L., Wong, G.K., Characterization of the gut microbiome using 16S or shotgun metagenomics. *Front. Microb.*, 7, 459, 2016 Apr 20.
6. Ranjan, R., Rani, A., Metwally, A., McGee, H.S., Perkins, D.L., Analysis of the microbiome: Advantages of whole genome shotgun versus 16S amplicon sequencing. *Biochem. Biophys. Res. Commun.*, 469, 4, 967–77, 2016 Jan 22.
7. Cui, L., Morris, A., Ghedin, E., The human mycobiome in health and disease. *Genome Med.*, 5, 7, 63, 1–2, 2013.
8. Huseyin, C.E., O'Toole, P.W., Cotter, P.D., Scanlan, P.D., Forgotten fungi—The gut mycobiome in human health and disease. *FEMS Microb. Rev.*, 41, 4, 479–511, 2017 Jul 1.
9. Zhao, G., Wu, G., Lim, E.S., Droit, L., Krishnamurthy, S., Barouch, D.H., Virgin, H.W., Wang, D., VirusSeeker, a computational pipeline for virus discovery and virome composition analysis. *Virology*, 503, 21–30, 2017 Mar 1.
10. Czeczko, P., Greenway, S.C., de Koning, A.J., EzMap: A simple pipeline for reproducible analysis of the human virome. *Bioinformatics.*, 33, 16, 2573–4, 2017 Aug 15.
11. Handelsman, J., Rondon, M.R., Brady, S.F., Clardy, J., Goodman, R.M., Molecular biological access to the chemistry of unknown soil microbes: A new frontier for natural products. *Chem. Biol.*, 5, 10, R245–9, 1998 Oct 1.
12. Wooley, J.C., Godzik, A., Friedberg, I., A primer on metagenomics. *PloS Comput. Biol.*, 6, 2, e1000667, 2010 Feb 26.
13. Handelsman, J., Metagenomics: application of genomics to uncultured microorganisms. *Microbiol. Biol. Rev.*, 68, 4, 669–85, 2004 Dec.

14. Sharpton, T.J., An introduction to the analysis of shotgun metagenomic data. *Front. Plant Sci.*, 5, 209, 2014 Jun 16.
15. Head, S.R., Komori, H.K., LaMere, S.A., Whisenant, T., Van Nieuwerburgh, F., Salomon, D.R., Ordoukhanian, P., Library construction for next-generation sequencing: Overviews and challenges. *Biotechniques.*, 56, 2, 61–77, 2014 Feb.
16. Rintala, A., Pietilä, S., Munukka, E., Eerola, E., Pursiheimo, J.P., Laiho, A., Pekkala, S., Huovinen, P., Gut microbiota analysis results are highly dependent on the 16S rRNA gene target region, whereas the impact of DNA extraction is minor. *J. Biomol. Techniques.* 28, 1, 19, 2017 Apr.
17. Olson, N.D., Treangen, T.J., Hill, C.M., Cepeda-Espinoza, V., Ghurye, J., Koren, S., Pop, M., Metagenomic assembly through the lens of validation: Recent advances in assessing and improving the quality of genomes assembled from metagenomes. *Briefings Bioinform.*, 20, 4, 1140–50, 2019 Jul.
18. Ghosh, T.S., Gupta, S.S., Nair, G.B., Mande, S.S., *In silico* analysis of antibiotic resistance genes in the gut microflora of individuals from diverse geographies and age-groups. *PloS One*, 8, 12, e83823, 2013 Dec 31.
19. Hemarajata, P. and Versalovic, J., Effects of probiotics on gut microbiota: Mechanisms of intestinal immunomodulation and neuromodulation. *Ther. Adv. Gastroenterol.*, 6, 39–51, 2013.
20. Kirtzalidou, E. *et al.*, Screening for lactobacilli with probiotic properties in the infant gut microbiota. *Anaerobe*, 17, 6, 440–3, 2011.
21. Spinler, J.K. *et al.*, Human-derived probiotic Lactobacillus reuteri demonstrate antimicrobial activities targeting diverse enteric bacterial pathogens. *Anaerobe*, 14, 166–71, 3, 2008.
22. Cunningham, M. *et al.*, Shaping the future of probiotics and prebiotics. *Trends Microbiol.*, 29, 8, 667–685, 2021.
23. Bong, K.C. *et al.*, The effect of a multispecies probiotic mixture on the symptoms and fecal microbiota in diarrhea-dominant irritable bowel syndrome: A randomized, double-blind, placebo-controlled trial. *J. Clin. Gastroenterol.*, 46, 3, 220–7, 2012.
24. Chaucheyras-Durand, F. and Durand, H., Probiotics in animal nutrition and health. *Beneficial Microbes*, 1, 3–9, 1, 2010.
25. Cho, J.H., Zhao, P.Y., Kim, I.H., Probiotics as a dietary additive for pigs. *J. Anim. Vet. Adv.*, 10, 2127–2134, 2011.
26. Alakomi, H.-L. *et al.*, Effect of EDTA on Salmonella enterica serovar Typhimurium involves a component not assignable to lipopolysaccharide release. *Microbiol. (Reading England)*, 149, 8, 2015–2021, 003.
27. McDonald, P., Edwards, R.A., Greenhalgh, J.F.D., Morgan, C.A., Sinclair, L.A. *et al.*, *Animal Nutrition*, 7th, Pearson Books, England UK, Harlow, England, 2010.

28. Gueimonde, M. and Collado, M.C., Metagenomics and probiotics. *Clin. Microbiol Infect. Off. Publ. Eur. Soc. Clin. Microbiol. Infect. Dis.*, 18, 4, 32–4, 2012.
29. Cullen, C.M., Aneja, K.K., Beyhan, S., Cho, C.E., Woloszynek, S., Convertino, M., McCoy, S.J., Zhang, Y., Anderson, M.Z., Alvarez-Ponce, D., Smirnova, E., Emerging priorities for microbiome research. *Front. Microbiol.*, 11, 136, 19 Feb. 2020.
30. Gibson, G.R. and Roberfroid, M.B., Dietary modulation of the human colonic microbiota: Introducing the concept of prebiotics. *J. Nutr.*, 125, 6, 1401–12, 1995, https://doi.org/10.1093/JN/125.6.1401.
31. Davani-Davari, D., Negahdaripour, M., Karimzadeh, I., Seifan, M., Mohkam, M., Masoumi, S.J., Berenjian, A., Ghasemi, Y., Prebiotics: Definition, types, sources, mechanisms, and clinical applications. *Foods*, 8, 3, 92, 2019, https://doi.org/10.3390/FOODS8030092.
32. Delcour, J.A., Aman, P., Courtin, C.M., Hamaker, B.R., Verbeke, K., Prebiotics, fermentable dietary fiber, and health claims. *Adv. Nutr.*, 7, 1, 1–4, 2016, https://doi.org/10.3945/AN.115.010546.
33. Slavin, J., Fiber and Prebiotics: Mechanisms and health benefits. *Nutrients*, 5, 4, 1417, 2013, https://doi.org/10.3390/NU5041417.
34. Tzounis, X., Rodriguez-Mateos, A., Vulevic, J., Gibson, G.R., Kwik-Uribe, C., Spencer, J.P., Prebiotic evaluation of cocoa-derived flavanols in healthy humans by using a randomized, controlled, double-blind, crossover intervention study. *Am. J. Clin. Nutr.*, 93, 1, 62–72, 2011, https://doi.org/10.3945/AJCN.110.000075.
35. Gibson, G.R., Hutkins, R., Sanders, M.E., Prescott, S.L., Reimer, R.A., Salminen, S.J., Scott, K., Stanton, C., Swanson, K.S., Cani, P.D., Verbeke, K., Reid, G., Expert consensus document: The International Scientific Association for Probiotics and Prebiotics (ISAPP) consensus statement on the definition and scope of prebiotics. *Nat. Rev. Gastroenterol Hepatology*, 14, 8, 491–502, 20172017. https://doi.org/10.1038/nrgastro.2017.75.
36. Roberfroid, M., Gibson, G.R., Hoyles, L., McCartney, A.L., Rastall, R., Rowland, I., Wolvers, D., Watzl, B., Szajewska, H., Stahl, B., Guarner, F., Respondek, F., Whelan, K., Coxam, V., Davicco, M.J., Léotoing, L., Wittrant, Y., Delzenne, N.M., Cani, P.D., Meheust, A., Prebiotic effects: Metabolic and health benefit. *Br. J. Nutr.*, 104, S2, S1–S63, 2010, https://doi.org/10.1017/S0007114510003363.
37. Broekaert, W.F., Courtin, C.M., Verbeke, K., Wiele, T.V., Verstraete, W., Delcour, J.A., Prebiotic and other health-related effects of cereal-derived Arabinoxylans, Arabinoxylan-O ligosaccharides, and Xylooligosaccharides. *Crit. Rev. Food Sci. Nutr.*, 51, 2, 178–194, 2011, https://doi.org/10.1080/10408390903044768.
38. Walker, A.W., Ince, J., Duncan, S.H., Webster, L.M., Holtrop, G., Ze, X., Brown, D., Stares, M.D., Scott, P., Bergerat, A., Louis, P., McIntosh, F., Johnstone, A.M., Lobley, G.E., Parkhill, J., Flint, H.J., Dominant and diet-responsive

groups of bacteria within the human colonic microbiota. *ISME J.*, 20115, 2, 220–30, 2010, https://doi.org/10.1038/ismej.2010.118.

39. Louis, P., Flint, H.J., Michel, C., How to manipulate the microbiota: Prebiotics. *Adv. Exp. Med. Biol.*, 902, 119–42, 2016, https://doi.org/10.1007/978-3-319-31248-4_9.
40. Wichienchot, S., Thammarutwasik, P., Jongjareonrak, A., Chansuwan, W., Hmadhlu, P., Hongpattarakere, T., Itharat, A., Ooraikul, B., Extraction and analysis of prebiotics from selected plants from southern Thailand. *Songklanakarin J. Sci. Technol.*, 33, 5, 517–23, 2011.
41. Varzakas, T., Kandylis, P., Dimitrellou, D., Salamoura, C., Zakynthinos, G., Proestos, C., Innovative and fortified food: Probiotics, prebiotics, GMOs, and superfood. *Preparation Process. Religious, Cultural Foods*, 67–129, 2018, https://doi.org/10.1016/B978-0-08-101892-7.00006-7.
42. Azmi, A.F.M.N., Mustafa, S., Hashim, D. Md., Manap, Y.A., Prebiotic activity of polysaccharides extracted from gigantochloaLevis (Buluhbeting) shoots. *Molecules*, 17, 2, 1635–51, 2012, https://doi.org/10.3390/MOLECULES17021635.
43. Zeaiter, Z., Regonesi, M.E., Cavini, S., Labra, M., Sello, G., di Gennaro, P., Extraction and characterization of inulin-type fructans from artichoke wastes and their effect on the growth of intestinal bacteria associated with health. *BioMed. Res. Int.*, 2019, 25, 2019, https://doi.org/10.1155/2019/1083952.
44. Wang, Y., Prebiotics: Present and future in food science and technology. *Food Res. Int.*, 42, 1, 8–12, 2009, https://doi.org/10.1016/J.FOODRES.2008.09.001.
45. Grimoud, J., Durand, H., Courtin, C., Monsan, P., Ouarné, F., Theodorou, V., Roques, C., *In vitro* screening of probiotic lactic acid bacteria and prebiotic glucooligosaccharides to select effective synbiotics. *Anaerobe*, 16, 5, 493–500, 2010, https://doi.org/10.1016/J.ANAEROBE.2010.07.005.
46. Rengarajan, K.E. and Radhakrishnan, P., Screening for suitable prebiotic for probiotic strain by *in vitro* fermentation. *Biosci. Biotechnol. Res. Asia*, 13, 2, 1177–81, 2016, https://doi.org/10.13005/BBRA/2149.
47. Peng, M., Tabashsum, Z., Anderson, M., Truong, A., Houser, A.K., Padilla, J., Akmel, A., Bhatti, J., Rahaman, S.O., Biswas, D., Effectiveness of probiotics, prebiotics, and prebiotic-like components in common functional foods. *Compr. Rev. Food Sci. Food Saf.*, 19, 4, 1908–33, 2020, https://doi.org/10.1111/1541-4337.12565.
48. Guseva, E., Karetkin, B., Batyrgazieva, D., Menshutina, N., Panfilov, V., Online database for retrieval information about prebiotics and their activity. *Appl. Sci.*, 10, 9, 20202020, https://doi.org/10.3390/APP10093328.
49. Guseva, E., Batyrgazieva, D., Karetkin, B., Menshutina, N., Development of a user web-interface for working with the information database in the field of biotechnology: Prebiotics, probiotics and their activity. *International Multidisciplinary Scientific Geo Conference Surveying Geology and Mining*

EcologyManagement, SGEM, vol. 19, pp. 651–58, 2019, https://doi.org/10.5593/SGEM2019/6.1/S25.084.
50. Batyrgazieva, D., Guseva, E., Karetkin, B., Menshutina, N., Information database in the field of biotechnology: Prebiotics, probiotics and their activity. *International Multidisciplinary Scientific GeoConference Surveying Geology and Mining Ecology Management, SGEM*, vol. 18, pp. 291–98, 2018, https://doi.org/10.5593/SGEM2018/6.2/S25.039.

9

Prebiotics and Probiotics in Regulation of Metabolic Disorders

Manswama Boro, Sushruta Bhadra and Anil Kumar Verma*

Department of Microbiology, Sikkim University, Gangtok, Sikkim, India

Abstract

Symbiotic gut microbiota inhibits the gastrointestinal tract that helps to maintain balance and proper functioning of several prominent metabolic pathways in the gut. Dysbiosis of gut microbiota leads to several metabolic disorders, including obesity, diabetes, cardiovascular diseases, and liver diseases. The gut microbiota has proven to influence human health and diseases, particularly playing important roles in the development and onset of obesity and its related metabolic disorders that arise due to alteration in the gut microbial composition, leading to adiposity, pancreatic β-cell dysfunction, metabolic endotoxemia, systemic inflammation, and oxidative stress. Metabolic diseases, like T2DM and CVD, have turned into global public health concerns and are a major cause of death, and its development due to alterations in the gut microbial composition is significantly associated with unhealthy diet and lifestyle along with other environmental and genetic factors. Administration of probiotics and prebiotics has been proven by several researchers as an effective method to stabilize the gut microbial composition, to ultimately prevent and treat metabolic diseases. Probiotics are microbial strains that colonize the host gut and provide health benefits to the host, as well as maintains the microbial homeostasis in the host gut. Prebiotics does not contain microbial strains but only compounds that benefit in the growth of specific bacterial strains.

***Keywords*:** Probiotics, prebiotics, gut microbiota, obesity, diabetes and metabolic disorder

**Corresponding author*: akverma@cus.ac.in
Anil Kumar Verma: ORCID: 0000-0003-0561-1954

Rajesh K. Kesharwani, Tingirikari Jagan Mohan Rao and Raj K. Keservani (eds.) Prebiotics and Probiotics in Disease Regulation and Management, (239–270) © 2022 Scrivener Publishing LLC

Abbreviations

GI	Gastrointestinal tract
T2DM	Type II diabetes mellitus
CVD	Cardiovascular diseases
TMAO	Trimethylamine N-oxide
SCFA	Short-chain fatty acids
LPS	Lipopolysaccharides
HFD	High-fat diet
NAFLD	Non-alcoholic fatty liver disease
GLP	Glucagon-like peptide
T1D	Type 1 diabetes
TMA	Trimethylamine
ALI	Acute liver injury

9.1 Introduction

For proper metabolic functioning and for maintaining overall homoeostasis of the body, it is important to maintain healthy gut microbiota. Microorganisms, including bacteria, archaea, protozoa, viruses, and fungi, are part of the gut microbiota representing a complex ecosystem, which inhabits the gastrointestinal (GI) tract, and live in a symbiotic relationship with the host, that maintain human health by facilitating food digestion and nutrient absorption, protecting against pathogens, maintaining the intestinal mucosa layer and regulating the immune system. Therefore, the gut microbiota significantly regulates the host health, physiology, and pathophysiology. In recent decades, researchers have provided several important pieces of information that has helped understanding gut homeostasis regulation mediated by gut microbiota and how changes in the diversity and composition of the gut microbiota may lead to various metabolic disorders. Dysbiosis of the gut microbiota may cause various metabolic diseases, such as metabolic syndrome, obesity, type II diabetes mellitus (T2DM), cardiovascular diseases (CVD), and neurodegenerative diseases [1]. Researchers have defined the different factors of metabolic disorders commonly related to obesity as metabolic syndrome, even though the symptoms differ in number and criteria. Metabolic syndrome comprises of obesity, increased blood glucose levels (causing T2DM, impaired fasting glucose, impaired glucose tolerance, and insulin resistance), decreased lipid homeostasis (causing hyperlipidemia), and CVD (hypertension and fibrolysis disorders) [2].

In the human gastrointestinal tract, the most dominant bacterial phyla belong to the gram-negative Bacteroidetes and the gram-positive Firmicutes. The most abundantly found Bacteroidetes genera is *Bacteroides* out of ~20 genera whereas, the phylum Firmicutes consists of >274 genera, including *Bacillus*, *Lactobacillus*, *Mycoplasma*, and *Clostridium*.

The use of probiotics and prebiotics for the maintenance of microbial homeostasis in the GI tract for the prevention and treatment of metabolic diseases have attracted considerable interest. Many studies in animal models and human subjects have been conducted to correct gut dysbiosis by targeting the gut microbiota with probiotics and prebiotics. The intestinal microbiome produces metabolites, such as trimethylamine N-oxide (TMAO), short-chain fatty acids (SCFA), bile acids, lipopolysaccharides (LPS), and peptidoglycan, which influence cardiometabolic diseases and can be effectively treated by probiotic treatment [3]. Metabolic endotoxemia and gut barrier permeability is prominently involved in the development of obesity-associated metabolic diseases, which can be improved by probiotic and prebiotic treatment by modulating glucose, lipid, and inflammation homeostasis.

There are several definitions for probiotics and prebiotics. In simple terms, they are a microbial strain or group of microbial strains that colonize the gut of a host animal or human and provide health benefits to the host body by improving the microbial balance in the gut. Live active bacterial cultures such as *lactobacilli*, *lactococci*, or *bifidobacteria* in preparations are commonly used as prebiotics and probiotics for consumption [4].

9.2 Probiotics

The term "probiotics" originates from Greek and means "for life." Elie Metchnikoff first defined probiotics in the early 1990s and is known as the father of the probiotics concept. Metchnikoff referred to the beneficial properties of fermented milk with *Lactobacillus* consumed by the indigenous, long-lived Bulgarian population and linked it to its ability to reduce toxin-producing bacteria and increase host longevity [5]. Later, in the early 1990s, Henry Tissier suggested oral administration of live *Bifidobacteria* to infants with diarrhea to restore healthy intestinal flora after observing that the microbial concentration of *Bifidobacteria* in the milk of infants with diarrhea was significantly low compared with healthy infants [5, 6].

In recent years, the use of probiotics in diarrheal disorders and several clinical conditions have provided encouraging results, which has generated considerable interest in researchers to use probiotics for the treatment of different metabolic diseases. Studies have proven that probiotics has the ability to treat and prevent obesity and associated metabolic disorders in animal models and humans, where it can be seen that probiotics have been in use in the field of agriculture for several decades for their growth-promoting activities [7].

Microbial strains can be considered probiotics if they are safe, effective, and have scientifically proven properties, including the ability to improve the health of their human host by colonizing in the human colon and maintaining colon microflora and immune responses that can help prevent infections, lower cholesterol, inhibit cancer development, and promote the synthesis of vitamins and cytokines. Probiotics should be safe, must not carry vectors with the ability to transfer factors of antibiotic resistance and adapted pathogenicity, and they must be able to live and proliferate in intestinal conditions in the presence of acidic pH, intestinal enzymes, and bile salts [8]. To consider and identify a microbial strain as a probiotic, it must have some general characteristics to facilitate its colonization in the gastrointestinal tract, such as tolerance to acidic pH, bile salt resistance, and the ability to adhere to the host gut epithelium. The symbiotic relationship between probiotics and the host epithelium promotes several mechanisms to maintain gut homeostasis that can be coupled with the health-promoting effects of the probiotic strains for the host. Much of the mechanisms are not clearly known, while some of these mechanisms are under study including the ability of the probiotics strains to modify gut microbiota composition, prevention of gut barrier dysfunction by strengthening the epithelial cells of the host intestine, ability to adhere to the gut mucosa, secretion of microbial metabolites that promote host health, production of antimicrobial metabolites, and host immune system modulation [9].

Some common probiotic bacterial strains are *Bifidobacterium, Enterococcus, Lactobacillus, Saccharomyces boulardii, Escherichia coli Nissle 1917, Lactococcus, Leuconostoc, Pediococcus,* and *Streptococcus* [8]. Change in the gut microbial community is associated with various metabolic disorders. Probiotics are commonly known to alter and restore the microbial community. They are used as a treatment strategy and the specific mechanisms of action are not yet fully understood by researchers, although much research has been conducted in this area. There are numerous probiotic food products available in the market all over the world, few of them have been listed in Table 9.1.

Table 9.1 List of some commercially available probiotic products.

Probiotic product	Strain	Food type	Health benefits	Manufacturer
Activia	*Bifidobacterium lactis* DN 173 010/CNCM I-2494	Yogurt drink	Reduce minor digestive discomfort including bloating, gas, abdominal discomfort, and rumbling	Dannon® (France)
Align	*Bifidobacterium infantis* 35624	Capsules and chewable tablets	Restoration of the digestive system	Procter & Gamble (Ohio, USA)
Bacilac	*Lactobacillus acidophilus*, *Lactobacillus rhamnosus*	Freeze dried tablets	Normalizes gut microflora, effective in treating diarrhea	THT (Belgium)
Bifilac	*Bacillus mesentericus*, *Clostridium butyricum*, *Lactobacillus sporegens*, *Streptococcus faecalis*	Tablets	Gastrointestinal disorders, bacterial infections, immunity	Allianz Biosciences (India)

(*Continued*)

Table 9.1 List of some commercially available probiotic products. (*Continued*)

Probiotic product	Strain	Food type	Health benefits	Manufacturer
Culturelle	*Lactobacillus rhamnosus* GG	Capsules	Prevent the growth of harmful bacteria in the stomach and intestines; treating or preventing diarrhea	Culturelle® (USA)
Yakult	*Lactobacillus casei* strain Shirota	Yogurt drink	Increase beneficial bacteria in the intestine, regulates bowl movement, reduces infection, constipation and diarrhea, improves immunity	Yakult Honsha Co., Ltd. (Tokyo, Japan)
Florastor	*Saccharomyces boulardii* lyo CNCM I-745	Capsules	Promote good intestinal health	Biocodex (Creswell, OR)

9.3 Prebiotics

Gibson and Roberfroid describe prebiotics as indigestible polysaccharides or oligosaccharides that stimulate the growth and activity of selective bacterial strains in the colon, thus benefiting the host. Synbiotics are produced by combining prebiotics and probiotics, which provide more benefits than probiotics or prebiotics alone [10]. Prebiotics were examined by Gibson *et al.* on three criteria, that includes: resistance to gastrointestinal acids and enzymes; ability of gut microflora to ferment sugar; and the ability to stimulate the growth and activity of selective gut bacteria that is responsible for the health and well-being of the host [11]. These criteria were met only by fructooligosaccharides, galactooligosaccharides, and lactulose [11]. Again, Gibson and Roberfroid reviewed the concept of prebiotics and their health effects in 2010 [12]. In infant feeding, prebiotics significantly changes the gut microfloral composition and increase Bifidobacterial concentration in the faeces, which helps improve stool quality (pH, SCFA, frequency, and consistency), reduce the risk of infections, stomach flu, and allergic symptoms like atopic eczema, and improve health status [12]. The most-studied prebiotics are fructooligosaccharides (FOS), inulin, and oligofructose [10].

Consumption of food rich in prebiotics strongly benefits against obesity and related metabolic disorders, through many different action mechanisms. There are evidence that prove the ability of prebiotics and

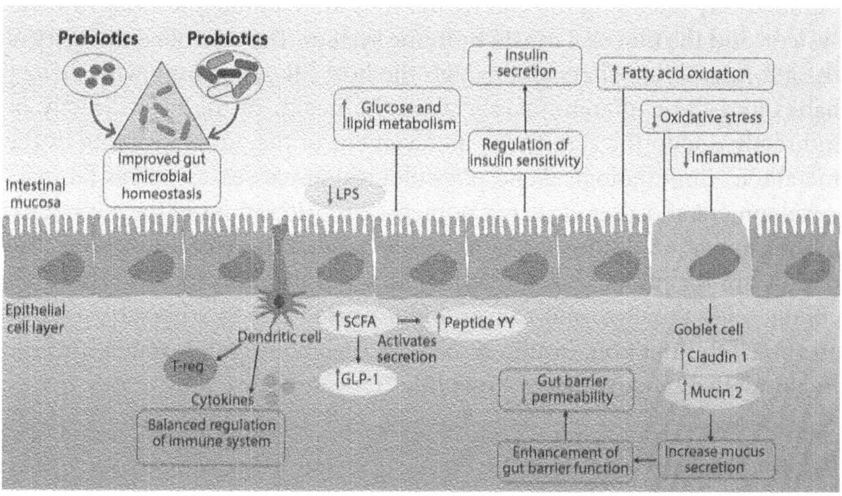

Figure 9.1 A summary of mechanisms by which supplementation of prebiotics and probiotics benefits human health in combating metabolic disorders.

the use of prebiotic therapy to positively regulate the composition of gut microbiota, promoting the growth and colonization of Lactobacillus and Bifidobacterium in the GI tract during obesity and, reducing the growth of pathogenic microorganisms to improve intestinal epithelial cell activities, and maintain glucose and lipid homeostasis, in oligofructose treated obese and diabetic mice and ob/ob mice treated with prebiotic carbohydrates. Gut microbial homeostasis brought about by prebiotic treatment was also responsible for the heightened glucagon-like peptide-2 (GLP-2) production, that affects intestinal barrier permeability, thus reducing disorders associated with obesity and hepatic inflammation [7] (Figure 9.1).

9.4 The Role of Gut Microbiota in Metabolic Disorders

An adult human gut may harbor microorganisms up to ten times the total number of somatic and germ cells [13] which may add to the large collective gene pool of the gut microbiota, that contains 100 to 150 times more genes than the genome of an adult human. The coevolution of these microorganisms with humans led to the establishment of a reciprocal relationship that strongly influences various host responses [14, 15].

Interactions and symbiotic relations between host gut epithelial cells and gut microbiota start right from birth and these interactions promote the maturation of several important parts of the functional systems of the human body including the enteric nervous system, the intestinal vascular system, and the mucosal innate immune system. The microbial diversity of the gut microbiota alters all through the host life span along with dietary habits and these alterations reflect on the health of the host directly or indirectly due to the significant involvement of the gut microbiota in the metabolic, immunological and physiological processes, as well as fat mass development and altered energy homeostasis. Alterations in the gut microbial composition, known as dysbiosis, is related to several disorders and diseases of the human body, that includes obesity, diabetes, CVD, non-alcoholic liver damage, and cancer, often caused due to adiposity, pancreatic β-cell dysfunction, insulin resistance, metabolic endotoxemia, chronic inflammation, and oxidative stress [6].

9.4.1 Obesity

The incidence of obesity has been increasing dramatically in developed and developing countries due to genes, unhealthy diet, and lifestyle.

Millions of people are obese around the world, creating a public health challenge. There are several pieces of evidence given by researchers about the role of gut microbiota in obese conditions. Intestinal microbiota can regulate adiposity and fat storage contributing to the regulation of obesity. Obese microflora has been found with a lower bacterial diversity as compared to lean microflora, with a low gene richness of faecal bacteria leading to adiposity, dyslipidemia, low-grade inflammation and reduced glucose homeostasis [16]. Alteration in the intestinal microbial diversity and composition is observed in obese conditions, often leading toan increase in Firmicutes and decrease in Bacteroidetes [2, 17]. Researchers have shown that obesity can be linked to an increase in theintestinal oxidative stress and abundance in SCFA producers such as *Eubacterium ventriosum* and *Roseburia intestinalis* in the gut microbiota [15].

There are several mechanisms followed by gut microbiota to regulate obesity and related metabolic disorders. In one of the mechanisms, it can be assumed that intestinal microbiota of obese individuals is able to produce energy from a given diet more efficiently compared to the intestinal microbiota of lean individuals, leading to increased levels of stored energy and adiposity. Production of SCFAs from dietary polysaccharides can be considered another mechanism that is followed by intestinal microbiota to control energy intake and intestinal metabolism. Bacterial fermentations of dietary polysaccharides and fibers result in production of SCFAs such as acetate, butyrate and propionate, which comprises >95% of the SCFA content that act as a source of energy for glucose metabolism and regulators of food satiety and intake. SCFAs activates the G protein-coupled receptors GPR41 and GPR43 on the colon epithelial cells promoting the secretion of peptide YY (PYY) and glucagon-like peptide (GLP)-1, that enhance nutrient absorption by restraining gut motility and delaying intestinal transit. Butyrate and propionate are able to protect against diet-induced obesity by reducing food intake capacity and insulin resistance in mice. Higher production of SCFAs has been associated with higher bacterial gene richness. Propionate-producer bacteria, such as *Akkermansia muciniphila*, have been considered effective in improving the metabolic homeostasis in mice. The function of SCFAs in maintaining the homeostasis of host metabolism is unclear, making it difficult to draw any conclusion. It has also been suggested that extensive use of antibiotics, which considerably affect the intestinal microbiota composition, may be significantly associated with gut microbial dysbiosis leading to weight gain and obesity in humans [16].

It is widely known that obesity may significantly lead to chronic low-grade inflammation and insulin resistance. Inflammation and higher expression of proinflammatory cytokines such as TNF-α and interleukins [IL]-1, IL-6,

IL-10, and IL-12 is associated with the actions of white adipose tissue and subsequently induce insulin resistance. High-fat diet (HFD)–induced disbalance in gut microbiota is considered one of the significant contributing factors of gut barrier dysfunction by either direct translocation of Gram-negative intestinal bacteria or LPSs secreted by Gram-negative bacteria, that leads to induction of metabolic endotoxemia, resulting in the generation of low-grade inflammation which may ultimately lead to insulin resistance. Thus, gut barrier dysfunction and invasion of bacteria and bacterial metabolites are factors that significantly contribute to insulin resistance and oxidative stress [7].

Gut barrier dysfunction in the intestines may create an opening for microbes and microbial molecules like LPS, peptidoglycans, and flagellin that may lead to metabolic endotoxemia observed in obesity and T2DM. Gut microbiota could regulate gut barrier permeability and metabolic endotoxemia during obesity through the endocannabinoid system (eCB), that comprises of endogenous bioactive lipids like anandamide that has greater affinity for cannabinoid receptor 1 (CB_1). Gut microbiota is also able to control the expression of intestinal alkaline phosphatase (IAP) enzyme that is involved in breaking down of dietary lipids, changing gut barrier functions and reduction in metabolic endotoxemia in obesity and T2DM [2].

9.4.2 Diabetes

The gut microflora has a major function in the regulation and metabolism of glucose in the host. T2DM, a widespread metabolic disorder in humans, is caused by impaired regulation and metabolism of glucose and is characterized by altered blood glucose levels, change in blood lipid profile, and increase in blood pressure [18]. Experimental studies have shown that 90% of all diabetes cases worldwide are due to the rapid progression of insulin resistance caused by alteration of gut microflora. The normal diet of a healthy person consists of a large amount of carbohydrates, which can increase glucose levels in the blood. However, blood glucose levels are controlled and maintained at a homeostatic level by the action of two host hormones, insulin and glucagon [18].

People suffering from T2DM exhibit elevated blood glucose levels or hyperglycemia due to increased resistance to insulin or inadequate secretion of insulin by the beta cells of the pancreas [19]. Most of the intestinal microflora belong to the Firmicutes, Bacteroidetes, Proteobacteria, and Actinobacteria families [20]. Experimental studies showed a shift in the ratio between Firmicutes and Bacteroidetes in subjects who were obese.

Obesity corresponds to an increased risk of T2DM, and obese patients have shown a progressive increase in insulin resistance and a decrease in insulin secretion at a fairly early stage [21]. Insulin secretion is also regulated by incretin hormones, which are intestinal peptides released into the bloodstream by enteroendocrine cells. These hormones stimulate insulin secretion and also promote the proliferation of pancreatic beta cells. The gut microbiota also takes part in modulating the secretion of incretins. These microorganisms are able to increase the number of enteroendocrine cells or are directly involved in the regulation of incretin secretion through the process of fermentation. Tests in rats showed that fermentation of indigestible carbohydrates such as fructooligosaccharides by the gut microorganisms improved incretin secretion in the subjects due to a doubling of the number of enteroendocrine L cells in the proximal colon. The metabolites produced by these gut microorganisms are also directly involved in increasing the incretin secretion. In rats, an increase in the incretin GLP-1 and improved insulin response and blood glucose control were observed when the gut microbiota of these subjects was enriched with sulfate-reducing bacteria. Sulfate-reducing bacteria abundantly produced the bioactive gas metabolite hydrogen sulfide (H_2S), which directly stimulated the GLP-1 response in the gut. Indole, produced by the dissimilation of tryptophan by bacterial groups belonging to the genera *Escherichia, Clostridium,* and *Bacteroides*, is another metabolite capable of modulating GLP-1 secretion [21]. Anaerobic fermentation of indigestible carbohydrates by gut saccharolytic microbes leads to SCFA production in the host colon and cecum. A large proportion of the SCFAs produced are acetate, butyrate, and propionate. These acids are able to regulate glucose metabolism by interacting with G protein-coupled receptors (GPRs) found on the epithelial, enteroendocrine, and immune cells of the intestine, as well as in adipose tissue, the pancreas, and the liver. Acetate, propionate and butyrate are able to bind to the GPR41 and GPR43 receptors of enteroendocrine cells and stimulate GLP-1 secretion [22].

9.4.3 Liver Disorders

Colon bacteria also have a considerable impact on liver diseases. 50% of patients with liver cirrhosis showed an overgrowth of pathogenic colonic bacteria in the small intestine [23]. Probiotics or beneficial gut microbes have shown the ability to improve liver disease. In individuals suffering from alcoholic liver damage or alcoholic cirrhosis, probiotics stimulate immune responses and decrease the production of inflammatory cytokines and reactive oxygen species (ROS) in the liver and GI tract. These beneficial microbes also help resist alcohol-induced hepatic steatosis by reducing lipogenesis and increasing β-oxidation of fatty acids [24]. It was observed that in individuals suffering from non-alcoholic fatty liver disease (NAFLD) the gut-liver homeostasis was altered due to dysbiosis of the gut microbiota. Observable changes in the gut-liver axis of individuals with NAFLD include disrupted gut barrier, increased transportation of bacterial endotoxins to the liver, change in the bile acid profile, and a decrease in SCFAs. NAFLD is a metabolic disorder caused by accumulation of excessive fat in the liver. Studies revealed that gut microbiota alteration associated with NAFLD displayed an abundant increase in Bacteroidetes and decrease in Firmicutes [25]. Cumulative studies disclosed that in NAFLD pathogenesis progresses with the exertion of toxic effects by the inflammatory cytokines, pathogenic endotoxins, and metabolites produced by the harmful microbes. SCFAs produced by the beneficial gut microbes have displayed direct involvement in acting against NAFLD. Propionate has displayed the capability to inhibit glucose production in the liver by down-regulating the expression of genes coding for gluconeogenic enzymes. Butyrate is involved in regulating intestinal barrier function by decreasing the permeability of the intestinal epithelium thereby preventing the portal transport of pathogenic endotoxins and LPS [26].

9.4.4 Cardiometabolic Disorders

Gut microbiota is significantly linked to cardiovascular conditions and is able to exhibit hypocholesterolemic and hypotriglyceridemic properties. High blood cholesterol and triglyceride levels can cause a number of heart diseases and complications such as heart attacks, strokes, and atherosclerosis. Diseases like atherosclerosis are also caused by dysbiosis of the gut microflora. Dysbiosis promotes the production of metabolites such as trimethylamine N-oxide (TMAO) in the gut and alters bile acid metabolism, which overall contributes to the development of atherosclerosis [27]. The gut microbiota is capable of regulating metabolism of cholesterol in the liver and can modulate systemic cholesterol levels by influencing the level of bile acid. Bile salts produced from the conjugation of primary bile acids with amino acids is capable of emulsifying fats to form micelles, which are then absorbed by the enterocytes. Certain gut microbes are capable of converting cholesterol into a non-absorbable reduced sterol known as coprostanol. This non-absorbable sterol is ultimately flushed out of the body through feces [28]. Promoting the growth of Lactobacillus and Bifidobacteria in the colon has also shown the ability to ameliorate heart disease and atherosclerosis. These groups of bacteria perform anaerobic fermentation to produce SCFAs. The SCFAs produced are able to inhibit hepatic cholesterogenesis and lipogenesis, resulting in lowering plasma triglyceride and cholesterol levels. The leukocyte population also display strong expression of Ffar2 receptors which recognizes SCFAs and establish metabolic conditions that promote the proper functioning of endothelial cells while reducing accumulation of monocytes and cholesterol in the endothelium. The lowered plasma cholesterol and triglyceride levels reduces the risks associated with various heart diseases [29].

9.5 Effect of Prebiotics on Metabolic Disorders

The gut microbiota has an important role in maintaining the health of a host by influencing metabolism and inflammation, and affecting the correlation of gut, brain and microbiota. Administration of prebiotics promotes the growth of health-promoting microorganisms in the host's gastrointestinal tract. These prebiotic compounds are indigestible, consumable fibers that improve host metabolic health directly or indirectly through anaerobic fermentation by the probiotic microorganisms. Although it is not clear, experimental studies in mouse models have revealed a number of possible mechanisms by which these dietary components contribute to the improvement of metabolic disorders [30].

9.5.1 Mechanism of Action

Prebiotics cannot be hydrolyzed by host digestive enzymes and are fermented only by a select group of colon bacteria. Fermentation of prebiotics produces a number of metabolites, including SCFAs like butyrate, propionate, and acetic acid, as well as hydrogen, methane, carbon dioxide (CO_2), vitamins, and amino acids [31]. The SCFAs produced play an important role in alleviating metabolic disorders by activating GPR41 and GPR43 receptors on the enteroendocrine L cells, immune cells, and adipocytes, that causes stimulation of secretion of GLP-1 and the secretion of leptin from adipocytes resulting in the regulation of lipid profile [32]. GLP-1 stimulates the pancreatic β-cells for higher insulin secretion and inhibit glucagon secretion from pancreatic islets. This results in increased uptake of glucose by peripheral cells and decreased production of glucose by hepatic gluconeogenesis. SCFAs also affect the autonomic nervous system or brain to suppress host appetite. Patients suffering from T2DM experiences increased levels of inflammatory markers, such as high-sensitivity C-reactive protein (CRP), tumor necrosis factor-alpha (TNF-α), and IL-6.

These inflammatory molecules influence insulin resistance and are overexpressed in tissues on which insulin acts.

A change in the SCFA profile is able to increase the anti-inflammatory response in the body, leading to a decrease in insulin resistance. Insulin resistance is also caused by microorganisms in the colon that can produce lipopolysaccharides (LPS). Toll-like receptor 4 (TLR4) in pancreatic islets is able to recognize LPS and, when activated, shows an increase in proinflammatory cytokine production that impairs the function of β-cells and reduces their viability. Activation of TLR4 results in a decrease in pancreatic duodenum homeobox-1 (PDX1) mRNA expression. It also leads to a decrease in insulin gene expression and decreased insulin concentration. SCFAs are able to counteract these deleterious effects by suppressing proinflammatory mediators and inducing the production of anti-inflammatory cytokines. SCFAs also display an anti-inflammatory effect by down-regulating adhesion molecules in endothelial cells, thereby inhibiting the migration of leukocytes to sites of inflammation. These mechanisms act together to maintain blood glucose homeostasis and regulate blood glucose levels through three primary methods: i) decreasing insulin resistance by reducing inflammation; ii) increasing insulin release by increasing secretion of the incretin hormone GLP-1 and decreasing hepatic gluconeogenesis by regulating glucagon hormone; iii) improving β-cell function and promoting their proliferation [32].

Prebiotics are also involved in the treatment of metabolic disorders such as hypercholesterolemia and hypertriglyceridemia, which are responsible for cardiovascular diseases. Elevated cholesterol level in the form of low-density lipoprotein (LDL) and triglycerides in the blood leads to various health problems such as liver damage, stroke, heart attack, and atherosclerosis. Prebiotics are capable of lowering lipid levels in blood serum through their hypocholesterolemic and hypotriglyceridemic effects [33]. There are two main mechanisms by which prebiotics can lower serum lipid levels: first, by decreasing cholesterol absorption and increasing cholesterol excretion, and second, by the activity of SCFAs produced by the fermentation of these compounds by beneficial gut microorganisms [29]. These indigestible food components are able to decrease the absorption of cholesterol in the intestine by promoting the thickening of the intestinal walls. The unabsorbed cholesterol is broken down in the liver, leading to a decrease in lipid levels. The SCFAs produced during the fermentation of prebiotics are also able to inhibit hepatic cholesterogenesis and lipogenesis, resulting in a decrease in plasma triglyceride and cholesterol levels. SCFAs lower luminal pH, resulting in a decrease in the amount of soluble bile acid. The decrease in solubility and absorption of bile acids causes increased excretion of fecal bile acid that results in decreasing cholesterol levels because available cholesterol in the liver is used to resynthesize bile acids to maintain bile acid levels [34]. Prebiotics also stimulate the growth of beneficial microbes known as probiotic microorganisms, which also have hypocholesterolemic and hypotriglyceridemic effects by assimilating cholesterol and binding to these microbial cells.

Prebiotics not only plays a significant part in combating metabolic disorders such as hypercholesterolemia and diabetes but also in the treatment of NAFLD, one of the most common metabolic disorders with a high incidence rate worldwide. Prebiotics are capable of inducing gut-mediated changes in luminal and peripheral metabolism. These changes include reducing bacterial-derived hepatotoxins, improving the gut epithelial barrier, reducing inflammation, reducing lipogenesis, and improving glycemic control. These changes exert a combined effect that contributes towards the improvement of NAFLD [35].

9.5.2 Prebiotics With Other Components

Prebiotics administered in consortium with a counter component such as probiotics are able to improve health benefits and resistance to metabolic disorders. These products that are created by combining prebiotics and probiotics are known as synbiotics. The development of synbiotics is primarily aimed at overcoming the potential difficulties in the survival of probiotics in the human colon [36]. Synbiotics are carefully designed products that contain a specific probiotic organism along with prebiotics that specifically support and enhance the growth of the introduced probiotic, giving it a competitive advantage over other microbial strains in the colon. These products are highly specific and promote the proliferation of the targeted probiotic strains even in a competitive environment, making them an efficient therapeutic consumable for the alleviation of numerous gut-related and metabolic disorders [37]. Extensive research has been conducted on synbiotics containing combinations of *Lactobacilli* and *Bifidobacteria* with prebiotics such as inulin, oligosaccharides, or dietary fiber [38]. Tests on subjects conducted over a 28-weeks period found that individuals treated with synbiotics had better fasting blood glucose levels and lower insulin resistance compared to placebo subjects. Fasting blood glucose decreased from 5.62 mmol/l to 5.16 mmol/l in the synbiotic-treated subjects and to 5.59 mmol/l in the placebo group. Insulin levels decreased from 71.39 mmol/l to 57.92 mmol/l in the synbiotic-treated group and from 75.63 mmol/l to 57.92 mmol/l in the placebo group. The synbiotic-treated group also displayed a significant decrease in triglyceride levels

Table 9.2 Symbiotic activity performed on test subjects against metabolic disorders.

Synbiotic combination	Synbiotic dosage	Subject condition	Observed outcome	Ref.
Lactobacillus sporogenes (1,107 CFU) and 0.4 gram inulin.	3 times a day in doses of 9 grams.	T2DM.	Reduction in serum insulin, triglyceride, high-sensitivity CRP and fasting glucose levels. Increase in HDL, glutathione and uric acid.	[58]
Streptococcus thermophilus and fructooligosaccharide (FOS).	500 mg per day.	T2DM.	Improvement in hemoglobin A1C levels and BMI.	[59]
Mixture of *Lactobacillus acidophilus*, *Bifidobacterium bifidum* and oligofructose.	NA	T2DM.	Reduction in fasting glycemia.	[60]
Lactobacillus acidophilus ATCC 4962 mixed with mannitol, inulin and FOSs.	1 gram of *Lactobacillus acidophilus* ATCC 4962 per day with 1.56 gram of mannitol, 1.25 gram FOS and 2.2 gram inulin.	Pigs with hypercholesterolemia.	Reduction in total cholesterol, triacylglycerol and LDL-cholesterol.	[61]

(*Continued*)

Table 9.2 Symbiotic activity performed on test subjects against metabolic disorders. (*Continued*)

Synbiotic combination	Synbiotic dosage	Subject condition	Observed outcome	Ref.
Bifidobacterium longum with FOS.	NA	Subjects with cirrhosis and minimal hepatic encephalopathy (MHE).	Reduction in ammonia and improvement in neuropsychological activity.	[62]
Mixture of 7 microbial strains that include *Lactobacillus casei*, *Lactobacillus rhamnosus*, *Lactobacillus acidophilus*, *Streptococcus thermophilus*, *Bifidobacterium breve*, *Bifidobacterium longum*, *Lactobacillus bulgaricus* with FOS.	Consumed as supplement twice daily for 28 weeks.	NAFLD.	Reduction in alanine aminotransferase (ALT), aspartate aminotransferase (AST), γ-glutamyltransferase.	[63]

from 2.58 mmol/l to 1.78 mmol/l compared to the placebo group, in which triglyceride levels decreased from 2.66 mmol/l to 2.54 mmol/l. Total cholesterol levels (TC) decreased from 3.84 mmol/l to 3.26 mmol/l in synbiotic-treated subjects, which was significantly lower compared to subjects in the placebo group, in whom TC levels decreased from 4.28 mmol/l to 3.92 mmol/l [39]. Other tests performed on healthy adults with a combination of *Lactobacillus salavarius* and fructooligosaccharide (FOS) showed greater reductions in total cholesterol, low-density lipoprotein (LDL) cholesterol, C-reactive protein (CRP), tumor necrosis factor-α (TNF-α), and interleukin-6 (IL -6) compared to the placebo group and the group treated with probiotics alone [38]. These synbiotics offer the potential for the development of new prebiotics targeting specific probiotic strains to improve human health (Table 9.2).

9.6 Effect of Probiotics on Metabolic Disorders

Probiotics are known for stimulating immune response, improving lactose tolerance, preventing diarrhea, reducing inflammation, and restoring gut dysbiosis associated with obesity. A single probiotic strain, even if of the same species, does not provide all the benefits associated with probiotics at once, and the beneficial effects tend to be strain-specific, contradicting the concept of a "universal strain."

Dysbiosis, i.e., change in gut microbiota composition, alters microbial interactions in the host causing inflammation and other diseases in humans. According to the researchers, homeostasis is maintained by limiting oxygen availability in the colon through epithelial hypoxia, creating a balance in the gut microbiota that produces metabolites that contribute to the host's immune system and nutrition. Probiotics help treat dysbiosis and maintain homeostasis of the gut microbiota through several mechanisms [8]. The exact mechanism by which probiotics treat metabolic diseases and establish metabolic homeostasis is not yet clearly known. A few researches conducted on the administration of probiotics for the treatment of metabolic disorders have been tabulated in Table 9.3.

The effects of probiotic treatment of metabolic disorders are complex and cannot be precisely determined. Probiotic treatment is majorly involved with the modification in the composition of gut microflora, although it remains unclear whether this modification is a cause or the result of probiotics competing for nutrients, metabolites, and proteins. Probiotics are associated with several components that contribute to their beneficial effects including the ability to control host response, pathogen

Table 9.3 List of some research on probiotic bacteria for the treatment of metabolic disorders.

Disease	Probiotic bacteria	Experiment model	Results and outcomes	Ref.
Obesity and related immune-metabolic disorders	*Lactobacillus rhamnosus* Lb102, *Bifidobacterium animalis* ssp. *lactis* Bf141	C57BL/6 mice	Selective changes in gut microbiota composition; reduced diet-induced obesity, visceral fat accretion and inflammation; improvement of glucose tolerance and insulin sensitivity.	[64]
Obesity	*Lactobacillus plantarum* KLDS1.0344 and *Lactobacillus plantarum* KLDS1.0386	C57BL/6J mice	Reduced liver lipid accumulation and improved lipid metabolism of adipose tissue; improved blood lipid levels and liver function; alleviated liver oxidative stress; improved gut microbiota, increasing acetic acid and butyric acid levels.	[65]
Type II diabetes	*Lactobacillus paracasei* TD062	Diabetic mice	Regulated levels of fasting blood glucose (FBG), postprandial blood glucose (PBG), glucose tolerance, hepatic glycogen and lipid metabolism; enhanced expression of genes that regulate glucose metabolism and the PI3K/Akt pathway.	[66]
	Lactobacillus plantarum SS18-5	Sprague Dawley rats	Lowered levels of hypoglycemia and regulated intestinal microbiota.	[67]

(*Continued*)

Table 9.3 List of some research on probiotic bacteria for the treatment of metabolic disorders. (*Continued*)

Disease	Probiotic bacteria	Experiment model	Results and outcomes	Ref.
Atherosclerosis	*Pediococcus acidilactici* R037	$ApoE^{-/-}$ mice	Induced tolerogenic DCs, which suppress Th1-driven inflammation and the proliferative activity of $CD4^+$ T cells.	[68]
	Lactobacillus plantarum ATCC 14917	$ApoE^{-/-}$ mice	Decreased atherosclerotic lesion formation by reducing the inflammatory process and lowering oxidative stress; modulated gut microbiota composition.	[69]
Hyperlipidemia and Atherosclerosis	*Lactobacillus mucosae* A1	$ApoE^{-/-}$ mice	Lowered chronic inflammation that resulted in decreasing metabolic endotoxemia; improved lipid metabolism and the structure of gut microbiota	[70]

inhibition, and interaction with the gut microbiota. These probiotic-associated components are constituents of cells such as various polymers (polysaccharides, peptidoglycans, DNA, teichoic acids), certain proteins, organic acids, fatty acids, bacteriocins and polyphosphates [40].

9.6.1 Role of Probiotics on Obesity

Development of obesity due to insulin resistance, oxidative stress, and chronic low-grade inflammation resulting from gut barrier dysfunction can be prevented and restored by the administration of probiotics by cytoskeletal modulation, normalizing expression of proteins that promotes intestinal permeability or promoting secretion of mucus. As it has been observed that gut microbiota composition of an obese individual significantly differs from that of a lean individual. Selective alteration of gut microbiota by administration of probiotics can be considered a potential therapy to control fat accumulation and obesity. Several strains of *Lactobacillus* and *Bifidobacterium* have been used for probiotic treatment of obesity in animal models, including *L. casei* Shirota (LAB13), *L. gasseri*, *L. rhamnosus*, *L. plantarum*, *B. infantis*, *B. longum*, and *B. breve* B3 [7]. Other bacterial probiotic strains with anti-obesity activity includes *Pediococcus pentosaceus* LP28, *Bacteroides uniformis* CECT 7771, *Akkermansia muciniphila*, and *Saccharomyces boulardii* Biocodex [7, 9]. In high-fat diet fed mice and rats, probiotics containing *Bifidobacterium* had beneficial affects including improved gut barrier functions that reduced endotoxemia; reduced levels of inflammation, insulin resistance, fat, and cholesterol accumulation [17].

In order to prepare probiotics for the treatment of obesity and its related metabolic disorders, it is important to improve research strategies; attain detailed knowledge and information regarding the interaction between the probiotic strain with the host gut microbiota; standardization of the probiotic therapy in terms of dosage and duration; effects of probiotics on target individuals based on age, and genetic information for the efficiency of the probiotic treatment; and the incorporation with foods products like fruit juice and yogurt to improve the effect of probiotic on body weight [7].

9.6.2 Role of Probiotics on Diabetes

Diabetes is currently one of the most common metabolic diseases and represents a major public health problem worldwide. Hyperglycemia results from decreased secretion of insulin in the blood caused by high oxidative stress, which damages pancreatic beta cells [41]. Experimental studies have shown the benefits of probiotics in blood glucose control through various probiotic bacterial strains such as *Lactobacillus acidophilus, L. casei, L. plantarum* TN627, *L. plantarum* DSM 15313, *L. gasseri* BNR17, *L. reuteri, L. rhamnosus*, and *Bifidobacterium lactis* [42]. Type 1 diabetes (T1D) is characterised by destruction of insulin producing pancreatic beta (β) cells by the immune system commonly during the early childhood [43]. Gut dysbiosis may progressively lead to T1D as the gut microflora closely interacts with the enteric mucosal immune system [43]. Thus, probiotics can be associated with improvement of gut dysbiosis and decline autoimmune response in the gut. T1D is often described by irregular function of the tryptophan-degrading enzyme indoleamine 2,3 dioxygenase 1 (IDO1), which lowers kynurenine levels and may contribute to autoimmunity in T1D. Administration of *Lactobacillus rhamnosus* GG may positively affect the metabolism of tryptophan and curb the actions proinflammatory cytokines in pediatric T1D [44]. Administration of the probiotic Immune Regulation and Tolerance 5 (IRT5), that consists of the microbial strains *Lactobacillus acidophilus, L. casei, L. reuteri, Bifidobacterium bifidium* and *Streptococcus thermophiles* to non-obese diabetic (NOD) mice with human T1D was able to significantly reduce the incidence of diabetes, decreasing insulitis and increasing pancreatic β-cell mass [45].

T2DM is a public health challenge and a common acute metabolic disease around the world, which can lead to several severe complications such as cardiovascular disease, diabetic retinopathy, neuropathy, and nephropathy [46]. Factors that may lead to T2DM include obesity, active substance deficiency, gene mutations, chronic inflammatory responses caused by insulin resistance pathogenesis, gut microbiota imbalance, heredity, and environmental T2DM [46]. However, the main cause of T2DM is irregular or decreased insulin secretion by pancreatic β-cells and development of insulin resistance by insulin-sensitive tissues [47]. The use of probiotics to manage blood pressure, lipid profile, fasting blood glucose and improve insulin resistance may be effective in the treatment of T2DM [46, 48]. Several mechanisms may be involved in probiotic treatment of T2DM, which may include: improving gut microflora, lowering lipopolysaccharide (LPS) levels, enhancing actions of incretins, reduction of stress on the endoplasmic reticulum (ER), improving peripheral insulin sensitivity and glucose tolerance, regulation of lipid metabolism, improvement in antioxidant levels, modulating the composition of SCFAs, and reduction of inflammatory response, autoimmune response, and oxidative stress [49]. Although further studies are needed, several studies have reported the positive use of probiotics in the treatment of T2DM, which could potentially provide a supportive alternative for the treatment of T2DM.

9.6.3 Role of Probiotics on Cardiovascular Disease (CVD)

Cardiovascular disease (CVD) affecting the blood vessels and heart is usually caused by hypercholesterolemia and dyslipidemia. The gut microbiome is able to produce metabolites from the host diet that affect the cardiovascular status of the host. The significant role of gut microbiome in CVD through various mechanisms such as the production of trimethylamine (TMA), SCFA and bile acids, have been demonstrated by several researchers [3]. Therefore, targeting specific gut bacteria and administering probiotics could potentially be used to treat CVD [3]. Probiotics are known to regulate several mechanisms and factors that contribute to the treatment of CVD (Figure 9.2). Atherosclerosis, an inflammatory disease of the arteries, is promoted in part by trimethylamine N-oxide (TMAO) by promoting macrophage foam cell formation in atherosclerotic lesions and disrupting lipid homeostasis [50]. TMA is produced by the gut microbiota from choline, phosphatidylcholine, or carnitinecontaining diet found in foods that are high in saturated or unsaturated fats. TMA is oxidized to TMAO by the enzyme flavin monooxygenase-3 (FMO3) after ingestion in the liver [3, 50]. Increased TMAO levels have been associated with major CVD and kidney diseases. Reduction in TMAO levels has been demonstrated by certain strains of probiotics in association with reduced development of atherosclerosis [50].

Arterial hypertension is a serious high blood pressure condition in the arteries from the heart to the lungs that may lead to stroke and heart failure. Human clinical trials of probiotics such as *Lactobacillus casei* and

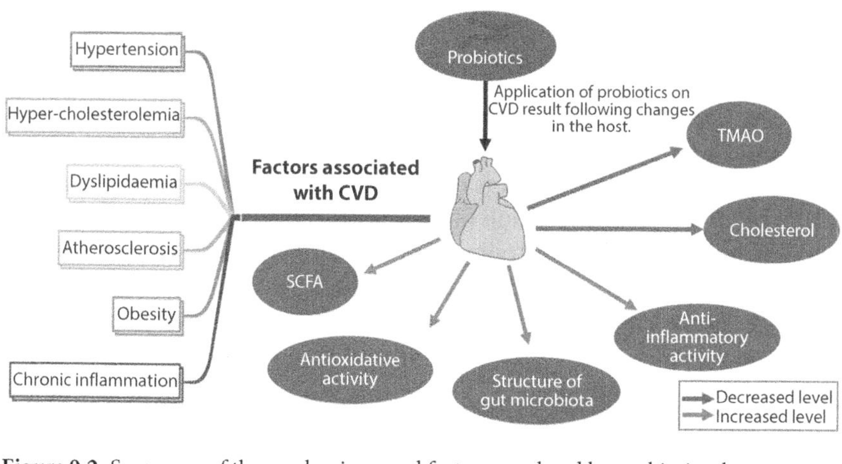

Figure 9.2 Summary of the mechanisms and factors regulated by probiotics that contribute to the treatment of CVD.

Lactobacillus plantarum on hypertensive patients, proved effective in reducing systolic/diastolic BP [51]. *Lactobacillus coryniformis* could significantly reduce endothelial dysfunction leading to hypertension caused by decrease in the bioavailability of nitric oxide (NO) due to lower enzymatic activity of endothelial NO synthase (eNOS) [51].

9.6.4 Role of Probiotics on Acute Liver Injury (ALI)

ALI can be caused by various causes such as drug abuse, biliary tract ligation, high fat and low choline diet, and viral infections. Probiotic *Lactobacillus casei* strain Shirota (LcS) can be actively used to treat ALI [52]. LcS was able to reduce liver and intestinal damage and decrease the Firmicutes to Bacteroidetes ratio; reduced the accumulation of various metabolites, increased d-glucose and l-methionine; and maintained the homeostasis of important metabolic and signalling pathways of the liver and gut [52]. Probiotics could be used to prevent and treat metabolic disorders by targeting the PPARγ-coactivator 1α (PGC-1α)-mediated signaling pathway [53]. The protective effect of the probiotic strain *Lactobacillus plantarum* is by targeting the PGC-1α signaling pathway in multiple organs against obesity, glucose intolerance, and dyslipidemia caused by high-fat diet (HFD). Under HFD feeding conditions, *L. plantarum* increases the expression of sirtuin 1 (SIRT1), PPARα, and PGC-1α in liver and adipose tissue, which improved bile acid synthesis and cholesterol homeostasis in liver, enhanced browning and thermogenesis of adipose tissue, and reduced accumulation of fat, all of which can be associated with enhanced homeostasis of gut microbiota [53].

9.6.5 Engineering Probiotics for Targeted Therapeutics

The next generation of biotherapeutics includes genetically engineered probiotics that target specific diseases. The mechanism by which probiotics work for disease treatment is often unknown, which ultimately hinders the preparation and production of therapeutic products. Therefore, genetic modification of probiotic strains with the ability to target a specific disease and thus have greater efficacy than wild strains, might be a promising strategy. Treatments with genetically modified probiotics may offer several advantages, such as less expensive formulations and significantly lesser negative side effects [54].

For proper functioning of metabolism, enzymes play one of the most important roles. Deficiency or absence of enzymes and dysfunction of enzymatic reactions disrupt metabolism and lead to metabolic disorders, including accumulation of toxins and decreased production of important products. Probiotics can be engineered to synthesize specific enzymes or target specific metabolic pathways to treat metabolic disorders [55].

Isabella *et al.* engineered a synthetic strain SYNB1618 by modifying *E. coli* Nissle 1917 to degrade phenylalanine (Phe) under anoxic conditions through high expression of PAL and L-amino acid deaminase (LAAD) to treat phenylketonuria (PKU) [56]. SYNB1618 was able to lower serum Phe levels in PKU model mouse and Phe treated healthy cynomolgus monkeys. Currently, SYNB1618 is being tested in clinical trials for its effectiveness and safety for human use. For the treatment of hyperammonemia, E. coli Nissle 1917 was engineered, in which the engineered probiotic SYNB1020 could biosynthesise L-arginine from NH_3 thereby reducing hyperammonemia. SYNB1020 decreased blood ammonia levels in mice and showed tolerability in non-human primates and human volunteers [57].

9.7 Conclusion and Future Prospect

The prevalence of metabolic disorders such as obesity, diabetes and CVD are increasing worldwide and reaching pandemic levels, posing a major public health problem and a major cause of death. These metabolic diseases are often caused by obesity, unhealthy high-fat diets, unhealthy lifestyles, hormonal imbalances, genetic disorders, and most importantly, changes in the composition and diversity of the gut microbiota that has a significant role in maintaining the general homeostasis in the host GI track and secrete several host health promoting factors for smooth running of host metabolism. The association between gut microbiota dysbiosis and metabolic disorders has been demonstrated in both animal models and humans, suggesting the administration of probiotics and prebiotics, to maintain the gut microbial homeostasis and present a new approach for the treatment and prevention of obesity and related metabolic disorders.

Evidences have suggested that different strains of bacteria are responsible for regulating and preventing metabolic disorders, although much research is still needed to understand the full mechanisms of action. There is very little data available in this field to draw clear conclusions on the mechanisms of action beyond the superficial knowledge of association of gut microbial homeostasis with treatment of metabolic disorders, which may lead to misinterpretation. The administration of probiotics and prebiotics for the treatment of metabolic diseases is still being intensively researched in order to understand the treatment dose, the duration of treatment and the effects of the different strains on the gut microbiota and the general health of the human host when the tests are conducted from the animal model to the human host. The administration of probiotics and prebiotics to maintain gut microbial homeostasis and improve metabolic disorders such as obesity, type 2 diabetes and cardiovascular diseases associated with gut permeability, metabolic endotoxemia and inflammation is, therefore, a significant future therapeutic approach that requires extensive human research.

Acknowledgment

The authors would like to thank the Department of Microbiology, Sikkim University for providing the computational infrastructure and central library facilities for procuring references.

References

1. Moszak, M., Szulińska, M., Bogdański, P., You are what you eat—The relationship between diet, microbiota, and metabolic disorders—A review. *Nutrients*, 12, 4, 1096, 2020.
2. Everard, A. and Cani, P.D., Diabetes, obesity and gut microbiota. *Best Pract. Res. Clin. Gastroenterol.*, 27, 1, 73–83, 2013.
3. Oniszczuk, A., Oniszczuk, T., Gancarz, M., Szymańska, J., Role of gut microbiota, probiotics and prebiotics in the cardiovascular diseases. *Molecules*, 26, 4, 1172, 2021.
4. Kerry, R.G., Patra, J.K., Gouda, S., Park, Y., Shin, H.S., Das, G., Benefaction of probiotics for human health: A review. *J. Food Drug Anal.*, 26, 3, 927–39, 2018.
5. Schrezenmeir, J. and de Vrese, M., Probiotics, prebiotics, and synbiotics—Approaching a definition. *Am. J. Clin. Nutr.*, 73, 2, 361s–4s, 2001.
6. Yoo, J.Y. and Kim, S.S., Probiotics and prebiotics: present status and future perspectives on metabolic disorders. *Nutrients*, 8, 3, 173, 2016.
7. Cerdó, T., García-Santos JA, G., Bermúdez, M., Campoy, C., The role of probiotics and prebiotics in the prevention and treatment of obesity. *Nutrients*, 11, 3, 635, 2019.
8. Plaza-Diaz, J., Ruiz-Ojeda, F.J., Gil-Campos, M., Gil, A., Mechanisms of action of probiotics. *Adv. Nutr.*, 10, suppl_1, S49–66, 2019.
9. Mazloom, K., Siddiqi, I., Covasa, M., Probiotics: how effective are they in the fight against obesity? *Nutrients*, 11, 2, 258, 2019.
10. He, M. and Shi, B., Gut microbiota as a potential target of metabolic syndrome: the role of probiotics and prebiotics. *Cell Biosci.*, 7, 1, 1–4, 2017.

11. Gibson, G.R., Probert, H.M., Loo, J.V., Rastall, R.A., Roberfroid, M., Dietary modulation of the humancolonic microbiota: Updating the concept of prebiotics. *Nutr. Res. Rev.*, 17, 2, 259–275, 2004.
12. Roberfroid, M., Gibson, G.R., Hoyles, L., McCartney, A.L., Rastall, R., Rowland, I., Wolvers, D., Watzl, B., Szajewska, H., Stahl, B., Guarner, F., Prebiotic effects: metabolic and health benefits. *Br. J. Nutr.*, 104, S2, S1–63, 2010.
13. Bäckhed, F., Ley, R.E., Sonnenburg, J.L., Peterson, D.A., Gordon, J.I., Host-bacterial mutualism in the human intestine. *Science*, 307, 5717, 1915–20, 2005.
14. Hur, K.Y. and Lee, M.S., Gut microbiota and metabolic disorders. *Diabetes Metab. J.*, 39, 3, 198–203, 2015.
15. Fan, Y. and Pedersen, O., Gut microbiota in human metabolic health and disease. *Nat. Rev. Microbiol.*, 19, 1, 55–71, 2021.
16. Kobyliak, N., Conte, C., Cammarota, G., Haley, A.P., Styriak, I., Gaspar, L., Fusek, J., Rodrigo, L., Kruzliak, P., Probiotics in prevention and treatment of obesity: a critical view. *Nutr. Metab. (Lond)*, 13, 1, 1–3, 2016.
17. Gérard, P., Gut microbiota and obesity. *Cell. Mol. Life Sci.*, 73, 1, 147–62, 2016.
18. Sharma, S. and Tripathi, P., Gut microbiome and type 2 diabetes: Where we are and where to go? *J. Nutr. Biochem.*, 63, 101–8, 2019.
19. Gérard, C. and Vidal, H., Impact of gut microbiota on host glycemic control. *Front. Endocrinol. (Lausanne)*, 10, 29, 2019.
20. Cunningham, A.L., Stephens, J.W., Harris, D.A., Gut microbiota influence in type 2 diabetes mellitus (T2DM). *Gut Pathog.*, 13, 1–3, 2021.
21. Golay, A. and Ybarra, J., Link between obesity and type 2 diabetes. *Best Pract. Res. Clin. Endocrinol. Metab.*, 19, 4, 649–63, 2005.
22. Le Bourgot, C., Apper, E., Blat, S., Respondek, F., Fructo-oligosaccharides and glucose homeostasis: A systematic review and meta-analysis in animal models. *Nutr. Metab. (Lond)*, 15, 1, 1–5, 2018.
23. Lo, R.S., Austin, A.S., Freeman, J.G., Is there a role for probiotics in liver disease? *Sci. World J.*, 874768 , 2014, 1–7, 2014.
24. Gu, Z., Liu, Y., Hu, S., You, Y., Wen, J., Li, W., Wang, Y., Probiotics for alleviating alcoholic liver injury. *Gastroenterol. Res. Pract.*, 2019, 1–8, 2019.
25. Bastian, W.P., Hasan, I., Lesmana, C.R., Rinaldi, I., Gani, R.A., Gut Microbiota Profiles in Nonalcoholic Fatty Liver Disease and Its Possible Impact on Disease Progression Evaluated with Transient Elastography: Lesson Learnt from 60 Cases. *Case Rep. Gastroenterol.*, 13, 1, 125–33, 2019.
26. Tokuhara, D., Role of the Gut Microbiota in Regulating Non-alcoholic Fatty Liver Disease in Children and Adolescents. *Front. Nutr.*, 8, 700058, 379, 2021.
27. Novakovic, M., Rout, A., Kingsley, T., Kirchoff, R., Singh, A., Verma, V., Kant, R., Chaudhary, R., Role of gut microbiota in cardiovascular diseases. *World J. Cardiol.*, 12, 4, 110, 2020.

28. Kazemian, N., Mahmoudi, M., Halperin, F., Wu, J.C., Pakpour, S., Gut microbiota and cardiovascular disease: Opportunities and challenges. *Microbiome*, 8, 1, 1–7, 2020.
29. Costa, G.T., Abreu, G.C., Guimarães, A.B., Vasconcelos, P.R., Guimarães, S.B., Fructo-oligosaccharide effects on serum cholesterol levels. An overview1. *Acta Cir. Bras.*, 30, 366–70, 2015.
30. de Cossío, L.F., Fourrier, C., Sauvant, J., Everard, A., Capuron, L., Cani, P.D., Layé, S., Castanon, N., Impact of prebiotics on metabolic and behavioral alterations in a mouse model of metabolic syndrome. *Brain. Behav. Immun.*, 64, 33–49, 2017.
31. Guarino, M.P., Altomare, A., Emerenziani, S., Di Rosa, C., Ribolsi, M., Balestrieri, P., Iovino, P., Rocchi, G., Cicala, M., Mechanisms of action of prebiotics and their effects on gastro-intestinal disorders in adults. *Nutrients*, 12, 4, 1037, 2020.
32. Puddu, A., Sanguineti, R., Montecucco, F., Viviani, G.L., Evidence for the gut microbiota short-chain fatty acids as key pathophysiological molecules improving diabetes. *Mediators Inflamm.*, 162021, 2014, 1–9, 2014.
33. Sabater-Molina, M., Larqué, E., Torrella, F., Zamora, S., Dietary fructooligosaccharides and potential benefits on health. *J. Physiol. Biochem.*, 65, 3, 315–28, 2009.
34. Shehata, M.G., El-Sahn, M.A., El Sohaimy, S.A., Youssef, M.M., Role and Mechanisms Lowering Cholesterol by Dietary of Probiotics and Prebiotics: A Review. *J. Appl. Sci.*, 19, 8, 737–46, 2019.
35. Parnell, J.A., Raman, M., Rioux, K.P., Reimer, R.A., The potential role of prebiotic fibre for treatment and management of non-alcoholic fatty liver disease and associated obesity and insulin resistance. *Liver Int.*, 32, 5, 701–11, 2012.
36. Pandey, K.R., Naik, S.R., Vakil, B.V., Probiotics, prebiotics and synbiotics-A review. *J. Food Sci. Technol.*, 52, 12, 7577–87, 2015.
37. Kearney, S.M. and Gibbons, S.M., Designing synbiotics for improved human health. *Microb. Biotechnol.*, 11, 1, 141, 2018.
38. Krumbeck, J.A., Walter, J., Hutkins, R.W., Synbiotics for improved human health: Recent developments, challenges, and opportunities. *Annu. Rev. Food Sci. Technol.*, 9, 451–79, 2018.
39. Eslamparast, T., Zamani, F., Hekmatdoost, A., Sharafkhah, M., Eghtesad, S., Malekzadeh, R., Hekmatdoost, A., Effects of synbiotic supplementation on insulin resistance in subjects with the metabolic syndrome: A randomised, double-blind, placebo-controlled pilot study. *Br. J. Nutr.*, 112, 3, 438–45, 2014.
40. Le Barz, M., Anhê, F.F., Varin, T.V., Desjardins, Y., Levy, E., Roy, D., Urdaci, M.C., Marette, A., Probiotics as complementary treatment for metabolic disorders. *Diabetes Metab. J.*, 39, 4, 291–303, 2015.
41. Liang, T., Wu, L., Xi, Y., Li, Y., Xie, X., Fan, C., Yang, L., Yang, S., Chen, X., Zhang, J., Wu, Q., Probiotics supplementation improves hyperglycemia,

hypercholesterolemia, and hypertension in type 2 diabetes mellitus: An update of meta-analysis. *Crit. Rev. Food Sci. Nutr.*, 61, 10, 1670–88, 2021.
42. Bock, P.M., Telo, G.H., Ramalho, R., Sbaraini, M., Leivas, G., Martins, A.F., Schaan, B.D., The effect of probiotics, prebiotics or synbiotics on metabolic outcomes in individuals with diabetes: A systematic review and meta-analysis. *Diabetologia*, 64, 1, 26–41, 2021.
43. Mishra, S., Wang, S., Nagpal, R., Miller, B., Singh, R., Taraphder, S., Yadav, H., Probiotics and prebiotics for the amelioration of type 1 diabetes: Present and future perspectives. *Microorganisms*, 7, 3, 67, 2019.
44. Mondanelli, G., Orecchini, E., Volpi, C., Panfili, E., Belladonna, M.L., Pallotta, M.T., Moretti, S., Galarini, R., Esposito, S., Orabona, C., Effect of probiotic administration on serum tryptophan metabolites in pediatric type 1 diabetes patients. *Int. J. Tryptophan Res.*, 13, 1–8, 2020.
45. Kim, T.K., Lee, J.C., Im, S.H., Lee, M.S., Amelioration of Autoimmune Diabetes of NOD Mice by Immunomodulating Probiotics. *Front. Immunol.*, 11, 1832, 2020.
46. He, J., Zhang, F., Han, Y., Effect of probiotics on lipid profiles and blood pressure in patients with type 2 diabetes: A meta-analysis of RCTs. *Med. (Baltimore)*, 96, 51, e9166, 2017.
47. Galicia-Garcia, U., Benito-Vicente, A., Jebari, S., Larrea-Sebal, A., Siddiqi, H., Uribe, K.B., Ostolaza, H., Martín, C., Pathophysiology of type 2 diabetes mellitus. *Int. J. Mol. Sci.*, 21, 17, 6275, 2020.
48. Kobyliak, N., Falalyeyeva, T., Mykhalchyshyn, G., Kyriienko, D., Komissarenko, I., Effect of alive probiotic on insulin resistance in type 2 diabetes patients: randomized clinical trial. *Diabetes Metab. Syndr. Clin. Res. Rev.*, 12, 5, 617–24, 2018.
49. Sun, Z., Sun, X., Li, J., Li, Z., Hu, Q., Li, L., Hao, X., Song, M., Li, C., Using probiotics for type 2 diabetes mellitus intervention: Advances, questions, and potential. *Crit. Rev. Food Sci. Nutr.*, 60, 4, 670–83, 2020.
50. O'Morain, V.L. and Ramji, D.P., The potential of probiotics in the prevention and treatment of atherosclerosis. *Mol. Nutr. Food Res.*, 64, 4, 1900797, 2020.
51. Vasquez, E.C., Pereira, T.M.C., Peotta, V.A., Baldo, M.P., Campos-Toimil, M., Probiotics as beneficial dietary supplements to prevent and treat cardiovascular diseases: Uncovering their impact on oxidative stress. *Oxid. Med. Cell. Longev.*, 2019, 3086270, 1–11, 2019.
52. Yan, R., Wang, K., Wang, Q., Jiang, H., Lu, Y., Chen, X., Zhang, H., Su, X., Du, Y., Chen, L., Li, L., Probiotic Lactobacillus casei Shirota prevents acute liver injury by reshaping the gut microbiota to alleviate excessive inflammation and metabolic disorders. *Microb. Biotechnol.*, 15, 247–261, 2021.
53. Kwon, J., Kim, B., Lee, C., Joung, H., Kim, B.K., Choi, I.S., Hyun, C.K., Comprehensive amelioration of high-fat diet-induced metabolic dysfunctions through activation of the PGC-1α pathway by probiotics treatment in mice. *PLoS One*, 15, 2, e0228932, 2020.

54. Aggarwal, N., Breedon, A.M., Davis, C.M., Hwang, I.Y., Chang, M.W., Engineering probiotics for therapeutic applications: Recent examples and translational outlook. *Curr. Opin. Biotechnol.*, 65, 171–9, 2020.
55. Zhou, Z., Chen, X., Sheng, H., Shen, X., Sun, X., Yan, Y., Wang, J., Yuan, Q., Engineering probiotics as living diagnostics and therapeutics for improving human health. *Microb. Cell Fact.*, 19, 1, 1–2, 2020.
56. Isabella, V.M., Ha, B.N., Castillo, M.J., Lubkowicz, D.J., Rowe, S.E., Millet, Y.A., Anderson, C.L., Li, N., Fisher, A.B., West, K.A., Reeder, P.J., Development of a synthetic live bacterial therapeutic for the human metabolic disease phenylketonuria. *Nat. Biotechnol.*, 36, 9, 857–64, 2018.
57. Kurtz, C.B., Millet, Y.A., Puurunen, M.K., Perreault, M., Charbonneau, M.R., Isabella, V.M., Kotula, J.W., Antipov, E., Dagon, Y., Denney, W.S., Wagner, D.A., An engineered E. coli Nissle improves hyperammonemia and survival in mice and shows dose-dependent exposure in healthy humans. *Sci. Transl. Med.*, 11, 475, eaau7975, 2019.
58. Asemi, Z., Khorrami-Rad, A., Alizadeh, S.A., Shakeri, H., Esmaillzadeh, A., Effects of synbiotic food consumption on metabolic status of diabetic patients: A double-blind randomized cross-over controlled clinical trial. *Clin. Nutr.*, 33, 2, 198–203, 2014.
59. sadat Ebrahimi, Z., Nasli-Esfahani, E., Nadjarzade, A., Mozaffari-Khosravi, H., Effect of symbiotic supplementation on glycemic control, lipid profiles and microalbuminuria in patients with non-obese type 2 diabetes: A randomized, double-blind, clinical trial. *J. Diabetes Metab. Disord.*, 16, 1, 1, 2017.
60. Moroti, C., Magri, L.F., de Rezende Costa, M., Cavallini, D.C., Sivieri, K., Effect of the consumption of a new symbiotic shake on glycemia and cholesterol levels in elderly people with type 2 diabetes mellitus. *Lipids Health Dis.*, 11, 1, 1–8, 2012.
61. Liong, M.T., Dunshea, F.R., Shah, N.P., Effects of a synbiotic containing Lactobacillus acidophilus ATCC 4962 on plasma lipid profiles and morphology of erythrocytes in hypercholesterolaemic pigs on high- and low-fat diets. *Br. J. Nutr.*, 98, 4, 736–44, 2007.
62. Malaguarnera, M., Greco, F., Barone, G., Gargante, M.P., Malaguarnera, M., Toscano, M.A., Bifidobacterium longum with fructo-oligosaccharide (FOS) treatment in minimal hepatic encephalopathy: A randomized, double-blind, placebo-controlled study. *Dig. Dis. Sci.*, 52, 11, 3259, 2007.
63. Eslamparast, T., Poustchi, H., Zamani, F., Sharafkhah, M., Malekzadeh, R., Hekmatdoost, A., Synbiotic supplementation in nonalcoholic fatty liver disease: A randomized, double-blind, placebo-controlled pilot study. *Am. J. Clin. Nutr.*, 99, 3, 535–42, 2014.
64. Le Barz, M., Daniel, N., Varin, T.V., Naimi, S., Demers-Mathieu, V., Pilon, G., Audy, J., Laurin, É, Roy, D., Urdaci, M.C., St-Gelais, D., *In vivo* screening of multiple bacterial strains identifies Lactobacillus rhamnosus Lb102 and Bifidobacterium animalis ssp. lactis Bf141 as probiotics that improve

metabolic disorders in a mouse model of obesity. *FASEB J.*, 33, 4, 4921–35, 2019.

65. Li, H., Liu, F., Lu, J., Shi, J., Guan, J., Yan, F., Li, B., Huo, G., Probiotic mixture of Lactobacillus plantarum strains improves lipid metabolism and gut microbiota structure in high fat diet-fed mice. *Front. Microbiol.*, 11, 512, 2020.
66. Dang, F., Jiang, Y., Pan, R., Zhou, Y., Wu, S., Wang, R., Zhuang, K., Zhang, W., Li, T., Man, C., Administration of Lactobacillus paracasei ameliorates type 2 diabetes in mice. *Food Funct.*, 9, 7, 3630–9, 2018.
67. Yang, F., Wang, J., Zhang, H., Xie, Y., Jin, J., Liu, H., Pang, X., Hao, H., Hypoglycemic effects of space-induced Lactobacillus plantarum SS18-5 on type 2 diabetes in a rat model. *J. Food Biochem.*, 45, 9, e13899, 2021.
68. Mizoguchi, T., Kasahara, K., Yamashita, T., Sasaki, N., Yodoi, K., Matsumoto, T., Emoto, T., Hayashi, T., Kitano, N., Yoshida, N., Amin, H.Z., Oral administration of the lactic acid bacterium Pediococcus acidilactici attenuates atherosclerosis in mice by inducing tolerogenic dendritic cells. *Heart Vessels*, 32, 6, 768–76, 2017.
69. Hassan, A., Din, A.U., Zhu, Y., Zhang, K., Li, T., Wang, Y., Xu, S., Lei, H., Yu, X., Wang, G., Anti-atherosclerotic effects of Lactobacillus plantarum ATCC 14917 in ApoE-/- mice through modulation of proinflammatory cytokines and oxidative stress. *Appl. Microbiol. Biotechnol.*, 104, 6337–50, 2020.
70. Jiang, T., Wu, H., Yang, X., Li, Y., Zhang, Z., Chen, F., Zhao, L., Zhang, C., Lactobacillus mucosae strain promoted by a high-fiber diet in genetic obese child alleviates lipid metabolism and modifies gut microbiota in ApoE-/- mice on a western diet. *Microorganisms*, 8, 8, 1225, 2020.

10

Developing Formulations of Prebiotics and Probiotics

Eknath D. Ahire[1*], Nisha Sharma[2], Prakash Chandra Gupta[2], Shubham Khairnar[1], Khemchand Surana[3], Bhavana Ahire[4], Vijayraj Sonawane[3], Umesh Laddha[1], Sneh Sonkamble[5], Rahul Sabale[1] and Sanjay Kshirsagar[1]

[1]*Department of Pharmacology, MET's, Institute of Pharmacy, BKC, Affiliated to Savitribai Phule Pune University, Adgaon, Nashik, India*
[2]*School of Pharmaceutical Sciences, Chhatrapati Sahu Ji Maharaj University, Kanpur, India*
[3]*Department of Pharmaceutical Chemistry, Shreeshakti Shaikshanik Sanstha, Divine College of Pharmacy, Satana, Nashik, India*
[4]*Department of Quality Assurance Techniques, NDMVP's, College of Pharmacy, Nashik, India*
[5]*Department of Pharmaceutical Chemistry, MET's, Institute of Pharmacy, BKC, Affiliated to Savitribai Phule Pune University, Adgaon, Nashik, India*

Abstract
Prebiotics and probiotics are currently commonly employed in yoghurts and fermented milks, which are the leading functional food products globally, due to their health benefits. The global functional food market was expected to be worth more than US$33 billion in 2003, with the European business at more than US$2 billion. Finding low-cost prebiotic raw ingredients, generating low-cost probiotics, and preserving probiotic viability after storage or during the manufacturing process of the functional food are key difficulties that industrial-scale probiotic and prebiotic production faces. In this overview, functional foods based on probiotics and prebiotics are introduced as a key biotechnological issue with plenty of space for innovation. The current state of the art is presented in a straight forward manner, addressing the foundations and challenges of generating new probiotic and prebiotic-based foods, as well as niches for future research that have been identified and investigated.

**Correponding author*: eknathahire05@gmail.com

Rajesh K. Kesharwani, Tingirikari Jagan Mohan Rao and Raj K. Keservani (eds.) Prebiotics and Probiotics in Disease Regulation and Management, (271–290) © 2022 Scrivener Publishing LLC

Keywords: Functional food, probiotics, prebiotics, synbiotics

10.1 Introduction

The important link between diet and health is now widely acknowledged. Although the basic function of food is to provide nutrients to meet metabolic needs, the use of food to improve health and well-being has become a more widely acknowledged concept in society during the course of the last three decades [1–3]. The concept of functional foods emerged as a result of a shift in how people think about food. A food is functional if, in addition to having enough nutritional content, it has a beneficial impact on one or more target functions in the body in a way that is necessary for general well-being and health or disease risk reduction [4]. In the late 1980s, Japan coined the term "functional foods" as a marketing slogan. In contrast, the global market has grown dramatically, with an estimated value of over US$33 billion in 2003, while the European market was valued at more than US$2 billion in the same year [5]. Functional meals rely on bioactive components, which are often found naturally in the product but often require the addition of a specific ingredient to maximize their therapeutic effects [1]. Probiotics, prebiotics, vitamins, and minerals are now common functional food components in fermented milk and yoghurts, sports drinks, infant meals, sugar-free sweets, and chewing gum [6, 7]. Prebiotics and Probiotics are key components of fermented milks and yoghurts, which make for the lion's share of the overall functional food market. As a result, the vast majority of research on functional foods has been on probiotics and prebiotics [5, 6, 8, 9]. This article gives a state-of-the-art assessment of probiotics and prebiotics, from the fundamentals to the concept of symbiosis and impediments to the development of new probiotic- and prebiotic-based foods. Finally, the important research niches in the topic are identified and investigated.

10.2 Probiotics

In the literature, probiotics are characterized in a variety of ways. As a result, probiotics were defined a decade ago as live microorganisms that improve the gut microbial balance of the host and so promote the host's health [10]. Fric [11] provides a more contemporary and complete definition: "Probiotics are non-pathogenic bacteria, primarily of human origin, that provide a health benefit to the host and enable the avoidance or amelioration of a range of diseases when given in sufficient proportions." The concept of probiotic microorganisms dates back to a century ago, when Nobel Laureate Ilya Metchnikoff observed that Bulgarian peasants lived long and healthy lives by consuming fermented milk products [2]. Metchnikoff proposed that the fermenting bacilli had a good effect on the gut microbiota when taken, because these microorganisms were theoretically able to establish themselves in the intestinal tract, reducing the pathogenic bacterial population [12]. However, subsequent research indicated that the microorganisms involved in milk fermentation are unable to establish themselves in the stomach [13, 14]. As a result, Metchnikoff's original hypothesis about how milk-fermenting microorganisms deliver health advantages to the host was fundamentally incorrect. Lactobacilli, bifidobacteria, and a range of nonpathogenic kinds of probiotics are among the most widely utilized today.

Lactobacillus rhamnosus GG, *Saccharomyces cerevisiae* Boulardii, *Lactobacillus casei* Shirota, and Bifidobacterium animalis are among the most extensively researched probiotics with demonstrated human health benefits [2, 7, 11, 15]. Table 10.1 provides a quick synopsis of significant probiotics documented in the literature and their impact on health. The majority of probiotics come from the Lactobacillus and Bifidobacterium families, with *S. cerevisiae* Boulardii being the only yeast with established probiotic properties. According to Saier and Mansour, probiotics have three methods for boosting human health [16, 17]. Supplying absorbed end-products of anaerobic fermentation of carbohydrates, such as organic acids, that can affect human mood, energy level, and even cognitive capacities; (ii) successfully battling with pathogens; and (iii) triggering host immune responses by generating particular polysaccharides. It's important to note that the health benefits of probiotics are strain-specific, not species- or genus-specific. As a result, no single probiotic strain, even from the same species, will provide all of the claimed benefits. In the same way, not all strains of the same species are equally successful in combating the same health problems [18, 19]. Nonetheless, one of the most prevalent benefits of the probiotics listed in Table 10.1 is the management of diarrhea, which is linked to pathogen competitive exclusion [2]. As a result, the ability of a microorganism to survive and colonise the gut via the upper gastrointestinal tract is a key factor in determining whether or not it should be classified as a probiotic [20, 21].

Table 10.1 Key probiotic micro-organisms reported in the literature.

Microorganism		Effect on human health
Lactic acid bacteria	*Lactobacillus rhamnosus* GG	Reduces the permeability deficiencies in the intestine induced by cow's milk or rotavirus infection. Rotavirus infection, which causes diarrhea, traveller's diarrhea, and antibiotic-associated diarrhea, may be shortened.
	Lactobacillus casei	Diarrhea is less severe and lasts less time. Stimulates the gut immune system, relieves Crohn's disease symptoms, and has powerful antibacterial capabilities.
	Lactobacillus casei Shirota	Virus or bacteria-caused diarrhea is prevented. In terms of lactose malabsorption, rotaviral diarrhea, antibiotic-associated diarrhea, and *Clostridium difficile* diarrhea, it has the best human health efficacy. Has a protective effect against the return of superficial bladder cancer following surgery.
	Lactobacillus acidophilus	Lactic acid is produced, which lowers the pH of the intestinal contents and helps to avoid invasive infections like *Salmonella* and *E. coli* strains. Antibody responses and seroconversion rates are also on the rise. Cholesterol levels in the blood are reduced.
	Lactobacillus johnsonii	Reduces the density of *Helicobacter pylori*, as well as inflammation and gastritis activity.
	Lactobacillus plantarum	Produces short-chain fatty acids, which reduce enzyme activity and so limit the formation of carcinogenic compounds.

(*Continued*)

Table 10.1 Key probiotic micro-organisms reported in the literature. (*Continued*)

Microorganism		Effect on human health
Bifidobacteria	*Bifidobacterium breve*	Activates the humoral immune system by increasing the generation of anti-rotavirus IgA or anti-influenza virus antibodies.
	Bifidobacterium bifidum	Pathogenic or putrefactive bacteria may be able to outcompete them for space and nutrition. The incidence of diarrhea is lower, but antibody responses and seroconversion rates are higher.
	Bifidobacterium infantis	Diarrhea and constipation are avoided.
	Bifidobacterium animalis	Normalizes the motility of the intestines in constipated people. In children and adults, it lowers the risk of acute diarrhea.
	Saccharomyces cerevisiae Boulardii	Prevents diarrhea and the development of pathogenic colitis and enterocolitis in travellers. Diarrhea caused by antibiotics is less likely to develop and lasts longer.

10.3 Prebiotics

The concept of prebiotics has also evolved significantly over time. A prebiotic is a nondigestible food component that promotes the growth and/or activity of one or a small number of bacteria in the colon, hence improving the host's health [22]. According to current research, a prebiotic is a selectively fermented meal that allows specific changes in the composition and/or activity of the gut microbiota that are beneficial to the host's welfare and health [23]. The important principle in each of these definitions is that prebiotics have a selective effect on the microbiota, resulting in better host health [24]. To be termed a prebiotic, a component must meet three criteria: (i) digesting resistance; (ii) fermentation by the large intestine bacteria; and (iii) a health-promoting influence on the microbiota [25].

Table 10.2 Main candidates for prebiotic status reported in the literature.

Carbohydrate	Chemical structure	Method of manufacture	Degree of polymerization
Inulin	β (2-1)-Fructans	Extraction from chicory root and *Agave tequilana*	2–65
Fructo-oligosaccharides	β (2-1)-Fructans	Transfructosylation from sucrose or hydrolysis of chicory inulin	2–10
Galacto-oligosaccharides	Galactose oligomers and some glucose/lactose/galactose units	Produced from lactose by β-galactosidase	2–5
Soya-oligosaccharides	Mixture of raffinose and stachyose	Extracted from soya bean whey	3–4
Xylo-oligosaccharides	β (1–4)-Linked xylose	Enzymatic hydrolysis of xylan. Enzyme treatments of native lignocellulosic materials. Hydrolytic degradation of xylan by steam, water or dilute solutions of mineral acids	2–4
Isomalto-oligosaccharides	α (1–4)-Glucose and branched α (1–6)-glucose	Maltose transgalactosylation by bacteria or enzymes. Sucrose production by enzymes	2–8
Pyrodextrins	Mixture of glucose-containing oligosaccharides	Pyrolysis of potato or maize starch	Various

Prebiotics must, therefore, enter the large bowel with virtually identical chemical and structural features in order to further selectively promote the microbiota. Prebiotics are short-chain carbohydrates with a polymerization degree of two or more that pancreatic and brush border enzymes cannot digest [24]. Table 10.2 lists the most important contenders for prebiotic status. Extraction from plant sources, microbial/enzymatic synthesis, and enzymatic breakdown of polysaccharides can all be used to make prebiotic oligosaccharides. Prebiotics of various types are widely accessible on the market and are made on a huge scale [26]. Prebiotics, in fact, has been reported to be inexpensive to manufacture [27]. Prebiotics are made from relatively low-cost raw materials, which may have influenced this view [28]. However, because most prebiotics are produced by enzymatic processes, synthesis and subsequent purification are not always inexpensive. In fact, various studies on new aqueous/organic mediums for enzymatic synthesis have been conducted in attempt to boost prebiotic yields [29, 30]. Palframan *et al.* [39] suggested adding a prebiotic index (PI) to an equation to provide a quantitative tool for comparing prebiotics' effect on probiotic bacteria proliferation. According to the following calculation, the PI score is based on the preferential stimulation of probiotic bacteria

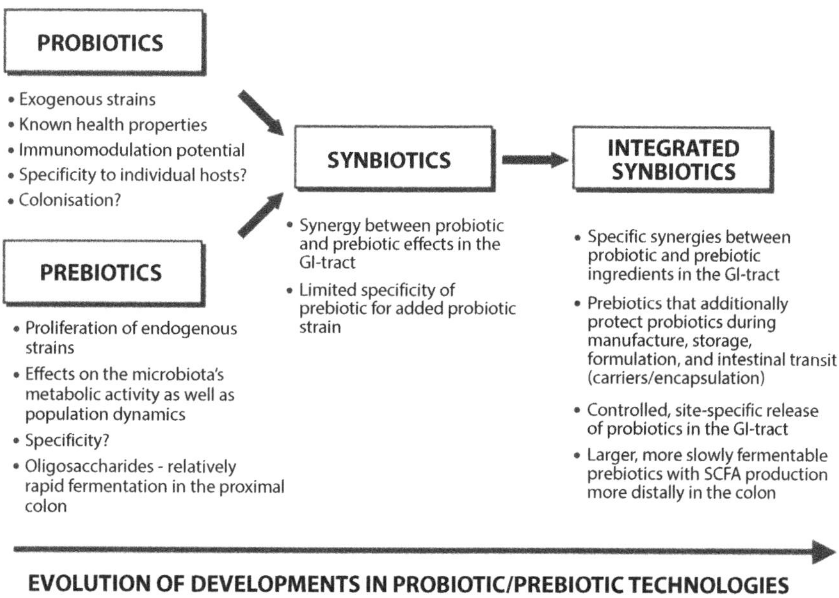

Figure 10.1 Steps involved in developments of prebiotics and probiotics.

(bifidobacteria and lactobacilli) over other microorganisms (Bacteroides and clostridia) due to the administration of a prebiotic [31, 33]. Figure 10.1 shows the various steps involved in the developments of prebiotics and probiotics.

10.4 Synbiotics

It is now common to find probiotic foods that also include prebiotics (for example, yoghurts and fermented milks). A "synbiotic" mixture is one in which the prebiotic concentration is less than 10 g kg1 [19, 35, 36]. Synbiotics have long been seen as a promising area for the development of innovative functional foods. The potential for probiotics and prebiotics to interact has been described as "clear" [37, 38, 40]. Synbiotics are a combination of probiotics and prebiotics that help the host survive and implant living microbial dietary supplements in the gastrointestinal tract [41]. *In vitro* gastrointestinal tract simulations are commonly used as an experimental platform for studying synbiotics (Table 10.3). One of the most important advantages of synbiotics is that probiotics last longer in the gastrointestinal tract [42]. As a result, the presented in vitro studies are primarily concerned with elucidating.

(i) Whether probiotics can metabolize the prebiotic component in simulated gastrointestinal settings, (ii) if pathogenic bacteria can metabolize the prebiotic component, and (iii) if the synbiotic can limit or reduce pathogenic bacteria development compared with a control without synbiotic. Despite the useful information gathered from *in vitro* experiments,

Table 10.3 Content of total dietary fiber in a variety of cereal grains.

Cereal	Total dietary fiber (g kg−1 dry matter)	Reference
Wheat	121	[55]
Rye	161	[55]
Barley	100	[52]
Sorghum	107	[52]
Rice	192	[55]
Corn	150	[52]
Oat	140	[52]

experts working on this type of study understand that more *in vivo* trials are required to confirm the efficacy of synbiotics [40]. In this connection, de Vrese and Schrezenmeir [19] pointed out that synbiotics may boost microbial survival and implantation only if the prebiotic and probiotic components are mutually reinforcing and really synergistic It is presently unknown if synbiotics will result in greater amounts of probiotic bacteria due to the prebiotic component [42]. In Wistar rats, for example, a symbiosis based on *Bifidobacterium longum* and oligo fructose increased faeces bifidobacteria proliferation by 1.4 log (CFU g1), whereas simply oligo fructose increased faecal bifidobacteria proliferation by 1.6 log (CFU g1) [43]. Morelli *et al.* [44] *Lactobacillus gasseri* (strain B21090), inulin, and unidentified oligosaccharides were used to study the proliferation of probiotic bacteria. Although the synbiotic was demonstrated to be successful in raising the population of faecal probiotic bacteria in human volunteers, the stimulation of probiotic bacteria by synbiotic treatment was not comparable to that obtained with the prebiotic alone. As a result, a comparison of the synbiotic's potential improved effectiveness over the prebiotic on its own is impossible. As a result, future *in vivo* research comparing the performance of synbiotics with their components should provide solid evidence for their true potential.

10.5 Challenges for New Probiotic and Prebiotic-Based Foods

Because of their purported health benefits, probiotics and prebiotics are becoming more widely employed in yoghurts and fermented milks [5, 6, 50]. Prebiotic synthesis using novel procedures and cost-effective supplies, (ii) low-cost probiotic production, and (iii) increasing probiotic vitality after storage Industrial-scale production of prebiotics and probiotics faces challenges during the functional meal manufacturing process as well as stomach transit. These significant issues will be covered further down [55].

Enzymatic treatment of low-cost source materials, such as sucrose, lactose, and plant derivatives, produces the majority of prebiotic oligosaccharides (Table 10.2). The majority of prebiotic oligosaccharides are produced by enzyme treatment of low-cost source materials, including sucrose, lactose, and plant derivatives [32]. Nonetheless, the present methods for obtaining oligosaccharides have very poor yields, increasing the expense of production [29, 51]. According to Panesar *et al.*, reducing the water concentration in the reaction medium can increase oligosaccharide yield [34].

In this context, Del Val and Otero [29] looked into the enzymatic synthesis of galacto-oligosaccharides from lactose in an aqueous/polyethylene glycol medium. They discovered that lowering the water content boosted both overall galacto-oligosaccharide yield and selective synthesis of 6-galactosyl lactose. Cruz-Guerrero *et al.* [30] used a hyper thermophilic -glycosidase to study the synthesis of galacto-oligosaccharides from lactose in an aqueous/acetone medium. They discovered that water activity influenced oligosaccharide yields significantly, with the maximum yield obtained at 0.57 and an initial lactose content of 8 g L1.as a result, enzymatic prebiotic biosynthesis in organic media is a promising study area for increasing prebiotic yields over standard aqueous media synthesis. When the synthesis medium comprises mostly of an organic solvent, the reviewed literature already concentrates on such research to create appropriate aqueous/organic volume ratios or aw/substrate concentration ratios. Non-dairy oligosaccharide manufacturing is another promising alternative for low-cost

Table 10.4 Some examples of probiotic microencapsulation coating materials.

Coating material	Probiotic	Reference
Alginate/starch with a high resistance	*Lactobacillus acidophilus* and *Bifidobacterium* spp.	[71]
Whey protein	Lactobacillus rhamnosus	[71]
Whey protein	Bifidobacterium longum	[70]
Cellulose acetate phthalate	Bifidobacterium pseudolongum	[70]
Alginate/sodium lauryl sulfate	*Lactobacillus delbrueckii*	[70]
Carrageenan/locust bean gum	Lactobacillus casei	[70]
Alginate	Lactobacillus acidophilus	[70]
Canola vegetable oil/caseinate/fructo-oligosaccharides/starch with a high resistance (or glucose syrup)	*Bifidobacterium infantis*	[72]
Alginate/gellan gum/fructo-oligosaccharides/peptides	*Bifidobacterium bifidum*	[48]

prebiotic manufacture on a large scale. Cereals have been studied in recent years to see if they may be used as prebiotic sources. According to Charal ampopoulos *et al.* [52], cereal grains contain at least two forms of naturally occurring oligosaccharides: galactosyl sucrose derivatives, stachyose, and raffinose, and fructosyl sucrose derivatives. Cereal grains, on the other hand, are high in dietary fiber, which is made up of a variety of complex polysaccharides that are not fully digested and metabolized in the small ilum and pass through to the colon. As a result, dietary fiber is a possible source of prebiotics in cereals [53]. Dietary fiber content in cereals like rice, rye, and corn can range from 150 to 190 g kg1 dry matter (Table 10.4). Dietary fiber is mostly made up of -glucans, xylans, xylo-oligosaccharides, and arabinoxylans. According to Crittenden *et al.*, xylo-oligosaccharides allowed many Bifidobacterium species and *Lactobacillus brevis* to grow at high yields [53].

They also discovered that *B. longum* strains could thrive with only arabinoxylan as a carbon source. Furthermore, -glucan hydrolysates have been shown to boost the growth of many Bifidobacterium strains as well as L. rhamnosus GG [52]. Moura *et al.* [54] used autohydrolysis techniques to selectively generate oligosaccharides with degrees of polymerization of 3–4 and 5–6 utilizing corn cobs as the raw substrate. Furthermore, the acquired oligosaccharides encouraged Bifidobacterium or Lactobacillus species growth to the same amount as commercial xylo-oligosaccharides. Corn, wheat, rice, and oats, for example, all have a high starch content (785, 650, 820, and 636 g/kg dry matter, respectively) [56]. Starch with a high resistance is found naturally in cereal grains; however, it is often removed during modern food preparation. Some of the industrial procedures for creating starch with a high resistance include partial acid hydrolysis, hydrothermal treatment, heating, retrogradation, extrusion cooking, chemical modification, and repolymerization [52]. Studies in animals and human volunteers have demonstrated that a portion of total starch is not digested in the small intestine and goes through to the colon, similar to the case with dietary fiber. Starch with a high resistance is the name given to this fraction, which has been described as a prebiotic [57]. Many Bifidobacterium strains, including *B. adolescentis*, *B. bifidum*, *B. breve*, *B. infantis*, *B. lactis*, and *B. longum*, were able to hydrolyze starch with a high resistance, according to Crittenden *et al.* [40] Only *B. lactis* (strain Lafti B94) was able to survive in conditions similar to those encountered after passing through the gastrointestinal tract. Finally, a synbiotic yoghurt including starch with a high resistance, and *B. lactis* was demonstrated [57]. Because much of the experimental work has been done in animals, and the existing human studies have been brief, evidence supporting starch with a high resistance as a prebiotic is currently limited. However, the scientists agreed that starch with a high resistance has a lot of potential as a prebiotic in humans and that more research is needed.

10.6 Production of Probiotics at a Low Cost

To meet the market's growing demand for probiotics, low-cost production of concentrated cultures of probiotics is a major problem [58]. Because most vitamins and amino acids are not biosynthetically synthesized by probiotic microbes, both amino acids and vitamins must be added to the culture medium for probiotic synthesis [59, 60]. The use of various agro-industrial residual effluents as probiotic growth media could be a starting point for lowering production costs on an industrial scale. Fruit and vegetable processing effluents often contain high levels of proteins, carbs, lipids, and vitamins in this regard. Monosaccharides, disaccharides, and oligosaccharides can also be discovered in effluents following cereal processing [61, 62]. A notable example of this form of effluent is wastewater from industrial corn processing. According to Gutierrez-Uribe *et al.*, the wastewater from the manufacturing process of commercial fresh masa and dry masa flour (also known as nejayote) has a considerable load of corn solids. The remaining 50% is made up of proteins, carbs, vitamins, and phytochemicals strong in phenolics and carotenoids. Nejayote includes arabinose, xylose, glucose, galactose, and D-glucuronic acid polysaccharides, as well as around 23% crude fiber, according to prior study (whose dietary fiber fraction may stimulate the growth of probiotics) [52, 53]. As a result, agricultural and industrial effluents such as cereal processing wastewater could be a rich source of prebiotic compounds. The possibility of using these effluents in the formulation of culture medium, either partially or totally, must be assessed [63–65].

10.7 Improving Viability of Probiotics

The vitality of probiotic microorganisms is critical to their quality, as it is required to reach and colonise the human large intestine [66, 67]. Probiotics must be viable during three critical stages: storage, production of functional foods, and stomach and small intestine transit. Therefore, the viability of probiotics is an issue of vital importance from both an economic and a technological viewpoint. In this regard, Ratnakomala and Widyastuti [68] observed that storage of a probiotic by freezing at −40°C decreased its viability from1.8 × 1015 to 1.6 × 1010 CFU mL−1, while a freeze-drying pretreatment followed by storage at 4°C decreased its viability from 8.9×1014 to 2.4×109 CFU mL^{-1}. Likewise, Lahtinen *et al.* [66] remembered that probiotics can go dormant during storage. They discovered that after 25 days of storage at 4°C in an oat-in-water suspension, Bifidobacterium strains can remain entirely inactive. These findings clearly show that storing probiotics might dramatically reduce their vitality. Freeze-drying probiotics in food matrices during storage and transit through the stomach and small intestine has been suggested to boost viability. For example, Saarela *et al.* [69] discovered that freeze-drying a Bifidobacterium strain in a matrix of low-fat milk or fruit juice boosted its survivability substantially. They discovered that during storage, viability in the juice matrix was higher than in low-fat milk, and that after storage, tolerance to acid and bile was better in cells with the low-fat milk matrix. The scientists concluded that viability should not be the only characteristic to consider when selecting a food matrix as a cryoprotectant for a probiotic, but also the ability to withstand harsh conditions after storage. As a result, investigating low-cost food matrices as cryoprotectants to increase bacterial viability after storage is a viable endeavour. Microencapsulation, on the other hand, is a potential technology that has recently been researched to improve the survivability of probiotic microorganisms. Microencapsulation is a technique for encapsulating solids, liquids, or gases in small, sealed capsules that can release their contents at controlled rates under controlled conditions [70]. Probiotics have been discovered to be better protected by microencapsulation throughout storage and the production process of a specific functional food, resulting in increased vitality in hot and acidic environments [70, 71].

Probiotic bacteria have been protected by spray-drying, spray-congealing, fluidized bed coating/air suspension, extrusion, coacervation/phase separation, and electrostatic techniques thus far. Anal and Singh provide a full explanation of various microencapsulation technologies [70]. The coating substance in which the probiotic is contained is a common material used in all microencapsulation procedures. Coating materials include water-soluble/insoluble polymers, waxes, fatty acids, and lipids. Table 10.4 lists some of the most common probiotics and coating materials utilized in probiotic microencapsulation. Prebiotics such as fructo-oligosaccharides or starch with a high resistance could be used in the coating. Chen *et al.* [48] used fructo-oligosaccharides in their coating formulation for *B. bifidum* microencapsulation. When compared to microcapsules coated only with alginate, they discovered that a formulation comprising prebiotics, gellan gum, and peptides significantly enhanced probiotic viability.

Crittenden *et al.* [72] used prebiotics in the coating formulation for B. infantis microencapsulation. After 5 weeks in an open container at 25°C and 50% relative humidity, they discovered that a mixture of canola vegetable oil, caseinate, fructo-oligosaccharides, and starch with a high resistance (or glucose syrup) enhanced the survivability of the prebiotics by ten orders of magnitude compared to free cells. As a result, new coating materials and microencapsulation techniques are being investigated as an important research focus. The available research appears to be focused on developing low-cost, abundant coating materials, as well as optimizing coating material formulas (e.g., optimum prebiotic percentages).

10.8 Conclusions

In summary, probiotic and prebiotic-based functional foods are an important biotechnological subject with a lot of room for innovation. We found three major obstacles to industrial production of probiotic and prebiotic-based functional meals in this paper: (i) the advancement of prebiotic synthesis techniques; (ii) the decrease of probiotic production costs; (iii) probiotic viability is improved through storage, the production of functional meals, and transit via the upper gastrointestinal tract. A multidisciplinary strategy is required in order to solve such obstacles. The following are some of the alternatives considered in this article. Prebiotics are made in two-liquid-phase systems with the addition of an organic solvent, which boosts prebiotic yield. Such multiphase systems may also increase the production of prebiotics by varying the degree of polymerization. Production of oligosaccharides from nondairy, low-cost raw materials, with cereals looking to be the most tempting option due to the presence of naturally occurring oligosaccharides such as galactosyl sucrose derivatives, stachyose, and raffinose, as well as fructosyl sucrose derivatives. In addition, cereal grains are high in dietary fiber and starch, both of which can be converted into starch with a high resistance. Corn-processing effluents appear to be a very interesting option for probiotic production from agroindustrial effluents, with their high concentrations of nonstarch polysaccharides, starch, protein, sugars, vitamins, phytochemicals rich in phenolics and carotenoids, as well as polysaccharides of arabinose, xylose, glucose, galactose, and D-glucuronic acid. As a result, this type of effluent could be used in whole or in part to manufacture low-cost culture media. Probiotic viability can be increased by adopting low-cost food matrices or microencapsulation techniques. As a result, freeze-drying research on matrices like milk and fruit juice could potentially boost probiotic viability by acting as cryoprotectants. On the other hand, microencapsulation has been discovered as a promising technique for safeguarding probiotics during storage, creation of a specific functional meal, and transit through the upper gastrointestinal tract.

Acknowledgment

The authors thank the METs, Institute of Pharmacy, BKC, affiliated under Savitribai Phule Pune University, Nashik, Divine College of Pharmacy Satana and Sandip Institute of Pharmaceutical Science for their constant support and providing all facilities to complete this work. We also thank the Ministry of Tribal Affairs Govt. of India for providing financial assistance in the form of fellowship (award no 202021-NFST-MAH-01235).

References

1. Korhonen, H., Technology options for new nutritional concepts. *Int. J. Dairy Technol.*, 55, 79–88, 2002.
2. Vasiljevic, T. and Shah, N.P., Probiotics – from Metchnikoff to bioactives. *Int. Dairy J.*, 18, 714–728, 2008.
3. Wiseman, A. and Woods, L., Addition of designer enhancers to functional-foods: Need also for redesigned biocatalysts in fail-clean strategies of bioprocessing? *J. Chem. Technol. Biotechnol.*, 76, 1038–1040, 2001.
4. Roberfroid, M., Functional food concept and its application to prebiotics. *Dig. Liver Dis.*, 34, S105–S110, 2002.
5. Menrad, K., Market and marketing of functional food in Europe. *J. Food Eng.*, 56, 181–188, 2003.
6. Stanton, C., Gardiner, G., Meehan, H., Collins, K., Fitzgerald, G., Lynch, P.B. *et al.*, Market potential for probiotics. *Am. J. Clin. Nutr.*, 73, 476S–483S, 2001.
7. Heller, K.J., Probiotic bacteria in fermented foods: Product characteristics and starter organisms. *Am. J. Clin. Nutr.*, 72, 374S–379S, 2001.
8. Senok, A.C., Ismaeel, A.Y., Botta, G.A., Probiotics facts and myths. *Clin. Microbiol. Infect.*, 11, 958–966, 2005.
9. Prado, F.C., Parada, J.L., Pandey, A., Soccol, C.R., Trends in non-dairy probiotic beverages. *Food Res. Int.*, 41, 111–123, 2008.
10. Kaur, I.P., Chopra, K., Saini, A., Probiotics: Potential pharmaceutical applications. *Eur. J. Pharm. Sci.*, 15, 1–9, 2002.

11. Fric, P., Probiotics and prebiotics – renaissance of a therapeutic principle. *Cent. Eur. J. Med.*, 2, 237–270, 2007.
12. Mercenier, A., Pavan, S., Pot, B., Probiotics as biotherapeutic agents: Present knowledge and future prospects. *Curr. Pharm. Des.*, 8, 99–110, 2002.
13. Caplice, E. and Fitzgerald, G.F., Food fermentations: Role of microorganisms in food production and preservation. *Int. J. Food Microbiol.*, 50, 131–149, 1999.
14. Fuller, R. and Gibson, G.R., Probiotics and prebiotics: Microflora management for improved gut health. *Clin. Micriobiol. Infect.*, 4, 477–480, 1998.
15. Gomes, A. and Malcata, M.X., *Bifidobacterium* spp. and *Lactobacillus acidophilus*: Biological, biochemical, technological and therapeutical properties relevant for use as probiotics. *Trends Food Sci. Technol.*, 10, 139–157, 1999.
16. Saier, M.H. and Mansour, N.M., Probiotics and prebiotics in human. *J. Mol. Microbiol. Biotechnol.*, 10, 22–25, 2005.
17. Itsaranuwat, P., Shal-haddad, K., Robinson, P.K., The potential therapeutic benefits of consuming 'health-promoting' fermented dairy products: A brief update. *Int. J. Dairy Technol.*, 56, 203–210, 2003.
18. Shah, N.P., Functional cultures and health benefits. *Int. Dairy J.*, 17, 1262–1277, 2007.
19. De Vrese, M. and Schrezenmeir, J., Probiotics, prebiotics, and synbiotics. *Adv. Biochem. Eng. Biotechnol.*, 111, 1–66, 2008.
20. Gill, H. and Prasad, J., Bioactive components of milk: probiotics, immunomodulation, and health benefits, in: *Advances in Experimental Medicine and Biology*, Z. Bösze (Ed.), pp. 423–454, Springer, New York, NY, 2008.
21. Priebe, M.G., Vonk, R.J., Sun, X., He, T., Harmsen, H.J.M., Welling, G.W., The physiology of colonic metabolism. Possibilities for interventions with pre- and probiotics. *Eur. J. Nutr.*, 41, 1/2–1/10, 2002.
22. Gibson, G.R. and Roberfroid, M.B., Dietary modulation of the human colonic microbiota: Introducing the concept of prebiotics. *J. Nutr.*, 125, 1401–1412, 1995.
23. Roberfroid, M., Prebiotics: The concept revisited. *J. Nutr.*, 137, 830S–837S, 2007.
24. Steed, H. and Macfarlane, S., Mechanisms of prebiotic impact on health, in: *Prebiotics and Probiotics Science and Technology*, D. Charalampopoulos and R.A. Rastall (Eds.), pp. 135–161, Springer, New York, NY, 2009.
25. Macfarlane, S., Macfarlane, G.T., Cummings, J.H., Review article: Prebiotics in the gastrointestinal tract. *Aliment. Pharmacol. Ther.*, 24, 701–714, 2006.
26. Grajek, W., Olejnik, A., Sip, A., Probiotics, prebiotics and antioxidants functional foods. *Acta Biochim. Pol.*, 52, 665–671, 2005.
27. Venter, C.S., Prebiotics: an update. *J. Fam. Ecol. Consum. Sci.*, 35, 17–25, 2007.
28. Rastall, R.A., Gibson, G.R., Gill, H.S., Guarner, F., Klaenhammer, T.R., Pot, B. *et al.*, Modulation of the microbial ecology of the human colon by probiotics,

prebiotics and synbiotics to enhance human health: an overview of enabling science and potential applications. *FEMS Microbiol. Ecol.*, 52, 145–152, 2005.

29. Del Val, M.I. and Otero, C., Biphasic aqueous media containing polyethylene glycol for the enzymatic synthesis of oligosaccharides from lactose. *Enzyme Microb. Technol.*, 33, 118–126, 2003.
30. Cruz-Guerrero, A.E., Gómez-Ruiz, L., Viniegra-González, G., Bárzana, E., García-Garibay, M., Influence of water activity in the synthesis of galactooligosaccharides produced by a hyperthermophilic β-glycosidase in an organic medium. *Biotechnol. Bioeng.*, 93, 1123–1129, 2006.
31. Kelly, G., Inulin-type prebiotics – a review: part 1. *Altern. Med. Rev.*, 13, 315–329, 2008.
32. Iniguez-Covarrubias, G., Diaz-Teres, R., Sanjuan-Dueñas, R., Anzaldo-Hernandez, J., Rowell, R.M., Utilization of by-products from the tequila industry. Part 2: Potential value of *Agave tequilana* Weberazul leaves. *Bioresour. Technol.*, 77, 101–108, 2001.
33. Delzenne, N.M., Oligosaccharides: state of the art. *Proc. Nutr. Soc.*, 62, 177–182, 2003.
34. Panesar, P.S., Panesar, R., Singh, R.S., Kennedy, J.F., Kumar, H., Microbial production, immobilization and applications of β-D-galactosidase. *J. Chem. Technol. Biotechnol.*, 81, 530–543, 2006.
35. Boon, M.A., van't Riet, K., Janssen, A.E.M., Enzymatic synthesis of oligosaccharides: product removal during a kinetically controlled reaction. *Biotechnol. Bioeng.*, 70, 411–420, 2000.
36. Olano, A. and Corzo, N., Lactulose as food ingredient. *J. Sci. Food Agric.*, 89, 12, 1987–1990, 2009.
37. Vázquez, M.J., Alonso, J.L., Domínguez, H., Parajó, J.C., Xylooligosaccharides Manufacture and applications. *Trends Food Sci. Technol.*, 11, 387–393, 2000.
38. Goulas, A.K., Cooper, J.M., Grandison, A.S., Rastall, R.A., Synthesis of isomaltooligosaccharides and oligodextrans in a recycle membrane bioreactor by the combined use of dextransucrase and dextranase. *Biotechnol. Bioeng.*, 88, 778–787, 2004.
39. Palframan, R., Gibson, G.R., Rastall, R.A., Development of a quantitative tool for the comparison of the prebiotic effect of dietary oligosaccharides. *Lett. Appl. Microbiol.*, 37, 281–284, 2003.
40. Crittenden, R.G., Morris, L.F., Harvey, M.L., Tran, L.R., Mirchell, H.L., Playne, M.J., Selection of a *Bifidobacterium* strain to complement starch with a high resistance in a synbiotic yoghurt. *J. Appl. Microbiol.*, 90, 268–278, 2001.
41. Andersson, H., Asp, N.G., Bruce, A., Roos, S., Wadström, T., Wold, A.E., Health effects of probiotics and prebiotics: A literature review on human studies. *Scand. J. Nutr.*, 45, 58–75, 2001.
42. Rastall, R.A. and Maitin, V., Prebiotics and synbiotics: Towards the next generation. *Curr. Opin. Biotechnol.*, 13, 490–496, 2002.

43. Bielecka, M., Biedrzycka, E., Majkowska, A., Selection of probiotics and prebiotics for synbiotics and confirmation of their *in vivo* effectiveness. *Food Res. Int.*, 35, 125–131, 2002.
44. Morelli, L., Zonenschain, D., Callegari, M.L., Grossi, E., Maisano, F., Fusillo, M., Assessment of a new synbiotic preparation in healthy volunteers: survival, persistence of probiotic strains and its effect on the indigenous flora. *Nutr. J.*, 2, 1–11, 2003.
45. Figueroa-González, I., Hernández-Sánchez, H., Rodríguez-Serrano, G., Gómez-Ruiz, L., García-Garibay, M., Cruz-Guerrero, A., Antimicrobial effect of *Lactobacillus casei* strain Shirota co-cultivated with *Escherichia coli* UAM0403. *Rev. Mex. Ing. Quim.*, 9, 11–16, 2010.
46. Asahara, T., Nomoto, K., Shimizu, K., Watanuki, M., Tanaka, R., Increased resistance of mice to *Salmonella enterica* serovar *Typhimurium* infection by synbiotic administration of bifidobacteria and transgalactosylated oligosaccharides. *J. Appl. Microbiol.*, 91, 985–996, 2001.
47. Liong, M.T. and Shah, N.P., Optimization of cholesterol removal, growth and fermentation patterns of *Lactobacillus acidophilus* ATCC 4962 in the presence of mannitol, fructo-oligosaccharide and inulin: a response surface methodology approach. *J. Appl. Microbiol.*, 98, 1115–1126, 2005.
48. Chen, M.J., Chen, K.N., Kuo, Y.T., Optimal thermotolerance of *Bifodobacterium bifidum in* gellan-alginate microparticles. *Biotechnol. Bioeng.*, 98, 411–419, 2007.
49. Pan, X., Wu, T., Zhang, L., Cai, L., Song, Z., Influence of oligosaccharides on the growth and tolerance capacity of lactobacilli to simulated stress environment. *Lett. Appl. Microbiol.*, 48, 362–367, 2009.
50. Özer, D., Akin, S., Özer, B., Effect of inulin and lactulose on survival of *Lactobacillus acidophilus* LA-5 and *Bifidobacterium bifidum* BB-02 in Acidophilus-Bifidus yoghurt. *Food Sci. Technol. Int.*, 11, 19–24, 2005.
51. Crittenden, R.G. and Playne, M.J., Production, properties and application of food-grade oligosaccharides. *Trends Food Sci. Technol.*, 7, 353–361, 1996.
52. Charalampopoulos, D., Wang, R., Padiella, S.S., Webb, C., Application of cereals and cereal components in functional food: A review. *Int. J. Food Microbiol.*, 79, 131–141, 2002.
53. Crittenden, R., Karppinen, S., Ojanen, S., Tenkanen, M., Fagerström, R., Mättö, J. *et al.*, *In vitro* fermentation of cereal dietary fibre carbohydrates by probiotic and intestinal bacteria. *J. Sci. Food Agric.*, 82, 781–789, 2002.
54. Moura, P., Carvalheiro, F., Gírio, F., Loureiro, M.C., Esteves, M.P., *In vitro* fermentation of xylo-oligosaccharides from corn cobs autohydrolysis by *Bifidobacterium* and *Lactobacilllus* strain. *LWT - Food Sci. Technol.*, 40, 963–972, 2007.
55. Nyman, M., Siljestrom, M., Pedersen, B., Bach-Knudsen, K.E., Asp, N.G., Johansson, C.G. *et al.*, Dietary fiber content and composition in six cereals at different extraction rates. *Cereal Chem.*, 61, 14–19, 1984.

56. Snow, P. and O'Dea, K., Factors affecting the rate of hydrolysis of starch in food. *Am. J. Clin. Nutr.*, 34, 2721–2727, 1981.
57. Topping, D.L., Fukushima, M., Bird, A.R., Starch with a high resistance as a prebiotic and synbiotic; state of the art. *Proc. Nutr. Soc.*, 62, 171–176, 2003.
58. Mattila-Sandholm, T., Myllärinen, P., Crittenden, R., Mogensen, G., Fondén, R., Saarela, M., Technological challenges for future probiotic foods. *Int. Dairy J.*, 12, 173–182, 2002.
59. Altermann, E., Russell, W.M., Azcarate-Peril, M.A., Barrangou, R., Buck, B.L., McAuliffe, O. *et al.*, Complete genome sequence of the probiotic lactic acid bacterium *Lactobacillus acidophilus* NCFM. *Proc. Natl. Acad. Sci. U.S.A.*, 102, 3906–3912, 2005.
60. Ballongue, J., Bifidobacteria and probiotic action, in: *Lactic Acid Bacteria*, S. Salminen and A. Wright (Eds.), pp. 519–587, Marcel Dekker, New York, NY, 1998.
61. Federici, F., Fava, F., Kalogerakis, N., Mantzavinos, D., Valorisation of agro-industrial by-products, effluents and waste: concept, opportunities and the case of olivemill wastewaters. *J. Chem. Technol. Biotechnol.*, 84, 895–900, 2009.
62. Gutierrez-Uribe, J.A., Rojas-García, C., García-Lara SandSerna-Saldivar, O., Phytochemical analysis of wastewater (nejayote) obtained afterlime-cooking of different types of maize kernels processed intomasa for tortillas. *J. Cereal Sci.*, 52, 410–416, 2010.
63. Niño-Medina, G., Carvajal-Millan, E., Rascon-Chu, A., Marquez-Escalante, J., Santana-Rodriguez, V., Salmeron-Zamora, J., Maize processing waste water arabinoxylans: gelling capability and cross-linking content. *Food Chem.*, 115, 1286–1290, 2009.
64. Martínez-Bustos, F., Martınez-Flores, H.E., Sanmartín-Martınez, E., Sánchez-Sinencio, F., Chang, Y.K., Barrera-Arellano, D. *et al.*, Effect of the components of maize on the quality of masa and tortillas during the traditional nixtamalisation process. *J. Sci. Food Agric.*, 81, 1445–1462, 2001.
65. Rosentrater, K.A., A review of corn masa processing residues: generation, properties, and potential utilization. *Waste Manage.*, 26, 284–292, 2006.
66. Lahtinen, S.J., Gueimonde, M., Ouwehand, A.C., Reinikainen, J.P., Salminen, S.J., Probiotic bacteria may become dormant during storage. *Appl. Environ. Microbiol.*, 71, 1662–1663, 2005.
67. Tuomola, E., Crittenden, R., Playne, M., Isolauri, E., Salminen, S., Quality assurance criteria for probiotic bacteria. *Am. J. Clin. Nutr.*, 73, 393S–398S, 2001.
68. Ratnakomala, S. and Widyastuti, Y., Storage of probiotic *Leuconostoccitreum* TSD-10 by freezing and freeze drying. *Ann. Bogor.*, 7, 43–48, 2000.
69. Saarela, M., Virkajärvi, I., Alakomi, H.L., Sigvart-Mattila, P., Mättö, J., Stability and functionality of freeze-dried probiotic *Bifidobacterium* cell during storage in juice milk. *Int. Dairy J.*, 16, 1477–1482, 2006.

70. Anal, A.K. and Singh, H., Recent advances in microencapsulation of probiotics for industrial applications and targeted delivery. *Trends Food Sci. Technol.*, 18, 240–251, 2007.
71. Vidhyalakshmi, R., Bhakyaraj, R., Subhasree, R.S., Encapsulation 'the future of probiotics' – a review. *Adv. Biol. Res.*, 3, 96–103, 2009.
72. Crittenden, R., Weerakkody, R., Sanguansri, L., Augustin, M.A., Synbiotic microcapsules that enhance microbial viability during nonrefrigerated storage and gastrointestinal transit. *Appl. Environ. Microbiol.*, 72, 2280–2282, 2006.

11

Oral Health and Prebiotics

Khemchand Surana[1], Eknath D. Ahire[2*], Ritesh Pawar[3], Ritesh Khairnar[4], Sunil Mahajan[5], Sanjay Kshirsagar[2], Swati G. Talele[6], Nilima Thombre[2], Bhavana Ahire[7] and Raj K. Keservani[8]

[1]Department of Pharmaceutical Chemistry, Shreeshakti Shaikshanik Sanstha, Divine College of Pharmacy, Satana, Nashik, India
[2]Department of Pharmaceutics, MET's, Institute of Pharmacy, BKC, Affiliated to Savitribai Phule Pune University, Adgaon, Nashik, India
[3]Department of Pharmaceutical Chemistry, Poona College of Pharmacy, Pune, Maharashtra, India
[4]Department of Pharmaceutical Chemistry, St. John Institute of Pharmacy & Research, Palghar, Maharashtra, India
[5]Department of Pharmaceutical Chemistry, MGV's Pharmacy College, Panchvati, Nashik, India
[6]Department of Pharmaceutics, Sandip Institute of Pharmaceutical Sciences, Affiliated to Savitribai Phule Pune University, Nashik, India
[7]Department of Quality Assurance Techniques, NDMVP's, College of Pharmacy, Nashik, India
[8]Faculty of B. Pharmacy, CSM Group of Institutions, Prayagraj, Uttar Pradesh, India

Abstract
Oral infections are one of the most common and costly types of contamination in humans. While converting microbial ecology might also additionally make a contribution to enamel sickness, the idea of microbial ecological alternate as a method for stopping dental sickness is essential. New strategies inclusive of prebiotic processes to remove pathogenic contributors of the microbiota may be investigated. Prebiotics may be a powerful method to guide the increase of wholesome microorganism in each the intestine and oral microbiome. Abuse of antibiotics to deal with infections has been proven to increase resistant microbial strains, setting sufferers prone to pathogen overgrowth. Therefore, an available healing

**Corresponding author*: eknathahire05@gmail.com

Rajesh K. Kesharwani, Tingirikari Jagan Mohan Rao and Raj K. Keservani (eds.) Prebiotics and Probiotics in Disease Regulation and Management, (291–310) © 2022 Scrivener Publishing LLC

method to contamination is urgently needed. This new awareness has caused the emergence of prebiotics and/or probiotics with related healing fitness benefits. While the term "probiotics" pertains to purposeful foods, the term "prebiotics" typically refers to nondigestible materials that gain the host organism through selectively stimulating the increase and/or activity of 1 or a restricted quantity of microorganism. These used to outline meals ingredients. It improves the fitness of the host through getting rid of set up species within the colon. This prebiotic consist of inulin, fructooligosaccharides, galactooligosaccharides, and lactulose. A polyphenol-wealthy food regimen stands proud as one of the maximum promising strategies located in numerous human-consuming culmination and plants (for example, tea, coco, coffee, and raisins), which can be taken into consideration to gain dental health through decreasing oral microbes related to caries via antioxidant hobby. Chewing xylitol-sweetened gum has been proven to lessen the improvement of mutant streptococci inside the mouth. Xylitol is a robust prebiotic that can be discovered in a number fruits and vegetables. This indicates that this remedy might also additionally lessen oral mutans streptococci stages over time. Also, the anti-inflammatory houses of omega-three polyunsaturated fatty acids (PUFAs) have long been known. It will lessen periodontal sickness improvement through decreasing periodontopathic microorganism. It will raise phagocytic hobby even as lowering osteoclast hobby because of the anti-inflammatory action.

Keywords: Prebiotic, oral microbiota, polyphenol, xylitol, omega-3 fatty acids, nitrates

11.1 Introduction

11.1.1 Prebiotic

The term prebiotics became first described through Gibson and Roberfoid in 1995 as "the substrate this is selectively used by host microorganisms conferring a health benefit [1]. In 2010, Roberfroid *et al.* explicit prebiotic as it is a selectively fermented element that effects in particular changes, inside the composition and/or activity of the gastrointestinal microbiota, consequently conferring benefit upon host health. Prebiotics became evolved historically with intestine awareness; however, prebiotics has now been proposed for different use, along with regulating vaginal pH, controlling pores and skin infections, and optimizing healthy oral microbes. International Scientific Association for Probiotics and Prebiotics verified the definition and scope of prebiotics in 2017 and revised the concept as "a substrate this is selectively used by host microorganisms conferring a health benefit." This definition broadens the definition of prebiotics to encompass noncarbohydrate compounds, make use of out of doors of the gastrointestinal tract and plenty of classes aside from food [2].

Prebiotics offers a "new" way to manage the connection between nutrition and dental health. Although the effects of prebiotics on periodontal health are unclear, research shows that prebiotics encourages the development of beneficial microbes that are part of the oral microbiota. The development of probiotic microbes in the mouth is stimulated by certain oligosaccharide prebiotics. Glucomannans, for example, can be utilized for this, especially when hydrolyzed [3]. Prebiotics is beneficial in the treatment of oral disorders when used in conjunction with probiotics. Prebiotics are dietary supplements that are not digested. Their job is to boost the development and activity of beneficial bacteria while suppressing the growth and activity of potentially harmful bacteria. Prebiotics alter the microflora balance in the intestine in this way. The major aspect of prebiotic consumption is that it alters the microbial population density [4, 5].

Ideal prebiotics have the following characteristics:

- They are neither digested nor absorbed by mammalian enzymes or tissue.
- They encourage the development of certain probiotic organisms.
- They should be able to change the microbial flora and activity in the intestine.
- They should be able to change the host defense system's systemic features.

11.1.2 Prebiotic Selection Criteria

There are five major necessities for the categorization of nutritional additives consisting of prebiotics. Prebiotics are not digested (or are simplest in part digested) inside the better quantities of the alimentary canal, in line with the primary criteria. As a result, they attain the colon, in which they are fermented selectively via way of means of microorganism that can be helpful (a demand of the second criterion). The fermentation also can moreover bring about a growth in production or change inside the relative abundance of diverse short-chain fatty acids (SCFAs), elevated stool mass, a moderate cut price of colonic pH, a reduction of nitrous stop merchandise and fecal enzymes, and improvement of the immunological system, this is beneficial for the host (the requirement of the third criterion). Selective stimulation of growth and/or interest of the intestinal microorganism potentially associated with health protection and well-being is considered via way of means of a few different criteria. The very last criterion of the class assumes that a prebiotic have to be able to resisting food processing conditions and continue to be unchanged, nondegraded, or chemically unaltered, and available for bacterial metabolism inside the intestine. Huebner *et al.* tested several commercially available prebiotics for using various processing conditions. They placed no huge changes of the prebiotic interest of the tested substances in various processing conditions. Meanwhile, Ze *et al.* showed that it modified into feasible to modify the ability of the gut microorganism thru utilizing starch *in vitro*. The form of prebiotics has to be appropriately documented, and components used as pharmaceutical formulas, food, or feed additives have to be especially smooth to achieve at a commercial enterprise scale [6].

11.1.3 Prebiotics Mechanism of Action

Natural goods consist of prebiotics; however, they will additionally be introduced to meals. These components are intended to enhance the dietary and health advantages of the food. Inulin, fructooligosaccharides, lactulose, galactose, and b glucan derivatives are some of the examples. These compounds may act as probiotic carriers. They promote boom and now no longer include any microorganisms. Prebiotics are not digested through human enzymes and reach the colon in an almost undamaged state, wherein saccharolytic microorganism ferments them (e.g., *Bifidobacterium* genus). Prebiotics has a sizable effect at the makes up of the intestine microbiota and its metabolic pastime. This is attributed to modifications in lipid metabolism, elevated calcium absorbability, results at the immune system, and modifications in gastrointestinal function. It is probably providing a strength supply that simplest sure microorganism species can use and has a larger impact on microbiota composition and metabolism than those different parameters. Prebiotics' physiological outcomes and the types of microbes, which can make use of them as a supply of carbon and strength inside the intestine, are decided through their chemical structure. It became established that, despite the variety of carbohydrates that exhibit the prebiotic pastime, the impact in their management is an increased count of useful microorganism, maximum of the Bifidobacterium genus. The mechanism of prebiotics' effective impact on immune functioning is unknown. Several different fashions are suggested:

(1) Prebiotics can have an impact on the expanded synthesis of short-chain fatty acids (SCFAs), consisting of propionic

acid, that may have an effect on the motion of hepatic lipogenic enzymes.

(2) Fermentation-induced SCFA synthesis (especially butyric acid) has been observed as a modulator of histone acetylation, improving the supply of numerous genes for transcription factors.

(3) Controlling the era of mucin.

(4) FOS and several different prebiotics were proven to growth the wide variety of lymphocytes and/or leukocytes inside the intestine-related lymphoid tissues (GALTs) and the peripheral circulation.

(5) GALTs' improved IgA manufacturing might also additionally enhance intra-inflammatory macrophages' phagocytic pastime.

Prebiotics' foremost goal is to foster the improvement and pastime of useful microorganism inside the gastrointestinal system, which blesses the host's fitness. The intestine microbiota features as a barrier for pathogens thru techniques consisting of antagonism (the manufacturing of antimicrobial compounds) and opposition for epithelial adherence and nutrition. The majority of carbohydrate metabolism's quit merchandise are SCFAs, consisting of acetic acid, butyric acid, and propionic acid, which are then applied as a supply of strength through the host. Bifidobacterium or Lactobacillus might also additionally create chemical substances that restrict the increase of gastrointestinal pathogens and result in a lower in intestinal pH due to carbohydrate fermentation. Furthermore, microorganism of the Bifidobacterium genus displays resistance to the generated SCFAs and a decreased pH. An end result in their favor has an impact on the formation of useful intestine microorganism, prebiotics might also additionally resource inside the suppression of pathogen improvement. Prebiotics has been proven to suppress the increase of pathogens in a confined wide variety of studies. Bovee-Oudenhoven *et al.* investigated the usage of lactulose in the prevention of *Salmonella enteritidis* infections in rats in 1997 and 2003. Their findings confirmed that the acidity of the intestine generated through lactulose fermentation ended in reduced pathogen increase and improved pathogen translocation from the bowel. It has additionally been established that taking prebiotics enhances mineral absorption, specially magnesium and calcium [6].

11.2 Oral Microbiota in Health and Disease

To be ready to develop prebiotic interventions for applications in oral healthcare and to know their mechanisms of action and potential risks, it is essential to possess a transparent understanding of the oral microbiota and therefore their functions in oral health and disease. This can be not invariably easy, given the quality of the oral microbiota; about 700 species are detected within the human mouth and the resident microbiota of an individual could comprise thirty to one hundred species. The tongue may be an organism-laden organ. It is densely inhabited with secretion microbes, supragingival, and subgingival plaque microorganisms [7].

11.2.1 Functions of Resident Microbiota

The main focus of analysis has been the process of the microorganisms associated with their traits that are liable for disease; however, there is a magnified awareness that the resident microbiota doesn't play just a passive role, but actively contributes to the upkeep of health. The large, various resident microorganism communities that colonies tissue layer sites coexist with a host, with harmful effects as long as the host becomes immunocompromised, if the resident microbial populations are suppressed or if microorganisms reach sites to that they are doing not ordinarily have access (e.g. through trauma). Studies, principally bacteria, have shown that resident microbial populations contribute to hosting protection through a block of the organization by pathogens, development of cell structure and performance, development of the system, and modulation of inflammatory responses. The proof is accumulating to support an identical role for oral commensal bacterium within the development of the immune system, the upkeep of healthy oral tissue by influencing the expression of mediators, such as living thing adhesion molecule one (ICAM-1), E-selectin, and IL-8, modulating immune responses, and enhancing cellular physiological state mechanisms [8].

11.2.2 Microbiota Responsible for Oral Diseases

Caries and periodontitis are the most frequent oral illnesses, both of which are caused by a change in the local microbiota's equilibrium. The kinds and amounts of bacteria identified in plaque from locations with caries or periodontal disease differ from one another, and both are different from those found in healthy sites. Caries cause an increase in acidogenic and acid-tolerating bacteria, such as mutans streptococci and lactobacilli, though other bacteria with similar properties can also be found, including bifidobacteria, non-mutants streptococci, *Actinomyces* spp., *Propionibacterium* spp., *Veillonella* spp., and *Atopobium* spp. There is a rise in plaque quantity and a shift toward obligately anaerobic and proteolytic bacteria, many of which are Gram-negative and presently unculturable, in periodontal disorders. The combined actions of subgingival biofilms and the human responses to these various bacterial populations cause host harm during periodontal disease. A variety of publications provide good overviews of periodontal microbiology, demonstrating the enormous paradigm change that has happened, from focusing on the functions of individual pathogens to recognizing that periodontal disease is caused by an activity of successive consortia of organisms.

Other frequent oral illnesses are caused by the actions of microorganisms present in the oral microbiota. Oral candidiasis and denture-associated stomatitis can be caused by *Candida albicans* and other *Candida* species, which are found in low quantities in oral microbial communities. Oral bacteria, particularly Gram-negative anaerobes, produce malodorous metabolic end products (especially volatile sulfur compounds) that cause halitosis [8, 9].

11.2.3 Is Prebiotics Considered a Feasible Substitute for the Treatment of Oral Diseases?

Knowing which species can be regarded to promote health, and gaining some knowledge of their metabolic demands and interactions is vital for a reasonable approach to the production of oral prebiotics and the management of the resident microbiota. Endogenous nutrients, such as salivary proteins and glycoproteins, as well as gingival crevicular fluid, are catabolized by the indigenous oral bacteria. Controlling refined sugar intake has been utilized for many years to regulate the oral ecology and guard against caries, and it is clear that bad diet influences dental health as well as general health. Similarly, xylitol has been shown to inhibit acid generation by mutans streptococci, albeit this did not influence the efficiency of a chewing gum containing probiotics. Oral streptococci adhesion is reduced by algal lectins and cranberry juice. Cariogenic bacteria's viability and acid production can be reduced by cocoa polyphenols. While all of these employ (or recommend using) food/components to impact the oral microbiota, they are not prebiotics since they suppress possible pathogens rather than stimulating beneficial resident microbes [9].

We do not know much about the effect of dietary components on the composition of subgingival plaque. There is some evidence for the beneficial effects of promoting bifidobacteria and lactobacilli populations in the gut, which has been gathered over many years. Koll-Klais *et al.* discovered that homofermentative lactobacilli, particularly *L. gasseri*, were more common in healthy than periodontally diseased sites and that their presence was inversely related to clinical parameters associated with chronic periodontitis, as well as subgingival colonization by periodontal pathogens. *L. gasseri*, *L. salivarius*, and *Lactobacillus fermentum* were likewise shown to be more frequent in healthy locations, according to Hojo *et al.* *Bifidobacterium* spp. were recovered from 80% of periodontally healthy patients, whereas *Bifidobacterium adolescentis* was identified from 40% of healthy subjects and no periodontitis subjects, according to the same study. Bifidobacteria counts were notably high in a group of well cared for ex-periodontitis patients, suggesting that these bacteria are better able to colonize regions where plaque has been removed. Prebiotic therapy that increases the development of specific bifidobacteria and lactobacilli may thereby improve periodontal health. However, because lactobacilli and bifidobacteria are connected to caries etiology, it is difficult to see how boosting their development with prebiotics would not lead to an increase in the predominance of aciduric and acidogenic populations, which are linked to a higher risk of dental caries [8, 9].

11.2.4 Classification of Prebiotic

Nondigestible carbohydrates can be considered as prebiotic if they achieve the following criteria:

(A) resistance to gastric acidity and mammalian enzymes,
(B) susceptibility to fermentation by gut bacteria,
(C) ability to enhance the viability and/or activity of beneficial microorganisms [10–12].

Prebiotics are divided into three categories: established prebiotics, emergent prebiotics, and prebiotics with health-promoting properties (Table 11.1). Established prebiotics contain inulin, fructooligosaccharides (FOS), galactooligosaccharides (GOS), lactulose, and polydextrose. Emergent prebiotics is classified into isomaltoligosaccharides (IMO), xylooligosaccharides (XOS), and lactitol. Wheat bran-derived arabinoxylooligosaccharide (AXOS) xylooligosaccharides (XOS) and chicory root inulin derived (FOS) display prebiotic health-promoting application. Many earlier writers

Table 11.1 Prebiotic classified according to dietary fiber [23].

Sr. no.	Types of prebiotic	Food source
1.	Fructans (Inulin, Fructo-oligosaccharides)	Chicory, artichoke, garlic, onions, leek, asparagus, banana
2.	Resistant Starch	Green bananas, plantains, cooked and chilled potatoes, rice, cold oatmeal, beans, peas, lentils, and seeds
3.	Galactooligosaccharides	Chickpeas, beans, lentils, broccoli, brussel sprouts
4.	**β-Glucan**	Oatmeal, barley, mushrooms, yeasts, seaweed
5.	Polyphenols	Many different fruits, particularly berries, tea (black, green, or herbal), dark chocolate, red wine, globe artichokes, chicory, red onion, spinach, broccoli, herbs, spices
6.	Omega-3 fatty acids (EPA and DHA)	Fatty fish such as salmon, trout, sardines, herring, tuna

have demonstrated the health-promoting properties of mannitol, maltodextrin, raffinose, lactulose, and sorbitol (Figures 11.1 and 11.2). Other prebiotic, i.e., resistant starch-rich whole grains, are not absorbed in the small intestine of healthy people and are instead digested by the colon's natural microflora to form short-chain fatty acids (SCFA) (Tables 11.2 and 11.3) [12].

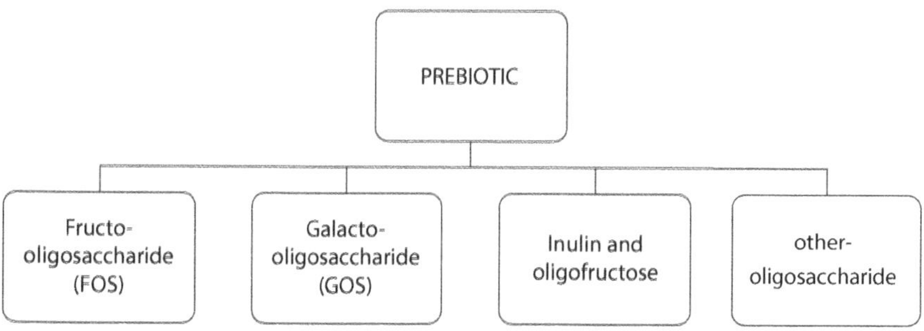

Figure 11.1 Prebiotic classified according to soluble fiber.

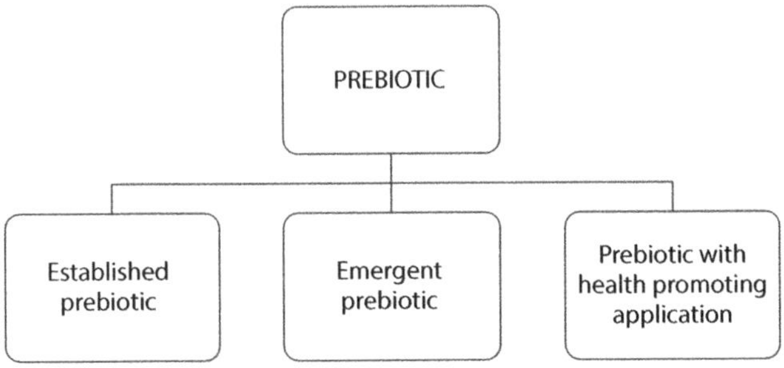

Figure 11.2 Prebiotics are classified according to their origin and chemical features.

Table 11.2 The list of nondigestible prebiotic [12].

1.	Insulin	9.	Starch-rich whole grains
2.	Xylitol	10.	Galactooligosaccharides (GOS)
3.	Lactulose	11.	Fructooligosaccharide (FOS)
4.	Mannitol	12.	Arabinoxylooligosaccharide (AXOS)
5.	Sorbitol	13.	Isomaltooligosaccharide (IMO)
6.	Raffinose	14.	Mannaoligosaccharide (MOS)
7.	Polydextrose	15.	Oligofructans
8.	Mannitol	16.	Xylooligosaccharides (XOS)

1) Polyphenol

Among the most popular treatments for these oral symptoms are fluoride supplementation in tap water, dietary sugar reduction, and expert mechanical removal of tooth plaque. Fluoridecan suppresses bacterial acid generation, block bacterial enzymes involved in sugar absorption, and prevent oral streptococci overgrowth, among other things. Despite this, natural alternative treatments are targeted at preserving oral health and avoiding microbial-related oral illnesses. A polyphenol-rich diet stands out as one of the most promising strategies [13]. Polyphenols, also known as phenolic acids or flavonoids, are found in several human-eating fruits and plants (for example, tea, cocoa, coffee, and raisins), that are thought to enhance dental health by suppressing oral microorganisms linked to caries through antioxidant activity. Oleanolic acid, oleanolic aldehyde, linoleic acid, linolenic acid, betulin, betulinic acid, 5-(hydroxymethyl)-2-furfural, rutin,

Table 11.3 Modes of Production of prebiotics [12].

Sr. no.	Prebiotic	Mode of production
1.	Lactulose	Alkali isomerization of lactose
2.	Pectin	Enzymatic hydrolysis of lemon peels
3.	Xylitol	Solid-Liquid extraction from lignocellulosic waste materials
4.	Inulin	Isolation from chicory root
5.	Mannan oligosaccharides	Enzymatic hydrolysis of mannose
6.	Fructooligosaccharides	Partial enzymatic hydrolysis of inulin
7.	Isomaltooligosaccharides	Enzymatic hydrolysis of starch/ transglucosylation of maltose
8.	Galactooligosaccharides	Trans galactosylation of lactose with *Aspergillus oryzae* β-galactosidase
9.	Soyabeanoligosaccharides	Extraction from soybean whey
10.	Oligofructans	Microwave hydrolysis of levan from Zymomonasmobilis
11.	Xylooligosaccharides	Enzymatic hydrolysis of xylan

beta-sitosterol, and beta-sitosterol glucoside have also been found to have antibacterial action against oral infections. The use of plant-derived products (i.e. extracts) with a high concentration of polyphenols is based on a method for mechanistic pathogen elimination, since these chemicals have anti-adhesive effects against certain oral bacteria (Figure 11.3) [14].

1.1) Tea

Tea is a liquid extract obtained from the dried leaves of the *Camellia sinensis* L. plant having the family Theaceae. Polyphenols, catechins, caffeine, amino acids, carbs, protein, chlorophyll, volatile chemicals, fluoride, minerals, and other unknown substances constitute tea's chemical composition. Epigallocatechin gallate, epicatechin gallate, epigallocatechin, epicatechin, gallocatechin, and (+)-catechins are the most interesting components of tea leaves when it comes to dental health. It shows antimicrobial and antiadhesion properties. The tea produces inhibitory action on bacterial

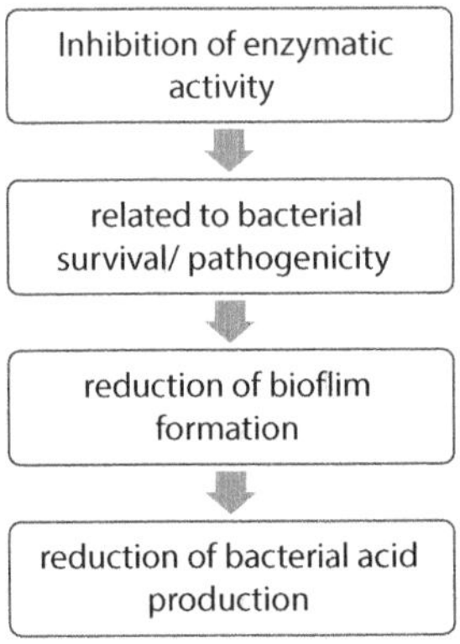

Figure 11.3 Mode of action of polyphenol on oral health.

growth, bacterial viability, glycosyltransferase activity, adherence, and salivary amylase activities [14].

1.2) Cranberry

S. mutans acid generation, adhesion, and biofilm development are all inhibited by cranberry components, making them effective anticaries agents. Cranberry constituents have an impact on glucan-binding proteins, extracellular enzymes, carbohydrate synthesis, and bacterial hydrophobicity. Cranberry components, particularly those that have a high molecular weight, are frequently recommended as bioactive agents for the prevention and/or treatment of oral disorders. Total bacterial and *S. mutans* counts in saliva were decreased after 42 days of using a mouthwash supplemented with a high molecular weight polyphenols cranberry fraction. It acts as antimicrobial, antiadhesion, and antibiofilm [14].

1.3) Cocoa

Cocoa is obtained from the Fruit of the cacao tree (*Theobroma cacao*) having the family Malvaceae. It acts as antimicrobial, antibiofilm activity. *S. mutans* and *Streptococcus sanguinis* biofilm development and acid production are greatly reduced by cocoa polyphenol pentamers. Extracts from cocoa mass have been found to have anticariogenic properties; however, they are not powerful enough to prevent sucrose from becoming cariogenic. Antibacterial and antiglycosyltransferase properties have been discovered in cacao bean husk extract (CBH). When the human dental plaque was exposed to CBH extract for 1 hour, the number of mutant's streptococci in the plaque was considerably decreased. When compared to rinsing with 1% ethanol alone, mouth rinses with CBH extract in ethanol, used before and after each meal and before sleeping at night for 4 days without performing other oral hygiene practices, reduced plaque deposition, and the number of mutant streptococci [14].

1.4) Coffee

It acts as an antiadhesion property. It is obtained from is its dried ripe seed of *Coffea arabica* having family Rubiaceae. The antiacidogenic actions of polyphenols from coffee against alpha-hemolytic streptococci imply that additional research into this beverage's potential application in the prevention of dental caries development is required [14].

1.5) Grapes and Wine

It shows the antimicrobial, antiadhesion, antibiofilm properties. The protective role of grapes and wine is an Inhibitory effect on lipopolysaccharide expression of *P. gingivalis*, antimicrobial activity against *S. mutans* and *P. gingivalis* of oleanolic acid, sodium salt of oleanolic acid, linoleic acid, and 5-(hydroxymethyl)-2-furfural [15].

1.6) Propolis

It shows the antimicrobial, antiadhesion, antibiofilm, antiacidogenic properties. Propolis has been demonstrated to have antibacterial action against a variety of oral bacteria and to prevent *S. mutans* and *S. sobrinus* from adhering to the glass. It was also discovered to be a strong inhibitor of the formation of water-soluble glucans (GTF-activity inhibitor). Propolis has been shown to have antimicrobial action against a variety of bacteria, including *S. mutants* and *Streptococcus sobrinus* [15].

2) Xylitol

Xylitol is a potent prebiotic that may be found in a variety of fruits and vegetables. Due to its unusual features, which make this polyol sugar industrially relevant, it has gotten a lot of attention from researchers. The FDA (Food and Drug Administration) has classed this pentose alcoholic sugar as generally recognized as safe (GRAS) [15]. Chewing xylitol-sweetened gum three to five times per day for at least 5 minutes after meals to lower mutans streptococci levels and limit plaque buildup and enamel demineralization. Additional *in vitro* and outdoor investigations are needed to confirm if xylitol can stop carious lesions from spreading. Caries management can benefit from xylitol-sweetened gum and, to a lesser extent, sorbitol-sweetened gum. Gum chewing is, for the most part, culturally acceptable in the United States, and most patients' daily routines are readily accommodated.

The US Food and Drug Administration has authorized xylitol for use in dietary supplements since 1963. It is not widely utilized, and it is not as well known as other sugar substitutes that are widely sold. Although evidence suggests that xylitol-sweetened gum is better than sorbitol-sweetened gum in terms of lowering caries risk, chewing sorbitol-sweetened gum multiple times per day is better than chewing sugared gum in terms of preventing caries. Xylitol works in chewing gum to inhibit caries development [16]:

- Since xylitol is not fermented by cariogenic plaque bacteria, it does not reduce plaque ph. Enamel demineralization is avoided, and plaque bacteria do not multiply, since plaque pH does not drop.
- Plaque deposition on the tooth surface is reduced by xylitol.
- Remineralization is improved when xylitol-sweetened gum is chewed since the pH of the plaque does not decrease.
- Chewing xylitol-sweetened gum has regularly been shown to suppress the proliferation of mutants' streptococci in the mouth. This shows that this treatment may result in long-term decreases in oral mutans streptococci levels.
- Chewing any gum increases the flow of saliva, which improves the plaque buffering action. This trait is not specific to xylitol-sweetened gum; the chewing sensation is considered useful on its own [17].

3) Omega-3 Fatty acid

Cod liver oil, fish oil, and marine creatures high in fat, such as tuna, sardines, herring mackerel, salmon, and menhaden, are common dietary sources of omega-3 fatty acid. Omega-3 fatty acids are found in greater abundance in oily seafood. Omega-3 fatty acids can also be found in flaxseed oil and nuts, particularly walnuts. To begin, therapeutic adjuncts administered exogenously may be designed to improve the microbial regulatory environment in the subgingival sulcus. Second, the inherent nature of these fatty acid inhibitors would have a role in the properties of microbial biofilms, their development, and the formation of species within them. Periodontitis is an irreversible chronic inflammatory illness characterized by gradual loss of both soft and hard structures. Periodontal disease is one of the most common human illnesses, making it a serious public health problem. It is impossible to entirely or predictably rebuild healthy periodontal architecture once it has been lost, the anti-inflammatory characteristics of omega-3 fatty acids, as well as their prospective application as a periodontal therapeutic adjuvant (Figure 11.4) [18].

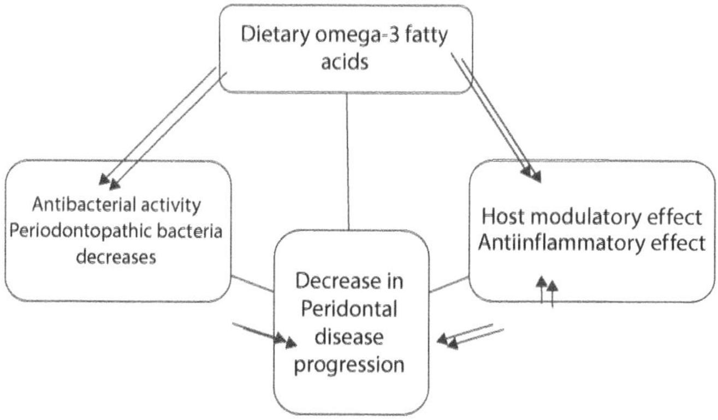

Figure 11.4 Mechanism of omega-3 fatty acid.

Inflammation of the periodontal tissues is caused by periodontopathic bacteria. Periodontitis is characterized by alveolar bone loss caused by the host's inflammatory response to primarily gram-negative bacteria. Omega-3 polyunsaturated fatty acids (PUFAs) have long been known to have anti-inflammatory effects. It will decrease the periodontopathic bacteria and decrease the periodontal disease progression. Due to the anti-inflammatory effect, it will increase phagocytic activity and decrease osteoclast activity [18].

11.3 Nitrate as Potential Prebiotic for Oral Health

The salivary glands aggressively concentrate plasma nitrate into saliva, resulting in salivary nitrate levels in the 100- to 500-M range during fasting (i.e., approximately 10 times higher than in plasma). This process produces a further increase in salivary nitrate concentrations after a nitrate-containing meal, up to 5–8 mM, which remains elevated for several hours because of the long half-life circulation of nitrate (Figure 11.5). Significantly, salivary nitrate, nitrite, and the oral microbiome's nitrate-reducing capabilities have all been postulated to help prevent caries within the mouth. In recent clinical research, 2 weeks of nitrate-rich lettuce juice drinking enhanced gingival health. Ultimately, 1 to 4 weeks of high doses of nitrate in the form of concentrated beetroot juice enhanced the number of health-associated nitrate-reducing bacteria in saliva in other clinical studies intervention trials. The findings of the present study show that nitrate supplementation at physiological salivary levels can prevent or diminish bacterial dysbiosis and

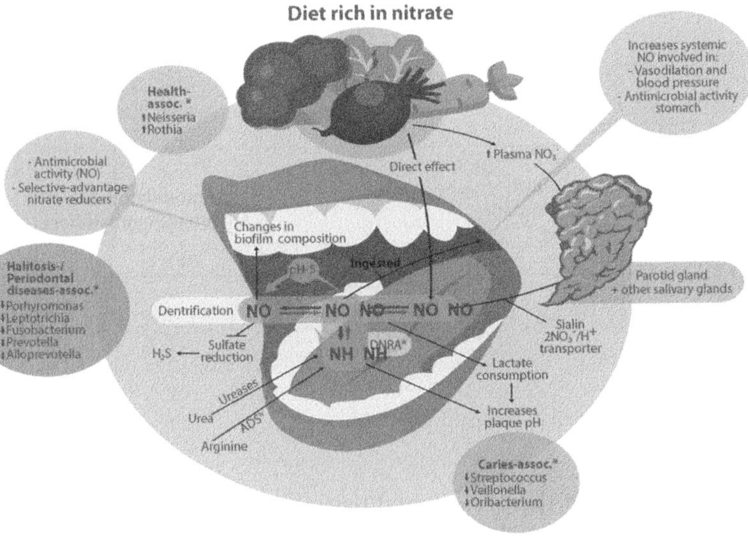

Figure 11.5 Diet rich in nitrate.

induce aerobiosis by increasing the numbers of health-associated bacteria while decreasing the levels of disease-associated bacteria. Furthermore, our findings reveal some of the processes underpinning nitrate's possible oral health benefits, such as lactate consumption or ammonia-mediated pH buffering. The salivary glands contain electrogenic Stalin $2NO_3$-/H+ transporters, which raise salivary nitrate to millimolar levels following a nitrate-containing meal, resulting in high nitrate concentrations for several hours [19].

An overview of nitrate's possible effects within the mouth. Based on this analysis and existing literature, here is a graphical overview of the topic. Food sources of nitrate (NO_3^-), such as leafy greens, beets, and carrots, enter the circulation, where plasma nitrate is condensed into saliva by sailing transporters in the salivary glands. Nitric oxide is an antibiotic molecule that has been found to change the composition of oral biofilms by limiting the development of particular species (e.g., periopathogenic species are sensitive to NO). Furthermore, acidic breakdown of nitrite to nitric oxide occurs at pH 5 and below (orange arrow), which may enhance the antibacterial impact when the pH declines owing to sugar fermentation. The bacterial dissimilatory nitrate reduction to ammonium (DNRA) pathway may also convert nitrite to ammonia (NH3), raising the local pH [20, 21].

11.4 Commercial Product of Prebiotic on Oral Health

1) O'BIOME prebiotic toothpaste
2) REVITIN toothpaste
3) BIOFLORA

11.5 Future Viewpoint

There is very little research on prebiotics and oral health. However, prebiotics may alter the sort of bacteria present in the mouth cavity by modifying the local microbiota. However, before we can undertake prebiotics studies, we need to learn more about the intricate formation and metabolism of oral biofilms in particular. Similarly, additional research is needed to investigate if the prebiotic-induced immunomodulatory benefits seen in the stomach are also beneficial in the oral cavity [22].

11.6 Conclusion

Prebiotics are an emerging field of microbiology with immense potential. Prebiotics are therapeutic agents with the least side effects as it is easily accepted by the body. They are of great interest to the researchers and their application as a therapeutic agent is a topic of extensive research to the scientists of the world. Prebiotics has been analyzed for the treatment and prevention of various diseases and disorders of the human body especially in the treatment of oral diseases and the results obtained are very encouraging. Prebiotics has turned out to be very promising in ensuring oral health and well-being.

Acknowledgement

The authors thank the METs, Institute of Pharmacy, BKC, affiliated under Savitribai Phule Pune University, Nashik, Divine College of Pharmacy Satana and Sandip Institute of Pharmaceutical Science, for their constant support and providing all facilities to complete this work. We also thank the Ministry of Tribal Affairs Govt. of India for providing financial assistance in the form of fellowship (award no 202021-NFST-MAH-01235).

References

1. Caglar, E., Kargul, B., Tanboga, I., Bacteriotherapy and probiotics' role on oral health. *Oral. Dis.*, 11, 3, 131–137, 2005.
2. Tester, R.F. and Al-Ghazzewi, F.H., Role of prebiotics and probiotics in oral health. *Nutr. Food Sci.*, 48 1, 16–29. 2018.
3. Grover, H.S. and Luthra, S., Probiotics–the nano soldiers of oral health. *J. Indian Acad. Clin. Med.*, 13, 1, 48–54, 2011.
4. Nanavati, G. *et al.*, Effect of probiotics and prebiotics on oral health. *Dent. J. Adv. Stud.*, 2021.
5. Reddy, R.S. *et al.*, Bacteria in oral health-probiotics and prebiotics a review. *Int. J. Biol. Med. Res.*, 2, 4, 1226–1233, 2011.
6. Markowiak, P. and Śliżewska, K., Effects of probiotics, prebiotics, and synbiotics on human health. *Nutrients*, 9, 9, 1021, 2017.
7. Siqueira, J.F. and Rôças, I.N., The oral microbiota in health and disease: An overview of molecular findings. *Oral. Biol.*, 1537, 127–138, 2017.
8. Devine, D.A. and Marsh, P.D., Prospects for the development of probiotics and prebiotics for oral applications. *J. Oral. Microbiol.*, 1, 1, 1949, 2009.
9. Jain, P. and Sharma, P., Probiotics and their efficacy in improving oral health: A review. *J. Appl. Pharm. Sci.*, 2, 11, 151–163, 2012.
10. Lugani, Y. and Sooch, B.S., Xylitol, an emerging prebiotic: A review. *Int. J. Appl. Pharm. Biol. Res.*, 2, 2, 67–73, 2017.
11. Al-Sheraji, S. *et al.*, Prebiotics as functional foods: A review. *J. Funct. Foods*, 5, 1542–1553, 2013.
12. Zanatta, C.A. and Ward, W.E., Prebiotics: Not only for gut health? Oralhealth Group, Canada, 2020.
13. Esteban-Fernandez, A. *et al.*, The role of wine and food polyphenols in oral health. *Trends Food Sci. Technol.*, 69, 118–130, 2017.
14. van Loveren, C., Broukal, Z., Oganessian, E., Functional foods/ingredients and dental caries. *Eur. J. Nutr.*, 51, 2, 15–25, 2012.
15. Kunova, G. *et al.*, In vitro fermentability of prebiotic oligosaccharides by lactobacilli. *Czech J. Food Sci.*, 29, Special Issue, S49–S54, 2012.
16. Ojansivu, I., Ferreira, C.L., Salminen, S., Yacon, a new source of prebiotic oligosaccharides with a history of safe use. *Trends Food Sci. Technol.*, 22, 1, 40–46, 2011.
17. Mussatto, S.I. and Mancilha, I.M., Non-digestible oligosaccharides: A review. *Carbohydr. Polym.*, 68, 3, 587–597, 2007.
18. Ahire, E.D. *et al.*, Role of omega-3 fatty acids in different neurodegenerative disorders, in: *Applied Pharmaceutical Science and Microbiology*, pp. 173–194, Apple Academic Press, London, 2020.
19. Rosier, B. *et al.*, Nitrate as a potential prebiotic for the oral microbiome. *Sci. Rep.*, 10, 1, 1–15, 2020.
20. Peeran, S.W. *et al.*, Therapeutic role of dietary omega-3 fatty acids in periodontal disease. *Univers. Res. J. Dent.*, 4, 2, 82–6, 2014.

21. Dahiwade, A.S. *et al.*, Probiotics and prebiotics: Current role in oral health. *JIDA: J. Indian Dent. Assoc.*, 8, 1, 11–17 2014.
22. Venema, K. and do Carmo, A.P., *Probiotics and prebiotics*, Caister Academic Press.[Google Scholar], Wageningen, 2015.
23 Gezer, C. and Okburan, G., Prebiotic dietary fibers for weight management, in: *Dietary Fibers*, IntechOpen, 2021.

Index